FIFTH EDITION

PHYSICAL

DIAGNOSIS

ILLUSTRATED

RALPH H. MAJOR, M.D.

Professor of Medicine and of the History of Medicine
The University of Kansas

MAHLON H. DELP, M.D.

Professor of Medicine
The University of Kansas

W. B. SAUNDERS COMPANY

Philadelphia & London

1956

PREFACE TO THE FIFTH EDITION

WITH THIS, the fifth edition of PHYS-ICAL DIAGNOSIS, it is a great pleasure to welcome Dr. Mahlon Delp as co-author. Dr. Delp, as resident in medicine, secured much material, both in illustrations and in factual data, for the first edition of this work. In the intervening years, he has been continuously active in teaching physical diagnosis and has become familiar with almost every line of this text. His suggestions for improvement have been invaluable.

In this Edition, many parts of the text have been rewritten, many additions have been made, and the order of certain paragraphs has been changed. The chapter on history taking and recording has been moved from the end of the book to the position of an early chapter—a suggestion made by numerous colleagues. Many new illustrations have been added and some old ones eliminated. These changes, we feel, have produced an obvious improvement in the work.

We are under especial obligations to our colleagues, Dr. Rosemary Schrepfer, Dr. Max Allen, Dr. Robert Bolinger, Dr. E. Grey Dimond, Dr. Fethi Gonlubol, and Dr. Ralph Edwards, for illustrations they have kindly permitted us to use. Our indebtedness to Miss Arline Nichols for her artistic drawings and to Mr. William McGrew and his associates for their excellent photographs is quite obvious to anyone reading this book.

THE AUTHORS

May, 1956

PREFACE TO THE
FIRST EDITION

THIS BOOK is a summary of some of the things I have learned in fifteen years' experience in teaching physical diagnosis to medical students. In it I have tried to emphasize, as Skoda did a century ago, that physical signs are produced by physical causes, and that these underlying physical causes must be understood before the physical signs can be properly appreciated.

I have deliberately avoided any chapters on roentgenology, electrocardiography, urine, feces, etc., for two reasons. First, this is a textbook of physical diagnosis, and second, these other subjects are far better presented in books written by experts in these fields. Where roentgenograms, electrocardiograms or pulse tracings are employed they are used only to make certain explanations clearer.

I have made free use of quotations, partly because of an interest in classic descriptions, and partly because of the excellence of many of these early accounts. I have also, in many instances, employed the illustrations used by the pioneers in certain fields of investigation, thinking for instance that Traube's original curve of pulsus alternans is of more interest than any one of the thousands of curves of this condition which have been made since.

If in this twentieth century I have seemed to hark back too much to the descriptions of the older masters, it is because I have been impressed with the remark of Osler, "And when you can, read the original descriptions of the masters who, with crude methods of study, saw so clearly." Also, since the descriptions of Biot's breathing, of Traube's semilunar space, of Skoda's resonance, and of other physical findings vary in different books, it is of interest to see what these men themselves wrote on these subjects.

I have drawn freely both in subject material and in illustrations from many sources for which I wish to express my indebtedness. The excellent texts of many writers have been drawn upon extensively, particularly those of Cabot, Rose and Elmer, Emerson, Norris and Landis, Pratt and Bushnell, Seifert and Müller, Edens and Letulle. In the sections on the heart I have been greatly aided by Hirschfelder's "Diseases of the Heart and Aorta," a book which in my judgment is one of the most clearly written and most interestingly presented treatises on cardiac diseases. The influence of Friedrich v. Müller on this book is clearly seen in its pages and the author considers himself unusually fortunate to have been a worker in his clinic in 1913, and again in 1933, twenty years later, to have followed the last course the master gave on physical diagnosis.

The illustrations have been taken from various sources but the majority are from patients seen in the University of Kansas School of Medicine. My colleagues, Dr. Edward H. Hashinger, Dr. Frank C. Neff, Dr. T. G. Orr, Dr. Arthur E. Hertzler, Dr. C. B. Francisco, and Dr. Nelse F. Ockerblad, have supplied me with many photographs for which it is a pleasure to express my appreciation. The photographs are in themselves a testimonial of my indebtedness to our photographer, Mr. D. M. Sams. The drawings are mainly the work of Miss Kay Bell, to whom my obligations are also obvious. I am under great obligation to Dr. George Walker for assistance in the preparation of phonograms and of the sound tracings which were made with a cathode-ray apparatus of his design and construction. Miss Opal Woodruff, librarian of the University of Kansas School of Medicine, has been of the greatest assistance in the location of certain references in the literature.

I am very grateful to my colleagues, Dr. Peter T. Bohan, Dr. Graham Asher and Dr. Galen Tice, who have been kind enough to look over sections of the manuscript and have aided me with many helpful suggestions. To Dr. Edward H. Hashinger, who has had the kindness and patience to review the entire manuscript, it is difficult to express adequate thanks. I have drawn very freely on "The Laboratory Notebook Method in Teaching Physical Diagnosis and Clinical History Recording" of Dr. Logan Clendening and have obtained even more assistance from him in the course of our conversations and discussions on the subject of physical diagnosis. If, after this enumeration of the aid I have received from so many sources, this treatise fails to prove a satisfactory outline of physical diagnosis, the fault is obviously mine.

In conclusion, this book is intended as a textbook of physical diagnosis, not as a yearbook or as an exhaustive encyclopedia. It attempts rather to indicate the paths of exploration a student should follow, and possibly suggests some byways that he may explore as the interest of the moment indicates.

RALPH H. MAJOR

CONTENTS

Chapter 9

INSPECTION, PALPATION AND PERCUSSION OF THE HEART   156

Chapter 10

AUSCULTATION OF THE HEART   171

Chapter 11

THE PULSE   195

Chapter 12

BLOOD PRESSURE   212

Chapter 13

PHYSICAL FINDINGS IN CARDIOVASCULAR DISEASES . . 221

Chapter 14

ABDOMEN AND GENITALIA 247

Chapter 15

THE EXTREMITIES 281

CHAPTER 1

INTRODUCTION

THERE ARE FOUR METHODS of physical diagnosis: inspection, palpation, percussion, and auscultation. Logically, the examination of the patient should proceed in this order. First, look at the patient—inspection; then touch him—palpation; then tap him—percussion; and lastly, listen to him—auscultation. Look, touch, percuss, listen. If one always follows this order, he will avoid many errors.

History. The importance of a rigid routine in examining patients cannot be overemphasized. Most errors in physical diagnosis are not the result of ignorance, but of haste and carelessness. Thoroughness in examination produces more correct diagnoses than sudden flashes of brilliancy. One should follow into the minutest detail every slight variation from the normal just as a detective follows every clue in unraveling a mystery. In many respects the methods of the physician are those of the detective, one seeking to explain a disease, the other a crime. Conan Doyle, the physician-author, was inspired to create the master-detective, Sherlock Holmes, by one of his teachers, Dr. Joseph Bell, whose uncanny powers of observation made an indelible impression upon the mind of the young medical student. The extent to which keenness of observation may be developed is illustrated by an anecdote told of Jean Nicolas Corvisart, who played an important and honorable role in the history of physical diagnosis. One day, while examining a portrait, Corvisart remarked, "If the painter has been accurate, the original of this picture died of heart disease." An investigation proved Corvisart's diagnosis to be correct. Voltaire's story *Zadig,* which every medical student should read, gives another and older story of how acuteness of observation can be developed.

The power of observation is developed by practice, by systematically following a routine which, with repeated use, becomes second nature. The physician should look long before he palpates, palpate long before he percusses, and percuss long before he listens. Frequently a student proceeds to place his stethoscope on the patient's chest as soon as the patient has undressed, without having percussed or even inspected him. In many respects a regulation forbidding a student to own a stethoscope until he has studied physical diagnosis for six months would be a wise measure.

Inspection, the first step in the examination of a patient, is also the oldest method. Just when it was first used we do not know, but probably at the time when the Neanderthal, or some other primitive man, emerged from the stage in which instinct was succeeded by reason and other mental processes. The most primitive man probably looked at his fellow in much the same way that we do today. Sometime back in those hazy historical epochs the discovery of inspection was made.

Leaving behind us those remote periods and coming down to the earliest times which have left a written record, we find the physician using inspection in the examination of his patients. The Papyrus Ebers, one of the most venerable medical treatises in the world, compiled about 1500 B. C., describes a great variety of disease conditions, including enlargement of the lymph glands, skin eruptions, pterygium of the eye and warts on the vulva, showing that the ancient Egyptian physician had trained his powers of observation and constantly used inspection in the diagnosis of disease. Hippocrates was a great master of inspection and saw so much with his eyes that when we read twenty-four hundred years later his description of certain diseases we can almost make an instantaneous diagnosis. "It has often been remarked that his clinical pictures of phthisis, puerperal septicemia, epilepsy, epidemic parotitis and some other diseases might, with a few changes and additions, take their place in any modern text-book" (Garrison).

There are isolated references to the use of percussion and auscultation in ancient times. Hippocrates used auscultation to a limited extent. He was familiar with the pleural friction rub, which he described as "squeaking like leather," in edema of the lungs he noted that, if one presses his ear against the chest and listens, "it boils inside like vinegar"; and he also described the well-known succussion splash since known as "Hippocratic succussion." Aretaeus the Cappadocian, in the second century of the Christian era, observed that in tympanites "if you tap with your hand the abdomen sounds." Johannes Platearius of Salerno in the twelfth century noted that, in ascites, the abdomen on per-

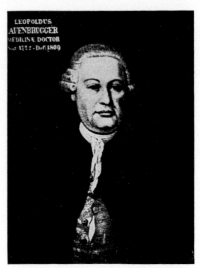

FIG. 1. Leopold Auenbrugger.

cussion gave the tone of a half-filled leathern bottle, while tympanites produced the tone of a drum. William Harvey, the discoverer of the circulation of the blood, observed that, when the blood was moved from the veins to the arteries, "a pulse is made which may be heard in the chest." These observations, however, remained isolated, unknown to and unappreciated by the medical profession.

For more than twenty-two hundred years, from the time of Hippocrates, nearly five hundred years before Christ, until the work of Auenbrugger in the latter part of the eighteenth century, the physician had at his disposal only inspection and palpation in the examination of patients. He made mistakes, but he must have made correct diagnoses too; otherwise, he could not have maintained his position as a leader of the society in which he found himself or upheld his reputation as a learned man. He looked at his patient's tongue, he noted whether he had fever, he felt and counted his pulse, but he knew little of the condition of his heart and lungs until the nineteenth century dawned, and percussion and auscultation were discovered.

Leopold Auenbrugger, the discoverer of percussion, was the son of an innkeeper in southern Austria. As a young lad, he assisted his father in his duties, one of which was to keep the guests' glasses well filled with wine. He learned from his father that he could tell a cask of wine was filled, half-filled or empty, by thumping on its end. This simple expedient gave him the germ of the idea which later led to his great discovery.

Leopold's father was ambitious for his son, gave him a good education and later sent him to Vienna to study medicine. He was an industrious student, a young man of charm, good sense and genial disposition. After graduation he rapidly achieved success in his profession and, when twenty-nine years of age, was appointed physician to the Spanish Military Hospital, the largest and finest hospital in Vienna. Ten years later, in 1761, he published in Latin his "Inventum Novum," in which the new art of percussion was described.

Auenbrugger states in his preface that "in making public my discoveries, I have been actuated neither by an itch for writing nor a fondness for speculation, but by a desire of submitting to my brethren the fruits of seven years' observation and reflection."

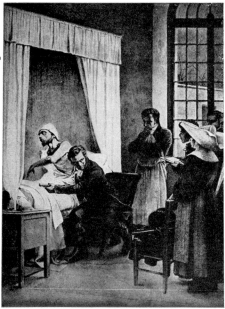

FIG. 2. Laennec examining a patient at the Necker Hospital.

For forty-seven years Auenbrugger's little book of ninety-five pages remained unnoticed. In 1808 Corvisart, the physician of Napoleon, translated it into French, only one year before Auenbrugger's death. Corvisart could easily have revamped the book and published it as his own, since Auenbrugger had been utterly neglected and forgotten. But with a fine sense of honor and integrity, he called attention to Auenbrugger's neglected treatise and wrote in his preface "It is he and the beautiful invention which of right belongs to him that I wish to recall to life."

Corvisart was destined to play another important role in the development of physical diagnosis. As one of the foremost teachers of medicine in Paris, he attracted many medical students, one of whom was René Théophile Hyacinthe Laennec. Corvisart recognized the industry, accuracy and brilliance of the young Laennec. He constantly encouraged him in his studies and taught him the value of percussion. The young student in turn was stimulated by the brilliance of his master's intellect and was deeply impressed and influenced by his high sense of integrity.

Laennec followed the usual course of the medical student of his day and, after living through many lean years, at last achieved a reputation as a careful, sane physician and slowly acquired a practice. One day while on his way to see a patient his attention was attracted by some small children who were playing on a long beam of wood in the court of the Louvre. One child was softly scratching the end of the beam with a pin, while the others, with their ears at the other end, were listening with delight to the sounds.

Laennec was thinking of his difficulties in examining a patient, a young woman who was suffering from heart disease. She was obese, and neither palpation nor percussion had aided him in his diagnosis. The sight of the children playing with the beam gave him an inspiration. Hurrying to the home of the patient, he asked for a sheet of

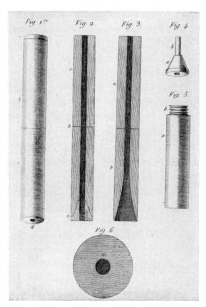

FIG. 3. Laennec's stethoscope.

paper, rolled it up tightly into a cylinder, applied one end to the chest and the other to his ear. To his joy, he heard the sounds of the beating heart as well as the breath sounds in the chest.

This was the discovery of auscultation. Laennec spent three years improving upon his roll of paper and listening to the chests of patients. He learned to turn wood and made first a solid cylinder of wood. This solid cylinder transmitted the heart sounds well, but gave poor results when applied to the lungs. He then bored a hole through the cylinder and found that he heard the sounds in the lungs better. He experimented with various kinds of wood—ebony, cedar, cane, beech and linden—but found little difference between them. At length he devised an instrument of wood exactly one foot in length consisting of two parts with a canal through the center, which could be taken apart for carrying and joined together before using. It also had an adapter which changed the size of the aperture on the end placed against the chest. Laennec used the smaller aperture when listening to the heart and the larger, bell-shaped aperture when auscultating the chest. After considering many names he finally

christened this instrument the stethoscope (στῆθος—stethos = chest; σκοπεῖν —skopein = to examine), the name it has carried ever since. His instrument, with slight modification, is still used extensively in European clinics (Fig. 3).

In 1819 Laennec published his famous "De l'Auscultation Médiate," in which this new method of examination was explained and its application to the diagnosis of diseases of the lungs and heart fully described. In this work he was compelled, because he was speaking in a new medical language, to coin a large number of new words, most of which are still in common use. Such terms as pectoriloquy, cavernous breathing, egophony, bronchophony and rales have gained universal currency. Rales was the term he gave to certain sounds bearing resemblance to the "râle des mourants," or the "death rattle."

Nine years after the publication of Laennec's work, Piorry, another French physician, invented *mediate percussion*. Although Auenbrugger was the father of percussion, it should be recalled that he practiced immediate percussion or direct percussion, striking the chest directly with the fingers and noting the sounds produced. Piorry, in his work "De la Percussion Médiate" (Paris, 1828), pointed out that better results could be obtained by placing a piece of ivory (plessimeter) over the chest and striking it with the index finger of the other hand. A percussion hammer soon appeared to take the place of the striking finger, but the experience of a century is in favor of using the finger as a plessimeter. Piorry states that "many English or American physicians who have done me the honor to attend my courses, have sought to simplify still further the procedure which I employ by using their finger as a plessimeter" and writes with disapproval of this method. The use of the plessimeter, however, has now been largely discontinued in favor of the fingers alone. A physician always has his fingers with him, but he may have forgotten his plessimeter. A friendly critic remarked that Piorry would certainly have done more for percussion if he had been preoccupied to a lesser degree with his plessimeters. Piorry also attempted to refine his percussion to the point where he could distinguish a liver sound, a spleen sound, a kidney sound, and so forth, an erroneous and fanciful idea, one, as Skoda remarked, which was "altogether unfounded in fact."

Piorry emphasized the importance of the tactile sense, the sense of resistance produced by the stroke. Every experienced examiner recognizes the importance of this tactile impression, and many of our most skillful diagnosticians percuss so softly as to emit no sound whatever, relying entirely upon this sense of resistance. Such skill is, however, the reward of persistent practice, and the beginner must rely at first, not upon his finger, but upon the sound produced by percussion.

Meanwhile the discovery of auscultation was enthusiastically acclaimed throughout the medical world; the new method came into general use; and the stethoscope became an accepted part of the physician's armamentarium. Josef Skoda introduced the new method in Vienna, which was rapidly becoming the medical center of the world, and filled his students and colleagues with a passion for the study of physical diagnosis. There has probably never been a clinic where patients were examined more carefully or more minutely. Skoda's aim in medicine seems to have been to see his physical findings in the patient confirmed by the subsequent autopsy, and his school is reproached with the criticism that they taught that the physician's purpose was not to heal, but to make correct diagnoses. Skoda was the chief priest of the school of "therapeutic nihilism" and his common remark, after he had diagnosed the patient's ailment and someone had inquired as to the treatment, is said to have been *"Ja, das ist einerlei"* (that's all the same).

Therapeutic nihilism has gone, although the scientific physician is still

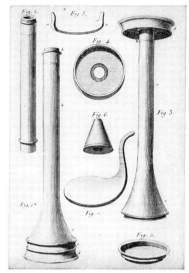

FIG. 4. Stethoscope and plessimeter of Piorry.

at times accused of it, and while we today do not agree that the chief duty of the physician is to make diagnoses and postmortems agree, we cannot but admire the accuracy and skill of the Vienna school of a hundred years ago. Every physician should try to make his diagnoses agree with a possible future postmortem—and then prevent that postmortem.

Skoda's "Abhandlung über Perkussion und Auskultation," which appeared in 1839, is one of the most remarkable books that has ever appeared on the subject. It represents the first thorough attempt to place the new discovery of percussion and auscultation upon a firm scientific footing and to apply physics in explaining the findings obtained by the new methods. Certain errors crept into this work, but his ideas were basically clear and logical. He treated the subject with a remarkable novelty of viewpoint and with an admirable spirit of scientific sincerity.

The following quotations from his book should be remembered by every student of physical diagnosis. "Percussion and auscultation cannot be learned except at the expense of time and pains." "The findings of percussion and auscultation depend never upon the

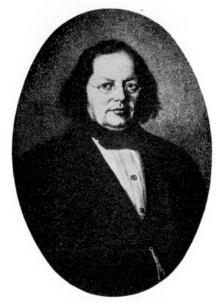

FIG. 5. Josef Skoda.

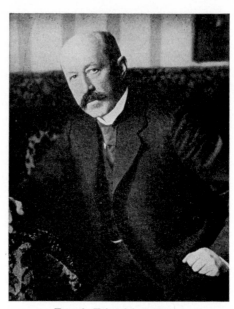

FIG. 6. Friedrich Müller.

disease itself, but always upon the changes produced in the organs." "Diseases which are entirely different may show the same findings on percussion and auscultation and vice versa, the same disease may show a great variety of findings when we percuss or auscultate, because sound depends not upon the chemical but upon the anatomical state of the organs." He emphasizes the fact that students must study the pathologic anatomy of the organs which show abnormal physical signs, closing with the remark that "everybody should be advised to spend no time or labor learning these methods of examination if he will not take the trouble to study pathology in the cadaver."

With the advent of Skoda's work the last great advance in the subject of physical diagnosis was made. The essential truths were established; it was now necessary to study these truths more carefully, to explain them and to thresh out some of the chaff that had been gathered in with the grain. This process began immediately and is still in progress.

The development of the new science of physics led to the epochal investiga-tions on sound by Savart in France, Tyndall in England and Helmholtz in Germany. Their studies and experiments upon sound had a direct bearing upon the subject of physical diagnosis. Helmholtz, famous as a physicist, was trained as a physician. "Medicine," he said, "was once the intellectual home in which I grew up; and even the emigrant best understands and is best understood by his native land."

In France, Mailliot in 1843 and Andry in 1845 wrote excellent books on physical diagnosis, while in England, Stokes in 1828 wrote one of the earliest treatises on auscultation in the English language, followed in 1843 by Walshe's book on physical diagnosis. In America, W. W. Gerhard wrote a text on physical diagnosis which appeared in 1842 and was the authoritative book on the subject until the work of Austin Flint. Flint's "Physical Exploration," published in 1856, remains today one of the best treatises on the subject and bears upon every page the imprint of the author's genius. In Germany, Gerhardt's "Lehr-buch der Auskultation und Perkussion," published first in 1866, remains a standard treatise. This was followed by the excellent texts of Guttmann, Eichhorst, Niemeyer, Traube, Wintrich and others.

Friedrich Müller of Munich, during his active career as teacher and investigator, was particularly interested in studying physical diagnosis. Each semester for forty years, until his retirement in 1934, he gave a course in percussion and auscultation. It has been the custom in many clinics for the chief of the medical department to turn over the courses in physical diagnosis to one of the younger assistants—as something almost unworthy of the chief's attention. To those who had the rare privilege of working in Müller's clinic it was always an inspiration to see this great master spending his time teaching the new students in medicine the rudiments of percussion and auscultation.

In no field of medicine is a true start more important or a false start more disastrous than in the study of physical diagnosis. There are no short cuts. It is learned only by practice, not a dull, dreary, monotonous practice, but practice with all the five senses alert. To quote Pasteur: "In the fields of observation chance favors only the prepared mind."

Continual practice in inspection, palpation, percussion and auscultation prepares the student to see more and to know. The effort is considerable, but no rewards are surer in medicine than those that come to the practiced eye, ear and finger.

As Osler said of medicine, so we may say that physical diagnosis "is to be learned only by experience; 'tis not an inheritance; it cannot be revealed. Learn to see, learn to hear, learn to feel, learn to smell, and know that by practice alone can you become expert."

"Many physicians have the idea that the art of percussion and auscultation is antiquated because they have been replaced by examination with the roentgen rays and the tuberculin test. They are, however, more necessary today than they were a hundred years ago, and they have not been superseded by the roentgen rays, for percussion and auscultation are now more necessary than ever, in order to interpret properly our x-ray pictures. The art of percussion and auscultation has gained greatly in accuracy, since the findings can be controlled by the roentgen pictures. Formerly the correctness or the errors of percussion could be demonstrated only by the autopsy. Today we can study the accuracy of our results in percussion on the living man and under natural conditions. It is also a great blessing that the roentgen plates have shown up the errors of an over-refined technique of percussion and auscultation" (Friedrich Müller).

BIBLIOGRAPHY

General Bibliography

Brust, Raymond W.: Physical Diagnosis. New York, Appleton-Century-Crofts Co., 1951.

Buck, Robert W.: The Essentials of Physical Diagnosis. Philadelphia, W. B. Saunders Co., 1934.

Cabot, Richard C.: Physical Diagnosis. Baltimore, William Wood & Co., 1934.

Dunphy, J. Engelbert and Botsford, Thomas W.: Physical Examination of the Surgical Patient. Philadelphia, W. B. Saunders Co., 1953.

Edens, Ernst: Lehrbuch der Perkussion und Auskultation. Berlin, Julius Springer, 1920.

Elmer, Warren P., and Rose, W. D.: Physical Diagnosis. St. Louis, C. V. Mosby Co., 1930.

Emerson, Charles P.: Physical Diagnosis. Philadelphia, J. B. Lippincott Co., 1929.

Flint, Austin: A Manual of Physical Diagnosis. Philadelphia, Lea & Febiger, 1934.

Foster, Nellis B.: The Examination of Patients. 2nd ed. Philadelphia, W. B. Saunders Co., 1928.

Gerhardt, C.: Lehrbuch der Auskultation und Perkussion. Tübingen, H. Laupp, 1900.

Külbs, F.: Leitfaden der Medizinisch-Klinischen Propädeutik. Berlin, Julius Springer, 1922.

Letulle, Maurice: Inspection, Palpation, Percussion, Auscultation. Paris, Masson & Cie, 1922.

Martini, Paul: Die unmittelbare Kranken-Untersuchung. Berlin, Springer, 1927.

Norris, G. W., and Landis, H. R. M.: Diseases of the Chest. 6th ed. Philadelphia, W. B. Saunders Co., 1938.

Pratt, Joseph H., and Bushnell, George E.: Physical Diagnosis of Diseases of the Chest. Philadelphia, W. B. Saunders Co., 1925.

Pullen, Roscoe L.: Medical Diagnosis, Applied Physical Diagnosis. Philadelphia, W. B. Saunders Co., 2nd ed., 1950.

Robertson, William E., and Robertson, Harold F.: Diagnostic Signs, Reflexes and Syndromes. Philadelphia, F. A. Davis Co., 1939.

Seifert, Otto, and Müller, Friedrich: Manual of Physical and Clinical Diagnosis, transl. by E. Cowles Andrus. Philadelphia, J. B. Lippincott Co., 1934.

Simon, P.: Manuel de Percussion et d'Auscultation. Paris, Felix Alcan, 1895.

Stern, Neuton S.: Clinical Diagnosis. New York, The Macmillan Company, 1933.

Bibliography of Chapter 1

Andry, F.: Manuel Pratique de Percussion et d'Auscultation. Paris, Ballière, 1844.

Bon, Henri: Laënnec. Dijon, Lumière, 1925.

Flint, Austin: Physical Exploration and Diagnosis of Diseases Affecting the Respiratory Organs. Philadelphia, Blanchard & Blanchard & Lee, 1856.

Gerhard, W. W.: Lectures on the Diagnosis, Pathology and Treatment of the Diseases of the Chest. Philadelphia, Haswell & Barrington, 1842.

Helmholtz, H.: Die Lehre von den Tonempfindungen. Brunswick, Friedrich Vieweg, 1870.

Laënnec, R. T. H.: De l'Auscultation Médiate. Paris, Brosson & Chaudé, 1819.

Laënnec, R. T. H.: Traité de l'Auscultation, Médiate. Paris, J. S. Chaudé, 1826.

Mailliot, L.: Traité Pratique de la Percussion ou Exposé des Applications de cette Méthode à l'Etat Physiologique et Morbide. Paris, Baillière, 1843.

Major, Ralph H.: Classic Descriptions of Disease. Springfield, Ill., Charles C Thomas, 1932.

Piorry, P.-A.: De la Percussion Médiate. Paris, J. S. Chaudé, 1828.

Skoda, Josef: Abhandlung über Perkussion und Auskultation. Vienna, Mosle & Braumüller, 1839.

Stokes, William: Two Lectures on the Application of the Stethoscope to the Diagnosis and Treatment of Thoracic Disease. Dublin, Hodges and McArthur, 1828.

Vierordt, Herman: Geschichte der Perkussion und Auskultation, Handbuch der Geschichte der Medizin. Jena, Neuburger & Pagel, 1903, p. 604.

CHAPTER 2

HISTORY TAKING AND RECORDING

HISTORY TAKING is an art. Certain persons seem endowed with the gift of extracting concise and accurate histories from patients. However, anyone, whether endowed with this gift or not, can learn to take accurate and satisfactory histories. One student may learn more readily than another, but it can be learned by anyone who possesses the necessary inquisitiveness, persistence and tact.

The history of a patient is absolutely essential to the physician who is attempting to make a diagnosis. In some diseases a physical examination is of great importance, while a laboratory examination is of little value; in other diseases the reverse obtains; but in all diseases the history is of great importance.

The value of a careful and accurate history has been stressed from the days of classical antiquity until today. Rufus of Ephesus remarked that "one must ask questions of the patient; for, with the aid of these questions one will recognize more exactly some of the things which are important in the disease, and one will treat it better." The essay of Rufus, "On the Interrogation of Patients" remains, after more than a millennium and a half, an excellent treatise on the subject. Since the days of Rufus, many essays, even small books, have been written on history taking. One of the best, in recent years, is the monograph by Herrmann, listed in the bibliography.

In angina pectoris the diagnosis is often made entirely from the history of pain under the sternum, a pain which gradually becomes more and more agonizing, radiates to the left arm and is accompanied by a sensation of impending death. In gallbladder disease the history of colicky pains in the right upper abdominal quadrant, radiating to the shoulder blade, often is more significant than all the findings on physical examination. In pulmonary tuberculosis, the history of loss of weight with night sweats and afternoon fever may be of greater value in the diagnosis than the physical findings. These examples could be multiplied indefinitely. Many experienced clinicians assert that in the diagnosis of many diseases the history of the patient's illness is of more importance than all the other methods of diagnosis combined.

A history should be thorough; therefore, all the details of the patient's past illnesses as well as of his present illness must be obtained. The historian must not, however, lose himself in this maze of details so completely that he fails to emerge with the information he went in to find. In antiquity the two most famous medical schools were at Cnidos and at Cos. The school of Cnidos developed physicians who were noted for their close attention to the details of illness, details which they described with such thoroughness that they often lost sight of the disease itself. They were famous for their meticulous and detailed descriptions of diseases as well as for the multiplicity of their diagnoses, many of which were mere enumerations of symptoms. The school of Cos, by contrast, as shown by the writings of its greatest luminary, Hippocrates, developed the art of distinguishing between the essential and the insignificant, and, although it went into great detail when necessary, it emphasized the important, minimized the unimportant and suppressed the irrelevant. The method of Cos lives on; that of Cnidos remains but a memory. This ability to distinguish between the relevant and the irrelevant may at times be almost an intuition, but it is usually the result of practice, thoroughness and experience.

In taking and recording a history we should note the absence of certain features as well as the presence of others. The absence of headache may be as significant as the impairment of vision. If we examine a patient who has pains in his legs and whom we suspect of having tabes dorsalis, the absence of any difficulty in gait is obviously significant. The absence of certain symptoms may be as important in arriving at a diagnosis as the presence of others, which, however, does not mean that every symptom which is absent should be recorded. Familiarity with the various and manifold symptoms of a disease will teach the student whether the absence of certain symptoms in a patient is of significance.

Order. The order in which a history should be taken is a matter of some dispute. There is general agreement that the patient should first be asked what ails him—the chief complaint. Regarding the next step, there is disagreement. Some physicians prefer to begin next with the patient's family history, then his past history and lastly his present illness. Such a procedure undoubtedly gives us an orderly account of his family and their disorders, his own past history with its record of illness leading up to his present illness, the whole in chronological sequence just as a historian writes a biography. There are, however, serious objections to this sequence when taking a patient's history.

A patient consults a physician because of pain, discomfort or apprehension which is troubling him at that particular moment. It is the present and not the past upon which his attention is focused. He has little interest in the ailments he had while a child and none at all in the diseases of his forefathers—although both may be important and aid the physician in his diagnosis. If the physician, on hearing that his chief complaint is "shortness of breath," asks him next what caused his father's death, the patient is unable to see any logical connection between the two questions and may immediately lose interest in the entire procedure as well as confidence in the physician. In this instance, and in practically all instances, it is better to ask the patient all the details regarding his shortness of breath. When this investigation has been completed, the examiner may ask, without any loss of interest on the part of the patient, "Is there any history of a similar illness in the family?" The patient is now assured of the examiner's interest in his ailment and is quite ready, willing and often eager to tell the physician all he knows about the illness of his parents and grandparents as well as all he remembers of his own past ailments.

Another advantage of taking the history of the present illness first, is that, when the physician knows the patient's present symptoms, he will be especially alert for any details of the patient's past life or for any information regarding his parents that may have a special bearing on his present illness. For these reasons, we prefer to take the history in the following order: First, chief complaint; second, present illness; third, personal history, fourth, family history; and, finally, the system review.

In recording the history the student may follow his own inclinations. He may record the history just as he has taken it or he may record it after he has written the chief complaint, in chronologic sequence beginning with the family history. Personally, we prefer the latter order, but tastes differ.

At the close of the history the student should always write a brief summary of the salient features. This procedure is one for which the attending physician is usually grateful, but it is of even greater value to the student. It teaches him to separate the relevant from the irrelevant, and indicates certain features of the physical examination which must be considered with special care.

Before proceeding to take the history of a patient, the examiner should know the name of the patient, his race, age, marital state and occupation. Age and occupation are particularly important. Certain diseases are diseases of youth, others are seen only in middle-aged or elderly persons. Tuberculosis is common in youth, but uncommon in old age; cancer is common in old age, but rare in youth. Certain occupations carry an increased hazard. Tuberculosis is not uncommon in stone masons and in typesetters, lead poisoning is more common in battery workers and in painters than in other persons, while bartenders often succumb to the temptations of their calling and suffer from alcoholism, with its complications of neuritis and cirrhosis of the liver.

Chief Complaint. This should be stated as briefly as possible and in the patient's own words. The complaint, however, and not the diagnosis should be recorded. The patient should be urged to tell what his symptoms are,

why he seeks relief, and not what the diagnosis of another physician has been. The chief complaint should not be recorded as "diabetes" or "heart trouble," but as "excessive urination" or "shortness of breath."

The statement that the chief complaint should be recorded in the patient's "own words" implies that these words should contain a clear expression of thought, a concise statement of his symptoms and not vague phrases such as "heart trouble," "lung trouble" or "kidney trouble."

Present Illness. The method which should be followed in obtaining a history of the present illness varies with the patient and with the illness from which he is suffering. The clinical clerk or physician should strive when possible to allow the patient to tell his story just as he wishes and to emphasize the features which he considers important. Some patients have the unfortunate tendency to ramble on and on and never give a clear or concise recital of their ailments. In such cases the examiner must, by skillful questioning, direct the story along the proper lines. He must take care, however, not to suppress the thoughts of the patient and to substitute his own instead. We are all familiar with the physician who can make the patient give the desired history, by laying undue emphasis on certain details and by suppressing others altogether. In percussing a patient's chest we should not, as Friedrich Müller remarked, percuss our ideas into it. Similarly, in taking a history we should not force our own thoughts into the patient's mind.

The most common complaint which causes the patient to seek medical advice is pain or its closely related symptom, discomfort. We should distinguish carefully between the two. A sharp pain in the stomach after eating has an entirely different significance from a dull heavy feeling in the abdomen. The other most common types of complaints are nervousness, loss of weight, and weakness. The history of the present illness must obviously vary with the complaint.

The following queries, however, are usually valuable.

DURATION. First, we should ask how long the patient has been ill. In other words: Is the trouble acute or chronic? Some diseases have a sudden onset with a rapid termination; others begin slowly and insidiously. In some diseases the patient can tell almost the exact minute he had his first symptoms; in others he cannot tell within a week or two when his symptoms first began.

If the patient has been ill for a month, he is not suffering from lobar pneumonia; if he was well yesterday, and quite ill today, his illness is not pernicious anemia.

LOCATION. The importance of the location of the pain or discomfort is obvious. If the pain is in the head, neck, chest, abdomen or extremities, this site directs our attention to a certain organ. Does the pain remain localized, or does it travel or radiate to some other region?

PROGRESS. The progress of the symptoms is closely related to their duration. Has the trouble developed rapidly or slowly? Have the symptoms become worse or better? Are they better at times and worse at others?

CHARACTER. It is important to learn the character of the pain or discomfort of which the patient complains. Is the pain sharp or dull? Is it really pain or is it discomfort? Does it appear suddenly and disappear quickly, or does it gradually increase in intensity and slowly subside?

RELATION TO PHYSIOLOGIC FUNCTION. It is important to ascertain the effects of certain normal activities upon the symptoms. What is the effect of posture? Are the symptoms worse when the patient is standing or sitting or lying down? What effect does exercise produce? Are the symptoms worse when the patient walks? The effect of posture or exercise upon symptoms due to disease of the circulatory or respiratory system is usually striking. Equally striking is the distress produced by exercise in patients with severe anemia.

The effects of eating in diseases of the digestive system should be noted. In some diseases, eating relieves the symptoms; in other diseases, it aggravates them.

The relation of sleep is important. Some symptoms appear while the patient is asleep and wake him from a sound sleep. In others, sleep brings relief from distressing symptoms.

EFFECTS OF DISEASE. The effects produced by disease vary greatly. Some diseases quickly produce prostration, loss of weight, failing appetite and extreme nervousness, causing the patient to appear quite ill and wretched. Other diseases, after days or weeks, produce little change in the patient's general condition or appearance. Certain diseases may produce little change for weeks or months and then quickly cause catastrophic symptoms and rapidly change the appearance of the patient.

After we have obtained the history of the onset of the present illness, its duration, location, progress and character, we should carefully inquire as to its effects. This can be quickly accomplished by inquiring about its general effects and then about its effects upon the systems of the body. Has the patient become weak and lost weight? Does he have fever, or chills or sweats? Has he headaches, shortness of breath, indigestion, loss of appetite, vomiting, distention of the abdomen, polyuria, painful urination or constipation?

Questions regarding the general effects of the symptoms are of extreme importance. In some diseases certain general effects follow the primary symptoms "as the night the day." Failure to pursue this line of inquiry may lead to serious errors of interpretation and of diagnosis.

It is important to know whether the patient has been treated for his ailment and also what the treatment was. Often a patient with a relatively minor complaint has taken some powerful drug and is suffering from the effects of the treatment rather than from the initial complaint.

The outline on page 13 should sug-

OUTLINE FOR HISTORY AND PHYSICAL EXAMINATION

A. Name of patient   M., F.   S; M; W; D.   Race   Telephone Number
   Address   Birthplace
   Age   Date

B. **Chief Complaint:** Brief, preferably in the patient's own words
C. **Present Illness:** Logically developed story of symptoms accurately described as to time of onset, mode of onset, duration, and reaction to symptoms
D. **Past Illnesses:**
    1. Diseases of childhood
    2. Serious illnesses
    3. Injuries
    4. Surgery and hospitalizations
E. **Personal History:**
    1. Marital status—duration, health of partner, compatibility, number of children, ages
    2. Habits: Alcohol, tobacco, sedatives or other medications, sleeping habits
    3. Occupation: Present and past work, exposure to occupational hazards, emotionally satisfactory or not
F. **Family History:** Father, mother, sisters, brothers, diabetes, hypertension, tuberculosis, apoplexy, nervous diseases, mental diseases, cancer, familial tendency
G. **System Review:**
    1. *Head:* Headaches, (duration, severity, character, location, etc.)
    2. *Eyes:* Vision, diplopia, inflammatory disease, when last examined
    3. *Ears:* Hearing, earache, discharge, tinnitus
    4. *Nose, throat, and mouth:* Tonsillitis, quinsy, glossitis
    5. *Respiratory:* Cough, expectoration, hemoptysis, pleurisy, date of recent chest x-ray, asthma
    6. *Cardiovascular:* Dyspnea, orthopnea, substernal pain, palpitation, leg cramps, edema
    7. *Gastrointestinal:* Appetite, distress before or after meals, foods craved, foods avoided, nausea, vomiting, hematemesis, melena, diarrhea, constipation, laxatives, color of stools, change in form of stool, jaundice, abdominal pain or colic
    8. *Genitourinary:* Frequency, nocturia, pain or burning on urination, hematuria, incontinence, dribbling, difficulty in starting stream, change in size and force of stream.
    9. *Menstrual:* Date of onset, interval, regularity, duration, amount of flow, date of last period, dysmenorrhea, menorrhagia, irregular bleeding, menopause, number of pregnancies, abortions, miscarriages, complications
    10. *Metabolic:* Normal weight, gain or loss
    11. *Neuromuscular:* Vertigo, paralysis, weakness in extremity, paresthesias, (numbness or tingling, syncope)
    12. *Neuropsychiatric:* Emotional stability or instability, history of nervous breakdown, environmental stress, memory defects

gest to the student the course to follow in taking a history. Hard and fast rules cannot be laid down. It is a problem for which there is no general solution. Each case demands its own procedure. The student should not cease his quizzing until he has extracted all the information possible from the patient, whether at the moment it seems relevant or irrelevant. The question of relevancy should wait for the summary.

The history of the present illness is the most important feature of the history, and often, also, the most difficult to obtain. The family history and the system review are less difficult to obtain, for here the questioning can follow a definite outline.

We have used the following plan in taking the family and personal history of patients, and it has proved very satisfactory. The student is given a mimeographed outline. This outline is followed in questioning the patient, and his answers are jotted down rapidly with a pencil. After the sheet has been filled out, the student uses it as a synopsis and writes out the account in full on the history sheets. This history taking can be accomplished rapidly, since no time is lost in the composition of sentences or in writing legibly at the bedside. This is greatly appreciated by the patient and also contributes to the accuracy of the history, since the student at the bedside has his attention fixed upon obtaining facts and postpones the worries of composition until he has returned to his desk.

Some criticize such a plan as stereotyped or mechanical. If abused, it can easily become so. If properly followed, it serves as a framework upon which to build an accurate, coherent and connected history. We should, however, emphasize to the student that it represents merely a skeleton outline and is the minimum of questioning. He should ask all the questions indicated on the outline and as many others as the occasion demands.

Personal History. The personal history as Herrmann has emphasized "should reveal the individual as a whole, his personality, his mental make-up." It is not sufficient to record merely his physical complaints, the various diseases from which he has suffered. It is important to know whether the patient is habitually depressed or elated, his reaction to his environment, to his social contacts, to his work, to his family and friends.

The patient's social, religious, and economic background, his education, his feeling of achievement or of frustration, all are important factors to evaluate. Patients, who are emotionally unstable, are particularly disposed to be on the alert for any symptoms that may, in their self-analysis, be the warning of an impending serious illness. We should never forget that many patients complaining of severe symptoms are anatomically or even physiologically sound. Their symptoms are not the result of organic disease but belong entirely to the class of psychosomatic disorders.

Habits. The habits of the patient may give important clues to diagnosis. There are certain diseases to which alcoholics are especially prone, certain diseases which attack especially a certain group of workers. The excessive use of tobacco and alcohol may produce a train of symptoms whose significance is entirely missed unless the patient's habits of smoking and drinking are known.

Such terms as "moderate smoker" or "moderate drinker" should be avoided as inexact and misleading. Moderation for one person may be excess for another. The patient's daily consumption of tobacco should be recorded in numbers of cigars, cigarettes or pipes smoked, and his daily consumption of alcohol in terms of the pints or quarts of wine, beer or whisky.

Many patients develop the habit of taking drugs for minor complaints, a practice which should be carefully noted. Patients often take irritating cathartics for constipation and develop a severe diarrhea which requires little treatment beyond a withdrawal of the offending drug.

System Review. The infectious diseases noted in the outline may all have a definite effect upon the patient's later health. The same holds true for the caption "surgery and hospitalizations."

If a patient is suffering from a *headache,* it is important to know where it is localized, also anything that increases its intensity or relieves it. The importance of inquiries regarding the *eyes* is obvious. Even the laity recognize the association of eye strain and headache.

The patient's history of disease of the *ears* and *throat* is of particular importance in affections which are the results of focal infection, particularly arthritis.

Inquiries regarding the history of the *cardiorespiratory* system are of great importance. A history of chronic cough with expectoration and hemoptysis is obviously suggestive of tuberculosis, while shortness of breath and palpitation of the heart, especially upon exercise, suggest the presence of a heart affliction. If this history of dyspnea is associated with the history of a past attack of rheumatic fever, the suspicion of heart disease becomes almost a certainty.

GASTROINTESTINAL. In diseases of the gastrointestinal tract the diagnosis is usually made from the history and the x-ray findings. Physical examination and laboratory examinations usually play minor roles. For this reason the history must be taken with extreme care. The outline indicates the type of questions to be asked.

GENITOURINARY. Abnormalities of urination are first considered. It is important to know whether the patient gets up at night to urinate and, if so, how often. The past history of possible gonorrhea, and particularly of syphilis, should be gone into with great care. The diagnosis of gonorrhea is usually obvious from the patient's history. The diagnosis of syphilis may be difficult from his account.

Family History. The family history is important in many diseases, particularly those of the nervous system, some of which are always hereditary. Diabetes shows a hereditary tendency, hemophilia is invariably passed on by the mother, migraine is transmitted usually by the mother to the children, allergic diseases are commonly hereditary, a cancer often stalks through generation after generation of the same family; neurasthenic parents beget neurasthenic children. Arterial hypertension shows a marked tendency to appear in certain families, and there are few diseases outside of hereditary nervous affections which show a more striking hereditary factor. The classic answer to the question of preventing arterial disease is "to be born of the proper parents." Life insurance actuaries have long since given preferential treatment to policy holders who are the children of long-lived parents. Physicians as a class need no indoctrination by the advocates of eugenics although they may question seriously the practicability of their program. While we have long bred cattle to produce the desired results, our young people will continue to mate and breed according to their own desires and not in the interests of the race or the strain.

In taking the family history it is important to note whether the father and mother are living and well. The health of the brothers and sisters should be ascertained.

The physician today appreciates, as never before, the role played by environment in the production of disease. Environment was previously considered only in the light of the patient's occupation. Today we realize that its scope is far more extensive and includes every phase of the patient's life—his success or failures in his work, his family life and marital relations.

Summary. The summary of the patient's history should include the chief complaint, the present illness, the family history and the personal history. The facts bearing upon the patient's illness should be briefly and clearly summarized. The summary is an epitome of the patient's illness and of all the facts in his past history and in his family history that may have had influence. In many respects it is the most difficult part of the history taking. It is a test of the observer's ability to see events in their proper perspective and to interpret them correctly.

Recording the Physical Findings. Just as history taking is an art, refined and perfected only after much experience, so the recording of the physical findings can be a clear-cut logical account of the patient's physical abnormalities, or a confused mixture of apparently contradictory findings which can mislead the reader as much as an erratic history. Just as the physical examination should proceed *a capite ad calcem* from head to foot—so the record should follow the same order, stressing and describing in some detail the important findings and not dwelling on important and trivial minutiae.

For the aid of the student of physical diagnosis we give an outline for a record, an outline which has, in our hands, proved eminently satisfactory over a period of years. We have also added the transcript of the record of the history and physical findings in an actual patient and not in a hypothetical case. We hope it may suggest to the student a logical method of approach, a method which in this somewhat baffling case led to a correct diagnosis.

OUTLINE FOR PHYSICAL EXAMINATION

Physical Examination:
1. *Vital signs:* Weight, height, temperature, pulse, respiration, blood pressure
2. *General inspection:*
   a. Posture
   b. Physique, constitution, nutritional state
   c. Severity and acuteness of illness
   d. Emotional state in reaction to illness
3. *Skin:* Complexion, texture, turgor, pigmentation, eruption, lesions
4. *Head:* Skull and scalp; configuration, scars
5. *Eyes:*
   a. LIDS: Edema, ptosis, width of palpebral fissures
   b. SCLERA: Jaundice, hemorrhage
   c. CONJUNCTIVAE: Pallor, injection, petechiae
   d. CORNEA: Scars, ulceration, arcus senilis
   e. PUPILS: Size, shape, equality, reaction to light and accommodation
   f. VISION: Acuity, visual fields by confrontation
   g. OPHTHALMOSCOPIC: Optic disks, vessels, exudate, hemorrhage
6. *Ears:*
   a. EXTERNAL: Tophi
   b. INTERNAL: Otoscopic examination, drum
   c. Auditory acuity
7. *Nose:* Shape, septum—deviation perforation, turbinates, congestion, discharge, polyps
8. *Mouth and Throat:*
   a. LIPS: Symmetry, cyanosis, cheilitis, herpes
   b. Pharynx and tonsils
   c. MUCOUS MEMBRANE AND GINGIVA: Pallor, ulceration, pigmentation
   d. TONGUE: Color, papillary atrophy, ulceration, deviation
   e. TEETH: Caries, missing teeth, dental repair
9. *Neck:*
   a. BLOOD VESSELS: Engorgement of veins, abnormal pulsations, scars
   b. THYROID: Enlarged, nodular, bruit
   c. TRACHEA: Position, midline or deviated, trachial tug
   d. LYMPH NODES: Anterior and posterior cervical, pre- and post-auricular, supra-clavicular
10. *Chest and Lungs:*
    a. GENERAL INSPECTION: Contour, symmetry, expansion, equality of expansion—rate and rhythm
    b. PALPATION: Tactile fremitus
    c. PERCUSSION: Kronig's isthmus—compare symmetrical areas
    d. AUSCULTATION: Character and intensity of breath sounds, relative duration of inspiration and expiration, rales, friction rub
    e. DIAPHRAGM: Determine level and excursion
11. *Heart:*
    a. INSPECTION: Point of maximal impulse, abnormal pulsations
    b. PALPATION: Point of maximal impulse, thrills, pulse rate, rhythm, volume, equality, vessel wall
    c. PERCUSSION: Retromanubrial dullness, right and left borders of heart
    d. AUSCULTATION: Heart sounds—intensity, 1st, A_2, P_2, character of cardiac rhythm; —murmurs, location, where loudest, duration, systolic or diastolic, effect of position change upon murmur
12. *Breasts:* Symmetry, nipple, ulceration, secretion, pigmentation, areola, tenderness, masses, axillary lymph nodes
13. *Abdomen:*
    a. INSPECTION: Contour, scars, dilated veins, peristalsis
    b. PALPATION: Distention, rigidity, tenderness, masses, liver, spleen, kidneys, bladder
    c. PERCUSSION: Shifting dullness, tympany, fluid wave, liver, splenic, or other dullness
    d. HERNIA: Femoral, inguinal
    e. LYMPH NODES: Inguinal
14. *Genitalia:*
    a. MALE: Discharge, penile lesions or scars, hydrocele, testicular atrophy or masses
    b. FEMALE: Inspection of external genitalia, pelvic examination, inspection of perineum, cervix, bimanual examination of uterus and adnexa

15. *Extremities:*
    a. UPPER: Hands—Color of palms, moisture of palms, clubbing of fingers, cyanosis of nails, joint swelling or deformity, shoulder, elbow
    b. LOWER: Mobility or deformity of joints, color and temperature of feet, posterior tibial and dorsalis pedis arterial pulsation, edema, varicose veins
16. *Back and Spine:* Mobility, curvature, vertebral tenderness to percussion
17. *Nervous System:*
    a. DEEP TENDON REFLEXES: Biceps, triceps, radialis, patellar, Achilles, Babinski
    b. CRANIAL NERVES: Recheck when indicated
    c. SENSORY EXAMINATION: When indicated
18. RECTUM: Sphincter tone, hemorrhoids, fissure, fistulae, masses, prostate
Diagnostic Impression:
Suggested Further Study:

ACTUAL HISTORY AND PHYSICAL EXAMINATION

G.S., a 52 year old, white male farmer entered this hospital for the first time on 16 February.

C.C. (Chief Complaint). "Pain and tingling of the arm and leg."

P.I. (Present Illness). The patient was relatively well and carrying on normal activities until twenty-four hours previous to this hospitalization. Just as the patient was seating himself at the table for the noon meal, he was suddenly seized with a severe, agonizing pain in the left elbow. Simultaneously, he noted a heavy pressure sensation in the substernal area and over the left chest. Faintness, nausea, and marked perspiration followed the onset of pain. The patient was assisted to bed by his wife—heat and massage to the arm was applied without relief. Three aspirin tablets were then taken and within about thirty minutes the patient was able to go to sleep.

After about three hours of rest the patient felt improved and went out of the house to water his stock. About one hundred yards from the house he developed a severe cramplike pain in the calf of the right leg followed quickly by a similar pain in the left thigh. In attempting to return to the house, the patient had great difficulty in walking because of great weakness and sensation of heaviness as well as tightness in the legs.

After the latter episode a physician was called; an opiate was administered and the patient was sent by ambulance to this hospital.

Although the patient was relatively well at the onset of this acute episode he had been a known diabetic for eight years. In 1947, the patient consulted his physician because of weakness and weight loss. A rigid diet, but no insulin was then prescribed; however, the patient did not do well. He continued to lose weight but was able to continue work until he developed a dermatitis and severe skin infection in 1953. With this infection his weight loss became very rapid; polyuria became severe, and hospitalization was required. At this time the patient's diet was readjusted and he was placed on 35 units of protamine-zinc insulin daily. Improvement was rapid—the patient gained thirty pounds and he was able to return to strenuous farm work. During 1954, the patient has noted frequent and annoying leg cramps particularly at night. On at least two occasions he has had pain in the left chest and shoulder while exerting. This pain on each occasion disappeared after a moment's rest. Only four months previous to this admission the patient was told by his physician he had high blood pressure and should "take it easy." No inquiry as to the level of the pressure was made. Small white pills to be taken twice daily were prescribed for the hypertension. After the initial prescription, the patient did not have it refilled.

The patient feels that he has not been physically able to carry on for four or five years; but financial stress and recently greater family burdens have forced him to disregard his symptoms. For months he has been much concerned about whether he had a "bad heart" and whether or not he would have to take insulin all his life, now that he had started taking it.

P.H. (**Past History**). The patient recalls only mumps and measles as childhood illnesses. At the age of 35 the patient had scarlet fever, and one year later he had severe influenza during a local epidemic. A farm accident resulted in an injury to the left hip at the age of 40, but there was no fracture. No operations. One hospitalization mentioned above.

Personal History. Married 30 years. One son age 27, living, and well. One daughter age 25 died accidental death eight months ago leaving a 4 year old daughter whom the patient has taken into the home. Family relationships are quite normal in the face of tragedy and illness. The son is married and living in another state. The wife is occupied in the home but assumes the usual responsibilities of a farm wife.

The patient has always been an independent farmer, worked hard, has owned his own farm for 20 years. His working day is usually twelve hours. The patient is a Protestant and attending church member. He rarely smokes, and has never used alcohol in any form.

At the time of the interview the patient was fairly comfortable, relaxed, and quite direct and reliable in answering.

F.H. (**Family History**). Father living and well at 82. The mother died at age 40 of "consumption." Three sisters are living and well. One sister died of diabetes. Maternal grandmother died of diabetes. No brothers. No nervous or mental diseases. No apoplexy. No cancer.

System Review

Head: Rare headaches; occasional vertigo past year.

Eyes: Left internal strabismus since birth, sight in this eye poor. Glasses for reading since 1946, last changed two months ago.

Ears: Otitis with draining right ear as child. No tinnitus, hearing good.

Nose, Throat, and Mouth: All teeth pulled because of "pyorrhea" fifteen years ago. Dentures fit well. No sore tongue, nor sore mouth.

Respiratory: Influenza about 1941 —severe. About two severe colds yearly. No asthma, pneumonia, pleurisy nor hemoptysis. No cough. Chest plate six months ago.

Cardiovascular: See above. Denies shortness of breath. Uses one pillow. No edema.

Gastrointestinal: Appetite very good. No food idiosyncrasies nor sensitivities. No nausea, vomiting, hematemesis. No indigestion. No constipation, but occasionally takes "laxatives." No diarrhea. No jaundice. No melena.

Genitourinary: Since beginning insulin there has been no polyuria. No nocturia. No frequency, urgency, nor hematuria. No alteration in size nor force of stream.

Metabolic: Weight has been fairly constant at 160 pounds for the past year. Maximum weight past 15 years 192 pounds, minimum weight 130 pounds in 1953.

Neuromuscular: See above. Tingling, numbness, and disturbed sensation in the left hand and both legs and feet have been mildly disturbing with this illness. There has also been coolness of the left hand and left foot.

Neuropsychiatric: The patient has apparently had no episodes of severe emotional instability.

He admits some difficulty in accepting the self-discipline necessary to control his diabetes and a tendency to be resentful of his misfortune. Reaction to stress of his daughter's tragic death seems to have been average.

Physical Examination

Vital Signs: Weight 162 pounds, height 67 inches, temperature 98.6°F., pulse 86, respiration 20, B.P. 160/90.

General Inspection: The patient is a well developed, well nourished, adult male apparently in no acute distress, pleasant and cooperative. He appears about the stated age of 52.

Skin: Normally free of eruption or unusual pigmentation.

Head: Normal skull, early baldness, no scars.

Eyes: Small bilateral xanthomatous lesions of lower lids, no ptosis. Left internal strabismus, otherwise extraocular movements normal. Conjunctiva normal. The pupils are round, regular, and react to light and accommodation. Fundus examination shows a grade III retinal sclerosis with silver wire arteries and arteriovenous nicking. No exudate nor capillary aneurysms noted. The disks are normal. Grossly visual fields are normal.

Ears: Externally normal. Canals clear. The right drum is scarred but intact, the left is normal. Hearing grossly normal.

Nose: No abnormalities noted although there is a mild deviation of the septum to the right.

Mouth and Throat: Lips normal, tongue red and somewhat slick. Artificial dentures. Alveolar ridges normal. Tonsils atrophic and uninfected.

Neck: No adenopathy. Thyroid palpable, but not enlarged. No abnormal pulsations. Trachea in midline.

Chest and Lungs: Normal contour, symmetrical. Expansion equal and normal. Respiratory rate normal. Fremitus normal. No unusual areas of dullness. Diaphragmatic position and excursion normal. Breath sounds normal. No rales.

Heart: P.M.I. 3 cm. to left of midclavicular line in 5th interspace. Forceful apex beat. Heart enlarged to left by percussion. No thrills. 1st heart tone diminished. A_2 greater than P_2. No murmurs. B.P. 160/90, pulse 86. Normal radial pulse on right. No radial pulse on left.

Breasts: Normal male.

Abdomen: Normal contour. Abdominal wall somewhat thickened by fat. Good muscle tone. No distention. No visible peristalsis. No rigidity. No tenderness. No abdominal masses. Liver palpable at right costal margin. Spleen not palpable. Kidneys not palpable. No scars. No hernia. Small shotty inguinal nodes.

Genitalia: Normal adult male genitalia, mild phimosis.

Extremities: The palm of the left hand obviously pale compared to right. Left hand cool compared to the right. Left foot cool and pale compared to right. Absent radial and ulnar pulsation on the left. Absent popliteal, dorsalis pedis and posterior tibial pulse on the left. No joint disease. Mild weakness in the left arm and left leg.

Back and Spine: No deformity.

Neurological: Normal deep tendon reflexes. No Babinski. Gait not tested. Mild weakness of left arm and leg. Moderate reduction in vibratory sensation in both lower extremities.

Rectal: Very spastic sphincter, external tags. Prostate normal in size and consistency.

Diagnostic Impression

Diabetes mellitus.
Arteriosclerotic heart disease.
Myocardial infarction.

Embolization of aorta and both common iliacs from mural thrombus in left ventricle.

BIBLIOGRAPHY

Daremberg, Ch. and Ruelle, Ch. Émile: Oeuvres de Rufus d'Éphèse. Paris Imprimerie Nationale, 1879, p. 195.

Herrmann, George R.: Clinical Case-Taking. St. Louis, C. V. Mosby, Co., 1949.

Wolf, Stewart: Talking with the Patient. Monographs in Medicine Series 1, Baltimore, Williams & Wilkins Co., 1952, p. 1.

CHAPTER 3

PAIN

PAIN IS ONE of the most common complaints that call the physician to the patient. Though it is a subjective rather than a physical finding, pain bears such an intimate relationship to physical diagnosis that a brief consideration of it is important. Pain directs the attention of the examiner to certain parts of the patient's body, and though it cannot be seen, palpated, percussed or heard, it may be elicited by palpation and percussion; and certain findings in physical diagnosis are seen, palpated and heard only in the presence of pain.

The tissues and organs supplied by the autonomic nervous system are not sensitive to pain in the ordinary sense. We can cut, burn or tear such organs as the heart, stomach, intestines, liver or kidneys without producing any sensation. William Harvey described the case of the eldest son of Viscount Montgomery who had a large open cavity in his side exposing the heart. He carried him to King Charles to "behold this wonderful case." "And his most excellent majesty, as well as myself, acknowledged that the heart was without the sense of touch; for the youth never knew when we touched his heart, except by the sight or the sensation he had through the external integument." Many surgeons in the days before anesthesia noted the insensitiveness of the viscera to pain or touch. Sir James Mackenzie has decribed an abdominal operation performed without anesthesia in which he broke up adhesions and resected the intestines without producing pain. He observed, however, that the patient had pain with each peristaltic movement of the upper part of the resected bowel, but that the pain was felt in the umbilicus some 12 inches from the point where the pain was produced. In abdominal operations today under a local anesthetic the surgeon observes that he can cut and handle the viscera without eliciting any pain or even sensation. When, however, the mesentery is pulled it produces severe pain immediately.

In considering the location of pain and its relation to lesions of various organs, it is of fundamental importance to note two classes of pain, local pains and referred pains. *Local pains* are pains felt over or in the vicinity of a pathologic process. *Referred pains* are pains which are not felt at the area of the disease process, but are referred and felt at some distant point on the body or extremities. Referred pains have been known to physicians for generations, but a clear understanding of them came first

21

with the fundamental investigations of Henry Head.

Head began his investigations with the study of pain in herpes zoster, finding that the distribution of the lesions on the skin correspond with the areas of cutaneous pain or tenderness occurring in certain visceral diseases. Since the lesions of herpes zoster produce cutaneous pain in the skin areas supplied by the sensory nerves whose ganglia are inflamed, Head postulated that the cutaneous pain felt in visceral disease was located in the areas whose sensory nerves enter the cord at the same segment which supplied nerves to the viscera concerned. In disease of an organ, impulses pass from its nerves to a segment of the cord and are felt as pain on the skin areas whose sensory nerves enter the same cord segment. With infinite patience Head succeeded in outlining the areas of the body corresponding to these segments of cord. These have since been known as Head's areas. Later investigations have produced certain divergences of view and exposed certain errors, but the essential correctness of Head's ideas has been definitely established.

The studies of Joseph A. Capps, which extended over a period of more than twenty years, have shed much light upon pain in the pleura, pericardium and peritoneum. Capps' investigations have cleared up many points which were obscure and reconciled many apparently conflicting views in regard to pain in diseases of these serous structures.

An extended consideration of the subject of pain is outside the scope of this book, but a brief consideration of some of its more evident and better understood manifestations is of great aid in the interpretation of disease, and assists us in localizing various lesions.

HEAD

Pain in the head is often due to a local condition. *Frontal sinusitis* usually causes pain in the forehead, while *maxillary sinusitis* produces pain over the maxillary sinuses, although either may cause a general unlocalized headache. *Epidemic parotitis* or mumps produces pain over the enlarged parotid glands.

Trifacial neuralgia, or *tic douloureux,* causes intense pain over the areas supplied by the trigeminal nerve. This disease affects most commonly the infraorbital, or maxillary division of the nerve, then the mandibular, and last the ophthalmic. It is usually unilateral. The pain is sharp, stabbing, lightning-like and usually excruciating. Eating or drinking hot or cold foods, talking, washing the face or brushing the teeth may precipitate an attack. Patients observe that certain areas along the course of the nerves are more sensitive than others. These areas are commonly referred to as "trigger zones," since touching them sets off an attack. Neuralgia of the ninth nerve is uncommon, but is seen occasionally.

Pain over the *occiput* radiating forward over the scalp is caused by neuritis of the great occipital nerve.

Headache is one of the commonest symptoms seen in the practice of medicine. Its causes are numerous and varied. Among the common causes are eye strain, high blood pressure, anemia, brain tumors, various infectious diseases, and fever of any origin. Migraine, or sick headache, is a distinct clinical entity, a hereditary affliction, periodic in its appearance, usually accompanied by visual disturbances and often by vertigo, nausea and vomiting.

THORAX

Lungs. The lung itself is insensitive to pain. Marked inflammation of the lung parenchyma produces no pain unless the parietal pleura itself is involved. The pain of pneumonia is the pain of pleurisy.

In lobar pneumonia of the right lung the pain at the onset is sometimes located in the abdomen, leading the physician to suspect that the patient is suffering from acute cholecystitis or acute appendicitis. When the right upper or middle lobe is involved, the pain is often located in the right upper quadrant of the abdomen, while in involvement of the right lower lobe the pain may be felt in the right lower quadrant (Fig. 7). In cases of lobar pneumonia when the pain is located exclusively in the abdomen, the differential diagnosis between lobar pneumonia and acute cholecystitis or acute appendicitis may be difficult. Careful examination will, however, usually disclose suggestive or conclusive evidence of pneumonia in the chest with an absence of the characteristic findings of cholecystitis or appendicitis in the abdomen.

Conversely, gallbladder disease or disease of the liver when it extends to the diaphragm may simulate pneumonia. Galen (A. D. 160) was familiar with the confusion in such cases and wrote in

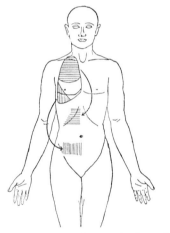

FIG. 7. Diagram showing projection of pain to the abdomen in pneumonia.

some detail about the differential diagnosis, pointing out that liver disease involving the diaphragm produced rapid respiration, local pain and coughing, but no brown sputum.

Pleurisy. The pain of pleurisy is situated usually over the area where examination shows the pleurisy to exist. This is due to the fact that the parietal pleura receives its innervation in part from the intercostal nerves which carry pain fibers. Diffuse involvement of the pleura usually causes more pain in the lower part of the thorax than in the upper part, probably because the excursions of the lungs are greater at the base than in the upper parts. The pain of pleurisy is probably transmitted only from the parietal pleura, since there is no evidence that the visceral pleura has nerves capable of transmitting pain impulses. Hence the pain of pleurisy is made more intense by deep or rapid breathing, which causes greater excursions of the lung against the inflamed parietal pleura. Occasionally in pleurisy where there is no pain, pressure over the inflamed area will produce pain.

DIAPHRAGMATIC PLEURISY. The pain in diaphragmatic pleurisy usually has a twofold distribution, a large local area of pain on the affected side of the lower part of the thorax, and upper part of the abdomen, and a second small area on the neck or the shoulder on the same side (Fig. 8). Capps has shown that the

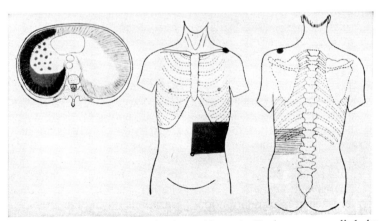

FIG. 8. Pain in diaphragmatic pleurisy. (Capps.) Dark area supplied by intercostal nerves, spotted area by phrenic nerve.

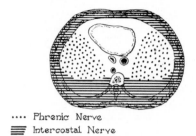

.... Phrenic Nerve
≡ Intercostal Nerve

Fig. 9. Nerve supply of diaphragm.

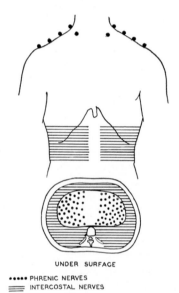

UNDER SURFACE

••••• PHRENIC NERVES
≡ INTERCOSTAL NERVES

Fig. 10. Diagram of torso showing areas to which diaphragmatic pain is referred.

diaphragm has a twofold sensory nerve supply. The peripheral rim of the diaphragmatic pleura is innervated by sensory branches from the intercostal nerves, while the central part is innervated by the phrenic nerve (Fig. 9). Inflammation of the outer margin of the diaphragm irritates the branches of the intercostal nerves, and the pain is felt in the corresponding spinal segment—in the lower part of the thorax, in the abdomen or in the lumbar region. Inflammation of the central part of the diaphragm irritates the phrenic nerve so that the pain is referred to the neck or shoulder which is supplied by nerves from the same spinal segment as the phrenic nerve. Each area of distribution is a typical example of referred pain (Fig. 10).

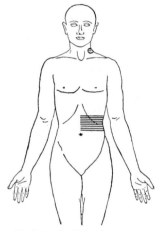

Fig. 11. Pain in left pleural effusion.

In *pleural effusions* the pain usually arises from pressure on the diaphragm and is felt in the shoulder when the central part of the diaphragm is involved, in the side or back when the outer part is involved, or in both locations when the entire diaphragm is involved (Fig. 11).

HEART

As William Harvey noted more than three centuries ago, the heart itself is insensible to pain. Yet some heart affections are accompanied by pain. A classic and outstanding example is angina pectoris.

Angina Pectoris. Angina pectoris was first clearly described by William Heberden in 1768. He noted, "The pain is sometimes situated in the upper part, sometimes in the middle, sometimes at the bottom of the os sterni, and often more inclined to the left than to the right side. It likewise very frequently extends from the breast to the middle of the left arm. . . . The pain sometimes reaches to the right arm as well as the left, and even down to the hands." John Hunter, a distinguished victim of this disease, describes the pain "as though the sternum was being drawn back to the spine." Matthew Arnold, another famous victim, described his sensations during the attacks as "though there were a mountain on my chest."

The areas over which the pain com-

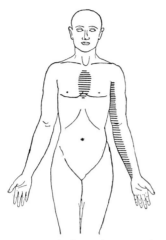

Fig. 12. Pain in angina pectoris.

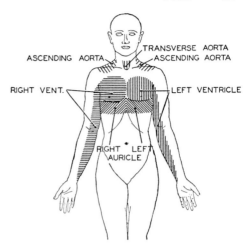

Fig. 13. Areas to which pain from various parts of the heart and aorta are referred. (After Hirschfelder.)

monly occurs in an attack of angina pectoris are seen in Figure 12. These areas are supplied with sensory nerves which enter the cord in the same segment with the autonomic nerves from the heart, particularly from the ventricles. The pain usually reaches the maximum intensity gradually and then gradually declines. It is unlike the lightning pains of tabes dorsalis which reach their maximum intensity almost instantly, at the moment of onset. The pain may appear only in the arms, or may appear first in the arms and then in the chest.

Pains arising from lesions of the ascending aorta are felt over both shoulders, while pains due to disturbances of the transverse arch are localized in the midline at or above the suprasternal notch. Pains on the right side of the chest and down the inner aspect of the right arm may be due to disease of the right ventricle. The pain in the right arm, which Heberden noted occasionally in angina pectoris, was probably due to lesions of the right coronary artery or of the circumflex branch of the left coronary artery.

In a dissecting *aneurysm* of the *thoracic aorta* there is usually excruciating pain, radiating from the midthoracic region to the anterior chest wall, down the back and even into the thighs or occasionally into the neck. The pain is often so intense it causes prostration and col-

lapse. Even if the patient recovers, the intense pain may last twenty-four to forty-eight hours.

The location of pain resulting from disease of the auricles, ventricles and aorta is shown in Figure 13.

Pericarditis. There has been much difference of opinion in regard to the frequency or importance of pain in pericarditis. Some authorities have stated that acute pericarditis is usually painless, while others consider precordial pain as the most characteristic complaint in pericarditis.

Mackenzie remarked, "This curious painlessness of pericarditis compared with pleurisy is one that has long puzzled me, and I have only a dim perception of how it may arise. I merely call attention to this fact in passing."

Capps, who has investigated this subject with especial care, has also come to the conclusion that simple, uncomplicated fibrinous pericarditis (Fig. 14) is painless. Pain in pericarditis is due to three complications: (*a*) a large effusion causing great tension on the pericardial sac with a resulting dull ache or sense of oppression over the heart; (*b*) an embarrassment of the coronary circulation causing myocardial involvement, producing a pain like that of angina pectoris; (*c*) an extension of the pericardi-

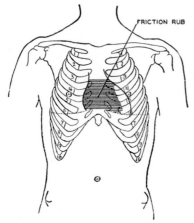

FIG. 14. Areas of friction rub in simple un-complicated fibrinous pericarditis—no pain. (After Capps.)

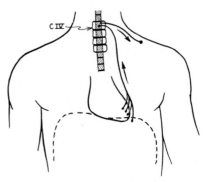

FIG. 16. Diagram showing reflexes of transmission of pain from diaphragm to shoulder (Capps). The nerve impulse starts at the diaphragm, passes upwards to the IV cervical segment, to which also the sensory nerves of the shoulder lead. The sensation of pain is reflected down these nerves to the shoulder.

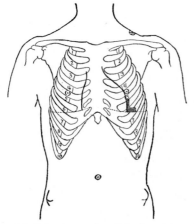

FIG. 15. Pain in pericarditis involving dia-phragmatic pleura.

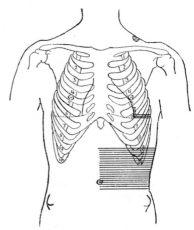

FIG. 17. Pain in pericarditis showing more extensive involvement of diaphragmatic pleura.

tis to the pleura producing a pleuroperi-carditis. When this extends to the dia-phragmatic pleura, the pain is felt in the neck or shoulder when the central part of the diaphragm is involved (Fig. 15). The path of transmission of these im-pulses is shown in Figure 16. If the lateral part of the diaphragm is involved as well, pain is felt in the region of the left shoulder and also in the abdomen around the umbilicus (Fig. 17).

Chronic adhesive pericarditis and per-icarditis with a small effusion produce no pain. Pain, if it is present, is due to involvement of the thoracic or dia-phragmatic pleura.

ABDOMEN

The hollow viscera of the abdomen are insensitive to heat and cold, and no pain is produced by cutting, clamping or burning them. The parietal peritoneum is, however, sensitive to irritation and to traction caused by pulling the organs. Irritation, distention or traction pro-duces pain which is conveyed directly to the cord by the splanchnic nerves. There is also evidence of a true somatic visceral pain produced by impulses from the viscera to the cord which are re-ferred to the corresponding segmental areas on the skin, in the same manner as the pain in angina pectoris.

The pain caused by a lesion of the parietal peritoneum is usually localized accurately on the abdominal wall near the lesion itself. If an inflammatory process involves the diaphragmatic peritoneum, the pain is never in the diaphragm, but is referred to the side or the shoulder or to both just as in inflammation of the diaphragmatic pleura. The pain in peritonitis, according to Hertzler, "be it categorically avowed, is due to irritation of the cerebrospinal nerve fibers lying in the parietal walls just beneath the parietal peritoneum or the diaphragm."

Peptic Ulcer. The pain in peptic ulcer is usually fairly sharply localized in the epigastrium. The characteristic "heartburn" of peptic ulcer is apparently due to gastric peristalsis. In gastric ulcer the pain usually follows immediately after eating; it is present during digestion and absent when the stomach is empty. In duodenal ulcer the pain is relieved by eating, the distress thus being absent during digestion and present when the stomach is empty. Pressure on the abdomen directly over the ulcer often elicits tenderness.

Appendicitis. The pain in a typical attack of appendicitis is located sooner or later quite accurately over the appendix (Fig. 18). At the onset the pain is often first in the epigastrium, then over the right side of the abdomen and later localizes definitely over the appendix. The early pain in the epigastrium is caused by spasm or edema of the appendix and is transmitted by the sympathetic fibers and referred to the epigastrium. The later "true" inflammatory pain is at the site of lesion and is transmitted directly by the pain fibers in the parietal peritoneum. Pressure almost invariably intensifies the pain. When the inflamed appendix lies behind the cecum, the pain is often most severe in the right lumbar region.

Gallbladder Disease. In acute inflammation of the gallbladder there is pain and tenderness on pressure directly over the gallbladder (Fig. 19). In attacks of gallstone colic, pain is felt over the gallbladder and over the upper part of the abdomen and the lower part of the thorax on the right side. Quite characteristic is the pain near the inferior angle of the right scapula and at times over the right shoulder (Fig. 20).

Capps states that in his experience gallbladder colic does not produce pain in the neck or trapezius region and that such pain indicates irritation of the undersurface of the diaphragm. Subscapular pain, he believes, is the only characteristic *referred* pain in gallbladder disease.

Intercostal Neuralgia. The pain produced by an intercostal neuralgia may

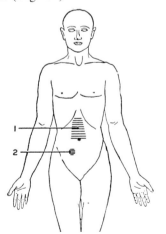

FIG. 18. Pain in appendicitis commonly first felt in epigastrium, later localized over appendix.

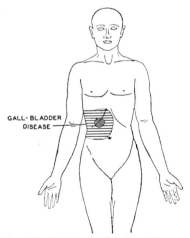

FIG. 19. Pain in gallbladder disease.

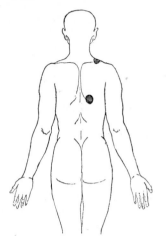

FIG. 20. Pain over the back in gallbladder disease.

simulate the pain of pleurisy, of gallbladder disease or acute appendicitis when the lower intercostal nerves on the right side are involved. The pain of intercostal neuritis is, however, usually more superficial than that of pleurisy, and on auscultation over the painful area no friction is heard. In intercostal neuritis there is also usually a cutaneous hyperesthesia over the area where pain is felt. The pain of intercostal neuritis is abolished by a subcutaneous injection of some local anesthetic into the painful area. This procedure is often of great value, particularly in differentiating between the pain of intercostal neuritis and that of gallbladder disease or appendicitis. It should not be forgotten, however, that a referred pain from visceral disease may be relieved by local anodynes and by local anesthesia, as shown so clearly by Weiss and Davis.

LIVER

The liver itself contains no pain fibers, but inflammations of the liver give rise to local pain over the liver due to involvement of the parietal peritoneum. When inflammatory processes of the liver and gallbladder extend upward and involve the diaphragm, the characteristic pain of diaphragmatic peritonitis is present. In cholangitis a sudden jar of the liver causes pain.

SPLEEN

Pain is not a prominent symptom in most affections of the spleen. In infarctions and acute inflammatory processes in the spleen a perisplenitis may result with involvement of the parietal and diaphragmatic peritoneum producing pain over the spleen, over the left hypochondrium and at times in the left shoulder. Infarction of the spleen is common in endocarditis.

KIDNEYS

Chronic Bright's disease, contrary to the common impression among the laity, is a painless affection. Acute nephritis, when the kidneys are enlarged, may at times produce severe pains in the lumbar region. Such pains are usually ascribed to tension on the kidney capsule caused by the swollen organ.

Kidney stones, which are relatively quiescent, may cause, as Osler observed from personal experience, a "constant localized, dull pain, the area of which could be covered on the skin of the back in the renal region by a penny piece, and which could be imitated exactly by deep firm pressure on a superficial bone." Attacks of renal colic may cause severe pain in this area and a radiation of the pain into the flank and into the testicle on the affected side (Fig. 21).

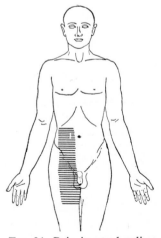

FIG. 21. Pain in renal colic.

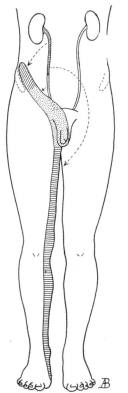

FIG. 22. Pain due to obstruction of ureter.

URETERS

The distribution of pain from a stone or kink in the ureter depends, of course, upon the location of the pathologic process. "The most common area of ureteral pain is in the lower quadrant on or below a line drawn between the anterior superior spines of the ilium, halfway between the midline and the spines. On the right side this is always inside and below McBurney's point and distinct from it" (Ockerblad and Carlson). Pain over the iliac crest originates in the upper part of the ureter, pain down the inner aspect of the thigh and leg originates in the middle part of the ureter, while suprapubic and genital pain arises in the lower part of the ureter (Fig. 22).

BLADDER

Acute cystitis produces pain in the suprapubic region, from whence it commonly radiates to the sacrum, perineum and penis. At the onset of the attack the pain may be limited to the lumbar region.

Bladder stones may produce discomfort in the pubic region. Frequently after micturition they cause a sharp pain which is referred to the end of the penis.

EXTREMITIES

The skin and subcutaneous tissues of the arms and legs are well supplied with pain fibers, and lesions here almost invariably produce local pains. The referred pains of angina pectoris in the arms have been already described. The "lightning pains" of tabes dorsalis are short, stabbing pains in the legs. These last only a second or two and pass as suddenly as they appear, leaving the skin and muscles tender. The pains appear at one time over a certain area of the leg, at another time over another area, and are pathognomonic of the disease. These pains are due to involvement of the sensory roots at the point of their entry into the cord.

Sciatic neuritis causes pain along the course of the sciatic nerve. This pain is felt on the posterior aspect of the thigh and leg. Diabetes is a common cause of sciatic neuritis. Similar pains are caused by pressure on the sacral plexus and nerves and are frequently present in sacroiliac disease and in carcinoma of the prostate.

ANESTHESIA

Anesthesias over certain areas of the body are often quite as significant as the presence of pain. The absence of sensation in a certain area when touched, pricked with a pin or touched by hot or cold objects indicates that there is either a lesion of the nerve itself or a lesion at the sensory ganglia or of that part of the cord which carries the sensory fibers.

Complete section of a nerve produces anesthesia over the area supplied by that nerve with a loss of motor power.

In *tabes dorsalis* the patient commonly has bands of anesthesia across the chest or abdomen which may be demonstrated on careful examination.

In *syringomyelia* there is dissociation of sensation, especially over the extremities, in which the sense of touch is retained, while that for pain, heat and cold is lost. Such patients may inadvertently burn their fingers from cigarettes or even burn their feet in a fireplace.

In the anesthetic form of *leprosy* the sensation of temperature and of pain may be lost. Father Damien, the martyr of Molokai, first realized that he had leprosy when he accidentally poured scalding water over his feet and felt no sensation of pain.

Anesthetic areas on the skin in patients suffering from *hysteria* are characteristic findings in many instances. Here the physician is often aided by the fact that the areas of anesthesia, which the patient shows, do not correspond to the anatomical distribution of any nerve.

Numbness or slight anesthesia of the hands is a common finding in *pernicious anemia*.

BIBLIOGRAPHY

Capps, Joseph A., and Coleman, George H.: An Experimental and Clinical Study of Pain in the Pleura, Pericardium and Peritoneum. New York, The Macmillan Company, 1932.

Capps, Joseph A.: Personal communication.

Hertzler, Arthur E.: Surgical Pathology of the Peritoneum. Philadelphia, J. B. Lippincott Co., 1935.

Jones, Chester M.: Digestive Tract Pain. New York, The Macmillan Company, 1938.

Ockerblad, N. F., and Carlson, H. E.: The distribution of ureteral pain. J. Urol. *39:*745, 1938.

Ortner, Norbert: Generalized Pain, transl. by Francis J. Rebman. New York, Medical Art Agency, 1922.

Pullen, Roscoe L.: Medical Diagnosis, Applied Physical Diagnosis. Philadelphia, W. B. Saunders Co., 2nd ed., 1950.

Rudolf, R. D., and Smith, A. G.: Observations on visceral pain. Tr. A. Am. Physicians *45:*264, 1930.

Schmidt, Rudolph: Pain, Its Causation and Diagnostic Significance in Internal Diseases, transl. by Karl M. Vogel and Hans Zinsser. 2nd ed. Philadelphia, J. B. Lippincott Co., 1911.

Weiss, Soma, and Davis, David: The significance of the afferent impulses from the skin in the mechanism of visceral pain. Skin infiltration as a useful therapeutic measure. Am. J. M. Sc. *176:*517, 1928.

CHAPTER 4

GENERAL INSPECTION

THE FIRST PROCEDURE on seeing a patient is a general survey or general inspection. Inspection is often aided by palpation. In order to conduct the proper inspection of the patient, the observer must have three things: a good light, the patient in a proper position, and a keen, observant eye. A poor light may cause the observer to miss entirely a definite jaundiced tint of the skin. An improper position of the patient may lead the observer to overlook completely a mass in the epigastrium—as, for example, the patient reclining on one elbow, with tense abdominal muscles. An observant eye is so necessary as to require no comment.

It is important that the patient be comfortable, but it is equally important that the examiner be in a comfortable position (Fig. 23). The examiner cannot do his best when in a strained or uncomfortable position.

The patient should be partially or completely undressed. Many cases of tuberculosis of the chest are missed because the physician did not insist upon the patient's removing his undershirt. Women, especially, may demur, but should have it impressed upon them that, since they came to be examined, clothing interferes with an accurate ex-

amination. An entirely impersonal attitude on the part of the examiner to nudity will usually aid in smoothing over any difficulties. Friedrich Müller relates that his father was once summoned before a hospital board on the charge that he had failed to respect a patient's privacy and had pulled down the sheets on the bed when examining her. His defense was that the disease was under the sheets and not on top of them. The board saw the point and dismissed the charges.

One of the first conditions the examiner should consider is the *psyche* or *mental* state.

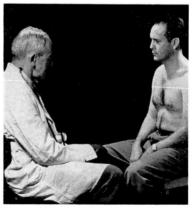

FIG. 23. Inspection of patient.

31

PSYCHE OR MENTAL STATE

Is the patient nervous, mentally alert and competent, or deranged, dull or stupid? Many nervous patients, particularly those suffering from Graves' disease, are unusually alert and "full of pep" and seem to be mentally quick and agile. Psychoneurotic patients are often emotionally unstable and cry easily. The account of their illness is often almost interminable, and they suffer pains in almost all the organs of the body. They often come with a list of complaints written down.

Some patients with certain forms of mental diseases such as manic-depressive insanity are phenomenally alert, their words being spoken with such swiftness that we can scarcely follow their thoughts.

Patients suffering from myxedema or hypothyroidism are noticeably dull, apathetic and torpid. Their mental reactions strike us instantly as being abnormally slow, their general torpidity reminds us perhaps of that of an alligator. The facial expression is characteristic. There is a dull, apathetic look and a lack of intelligence in the face. The eyes appear heavy and the face is swollen (Fig. 24). After thyroid therapy there is usually a striking change in the facial expression as well as in their mental reactions (Fig.

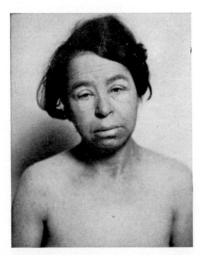

FIG. 24. Characteristic appearance in myxedema.

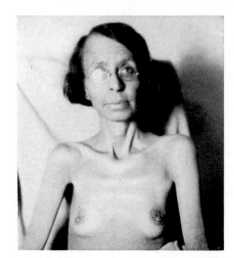

FIG. 25. Same patient after three months of thyroid medication.

25). This mental apathy and torpidity reaches its height in cretinism or congenital hypothyroidism. No one has described the cretin better than Balzac in his well-known novel "The Country Doctor."

"Much as the old cavalry officer had seen in the course of his soldier's career, he felt a thrill of surprise and horror at the sight of a human face which could never have been lighted up with thought —a livid face in which a look of dumb suffering showed so plainly—the same look that is sometimes worn by a child too young to speak, and too weak to cry any longer, in short, it was the wholly animal face of any old dying cretin. The cretin was the one variety of the human species with which the commandant had not yet come in contact. At the sight of the deep, circular folds of skin on the forehead, the sodden, fishlike eyes, and the head with its short coarse, scantily-growing hair—a head utterly divested of all the faculties of the senses—who could not have experienced, as Genestas did, an instinctive feeling of repulsion for a being that had neither the physical beauty of an animal nor the mental endowments of man, who was possessed of neither instinct nor reason, and who had never heard nor spoken any kind of articulate speech."

Certain patients in *depressed psychic states,* such as melancholia, impress us, not because of this torpor, but because of a lack of interest in their surroundings. Patients suffering from catatonia remind us more of statues than of men. Their faces are not dull or stupid as are those of cretins, but impassive, without expression, sphinx-like. Their eyes by contrast fairly gleam with intelligence and animation. They often impress one as persons who are keenly aware of the life going on about them, but are quite unable to take part in it.

Patients in coma due to diabetes or uremia are quite unconscious. Diabetic subjects in coma show a rapid, intense breathing, trenchantly described many years ago by Kussmaul as "air hunger" —a dyspnea with no cyanosis. Uremic coma is often accompanied by frequent convulsions. Patients who are unconscious after an attack of cerebral hemorrhage or "apoplexy" show stertorous breathing like a giant snoring, while hysterical patients, even after long attacks of unconsciousness, retain normal breathing and pulse rate, and persons overcome by too much alcohol or by an overdose of drugs may be totally unconscious. Here the diagnosis may be made from the alcoholic odor of the breath or from the history. It should be emphasized, however, that often a man, after drinking, may have been "slugged" and later, when carried to the hospital, diagnosed as "drunk" and die a few hours afterward from the results of a fractured skull.

Delirium may be the result of fever, of drugs such as belladonna, hyoscine, or barbiturate, or may be the predominant sign of a patient suffering from a mental disease. Alcoholic intoxication may lead to *delirium tremens,* a picture that suddenly appears at times in alcoholic patients who are suffering from an acute febrile disease, such as pneumonia. A patient suffering from delirium tremens talks incoherently and incessantly. He is constantly in motion. He sees rats, mice or other animals on the bed or floor, vermin which try to crawl over him and fill him with terror. A very interesting form of mental aberration seen most commonly but not exclusively in alcoholics is called *Korsakoff's syndrome,* in which the patients describe with great detail imaginary travels they have just finished, and imaginary persons whom they have just met.

POSTURE

The posture of a patient often gives a valuable diagnostic clue. Hippocrates, the Father of Medicine, laid great stress upon the position assumed by the patient in bed. He remarked that "to lie upon one's belly, when not habitual to the patient to sleep thus while in good health, indicates delirium or pain in the abdominal regions." Patients suffering from tabes dorsalis, from acute gastro-enteritis or from tuberculosis of the lumbar spine often assume this position.

The ancients observed that a patient suffering from pneumonia often lay on the affected side, a position which we often, but not invariably, see these patients assume. Aretaeus the Cappadocian, who practiced in the second century, noted that in these patients "it is comfortable to lie on the inflamed side, but on the opposite side painful." This observation was old in his day. Patients with pericarditis or heart

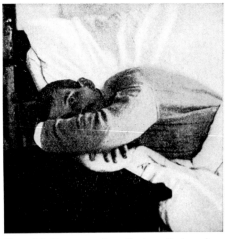

FIG. 26. Posture of patient suffering from pericardial effusion (Ebstein.)

trouble often appear most comfortable when lying on their right side and often when leaning their body over against a table (Fig. 26).

In tetanus the spine may be so bent backward that the body rests on the back of the head and the heels. This position is called *opisthotonos* (ὄπισθεν —opisthen = behind + τόνος—tonos = something stretched). When the body is bent forward it is called *em-prosthotonos* (ἔμπροσθεν emprosthen = forward + τόνος). Flexion of the body to one side is *pleurothotonos* (πλευρόθεν —pleurothen = side +τόνος); while at times the entire trunk and limbs may be rigid, *orthotonos* (ὀρθός—orthos = straight + τόνος). Opisthotonos was described by Hippocrates in tetanus.

Opisthotonos is frequently seen also in epidemic cerebrospinal meningitis and in tuberculous meningitis (Fig. 27).

Patients with congenital cardiac disease often are dyspneic and have severe pains in the legs when standing but obtain immediate relief when they assume a squatting position.

Patients suffering from serious cardiac disease usually assume a sitting posture in bed. These patients cannot lie flat in bed, and they even sleep in a sitting posture. The same posture is usually assumed by any patient suffering from embarrassment of respiration, whether due to heart disease, nephritis, pneumonia or asthma.

Many patients suffering from heart disease sleep at night, not in their beds, but sitting by the side of the bed with their arms resting on the bed and their heads buried in their arms. When a patient gives a history of sleeping, not in his bed, but propped up in his chair, such a history is almost pathognomonic of heart disease.

Patients suffering from severe pain often assume unusual attitudes to obtain relief. Figure 28 shows the position during sleep of a patient suffering from Buerger's disease. The subject of the position assumed by patients suffering from various diseases has been studied by Ebstein, whose article should be read by every student and physician interested in this subject.

MOVEMENTS

In health the body and the extremities are at rest except when moved by voluntary motions of the body. Involuntary movements are departures from the normal and may occur while the person is conscious or unconscious.

One of the most common types of involuntary movements occurring during consciousness is that which includes the so-called *tics* or *habit spasms*. These movements involve most commonly the eye muscles and the muscles of the face and neck. The person from time to time rolls his eyes around, from side to side or upward, or may suddenly squint his eye and then open it widely. Some persons make sudden terrifying facial grimaces or roll their heads about in an unexpected fashion. These tics, or habit spasms, as the latter name implies, are the result of habit and, like most habits,

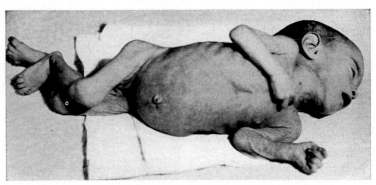

FIG. 27. Opisthotonos in child with meningitis.

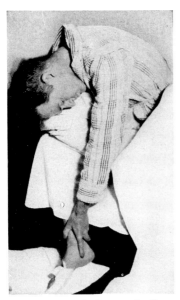

FIG. 28. Posture in Buerger's disease.

are difficult or even impossible to overcome.

The famous Dr. Samuel Johnson was a victim of habit spasms. His biographer Boswell has written a good account of the great lexicographer's tics. On one occasion a young girl asked him why he made "such strange gestures." "From bad habits," replied Dr. Johnson. "Do you, my dear, take care to guard against bad habits."

In *chorea,* or *St. Vitus' dance,* called first by Paracelsus *chorea Sancti Viti,* the patient makes sudden, unexpected and purposeless movements, usually of the arms and legs, but at times of the head or even of the whole body. This disease has been called *Sydenham's chorea* since Sydenham's masterful description of it. "The hand," Sydenham wrote, "cannot be steady for a moment. It passes from one position to another by a convulsive movement, however much the patient may strive to the contrary. Before he can raise a cup to his lips, he makes as many gesticulations as a mountebank." The disease, as Sydenham noted, "attacks boys and girls from the tenth year to the time of puberty." The first symptoms that parents often note is the awkwardness

of the children, who drop glasses and plates at the table. The name "St. Vitus' dance" came from the chapel of St. Vitus at Zabern, which sufferers from the "dancing mania" of the Middle Ages visited for cures. The "dancing mania" of the Middle Ages, an epidemic of religious excitement, was probably hysteria and entirely different from *chorea,* although the contortions of its victims resembled those of this disease.

In *Huntington's chorea,* a hereditary affliction, the movements are similar to those of Sydenham's chorea. In Huntington's chorea, however, the disease begins during adult life, becomes progressively worse and leads to mental deterioration.

Convulsions may occur with or without a loss of consciousness, show muscle spasms, and are seen in epilepsy, eclampsia, hysteria, tetanus, tetany, scarlet fever, encephalitis, typhoid fever, uremia and in poisoning, notably with strychnine. Clonic convulsions are those marked by an alternate contraction and relaxation of the muscles; tonic convulsions are those in which there is a persistent contraction of the muscles.

In *Jacksonian epilepsy* the spasm begins in a limited group of muscles in the face, arm or leg and may gradually extend to other muscles. The patient is conscious throughout and watches with both interest and apprehension the spread or march of the spasm.

GAIT

The gait of a patient gives information of great value. Several gaits are especially characteristic and often seen.

A patient suffering from *hemiplegia* usually drags the affected leg around in a semicircle while walking. An observant eye sees that the inner side of the toe of the shoe and the sole beneath it is worn away more on the affected foot than on the normal one. These patients, when walking, often hold the arm on the affected side slightly flexed and quite stiff, as contrasted with the free and easy movements of the normal side.

Patients with tabes dorsalis have a peculiar *slapping* or *flail-like gait*. They walk with their eyes on the ground, the feet wide apart, raising the legs quite high so their feet will clear the ground and then bringing them down with a peculiar slap, the heel usually striking the ground first, or the entire sole at the same time. "The normal man walks by faith, the tabetic by sight" (Osler). This gait has sometimes been compared with that of a man walking up-stream in shallow water. "If the patient is asked to close his eyes while standing upright, he immediately begins to sway and reel," as Romberg noted years ago. This has since been known as *Romberg's sign*.

Many patients suffering from *paralysis agitans* (Parkinson's disease) have a typical gait. They walk with their head and body sharply inclined forward, usually with sharp quick steps, and give the appearance of "running after their center of gravity." This gait, when once seen, impresses itself indelibly upon one's memory and may be sufficient to allow one to make what Traube called an "Augenblicksdiagnose," or "instantaneous diagnosis." It is a good example of what one recognizes, not because he has read a long description of it, but because he has seen it before (Fig. 29). It may be slight or absent in milder cases of paralysis agitans.

A *spastic gait,* a stiff, choppy sort of walking, is often seen in multiple sclerosis, in amyotrophic lateral sclerosis and in other nervous diseases involving lesions of the upper neuron. A slow, clumsy gait, as if the patient were stepping over obstacles, often accompanies peripheral neuritis. The *scissors gait* seen in spastic paraplegia is due to rigidity of the adductor muscles of the thigh. The name accurately suggests the appearance of the patient, who walks with his thighs close together like the blades of a scissors.

An *ataxic gait* is seen in cerebellar disease, in diseases of the labyrinth and in Friedreich's ataxia. These patients step irregularly, sway and reel like drunken men without, however, the stamping gait of the tabetic. An in-

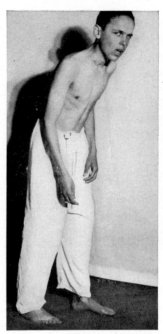

Fig. 29. Gait in postencephalitic Parkinson's disease.

teresting condition called *astasia-abasia* was described by Charcot in patients who had perfect control of their legs while lying in bed, but were unable either to walk or stand. This condition is produced by hysteria.

SPEECH

The character of the voice may aid in a diagnosis. The voice in a man suffering from infantilism is high pitched like that of a eunuch. In virilism, its antithesis, the voice of a boy of six may be deep and bass like that of an adult male. In aneurysm of the aorta the voice as well as the cough may have a brassy quality. In laryngeal paralysis the voice is usually feeble.

Diseases of the *larynx* with involvement of the vocal cords produce marked and obvious changes in the voice. In tuberculosis and syphilis of the larynx the voice is enfeebled, hoarse and rough. In carcinoma of the larynx the voice is markedly weakened, usually higher pitched than in tuberculosis or syphilis, and suggests a "stage whisper." Acute or chronic laryngitis causes hoarseness, enfeebled voice or even aphonia. A persisting hoarseness should always excite suspicion and should be carefully investigated.

Certain disturbances in speech are evidence of involvement of the nervous system and at times are so characteristic as almost to permit a diagnosis.

One of the most characteristic types of speech is the *"scanning speech,"* which, when present, is an important finding in multiple sclerosis. In this type of speech enunciation is slow and the patient hesitates at the beginning of words, then rushes on with the sentence, producing a peculiar staccato-like effect. It occurs also in Friedreich's ataxia.

In *paresis* the speech is slovenly and sticks, as it were, at certain consonants, particularly "l" and "r." The common test phrases which bring out these defects are "round the rugged rock the ragged rascal ran" and "third riding artillery brigade."

In a comparatively rare disease, *pseudobulbar paralysis,* the voice is dull, monotonous and without the normal modulations of tone. The patient speaks suddenly, almost explosively, and in order to pronounce a few words uses an immense amount of effort, which seems to exhaust him.

A patient with *delirium tremens* has a very tremulous speech; he stumbles over words and often mispronounces them. In *botulism* the patient suffers from an obvious paralysis of speech and complains of great difficulty in speaking. Articulation is indistinct, and there may be a complete loss of voice, or aphonia.

Aphonia, or loss of voice, must be distinguished from aphasia. A patient with *aphasia* or, more accurately, *motor aphasia* has a loss or defect in the power of expression by speech. The patient with aphasia has not lost his ability to speak, but has lost his ability to say what he wishes. He cannot speak the word he wishes spontaneously, but often can when the word he wishes has been supplied. A test often used is to show the patient a key. "What is it?" he is asked. "That is a . . . " "A ring?" "No." "A knife?" "No." "A key?" "Yes, that is a key."

Anarthria is the inability to articulate clearly. Aphonia, aphasia and anarthria are commonly the result of cerebral vascular lesions.

NUTRITION

Overweight. The state of nutrition is usually judged by considering whether the patient is overweight or underweight.

One of the most common causes of overweight is overeating. Many obese patients become so because of their appetites. Many fat people, however, do not eat excessively as compared with other people. However, they eat more food than they require and for that reason gain weight. Heredity, as is well known, plays an important role, so that many families show in successive generations this tendency to store fat.

Patients whose fat is the result of overeating usually show fat faces, with double chins, fat arms and a deposit of fat particularly about the abdomen. Such people often show a tremendous increase in girth, while the legs, although fat, seem unusually small by contrast, and appear quite inadequate to support the patient's weight. This type is especially seen in middle-aged persons (Fig. 30).

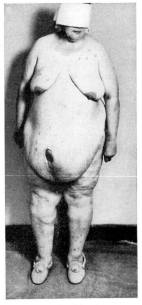

FIG. 30. Obesity.

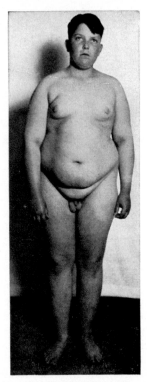

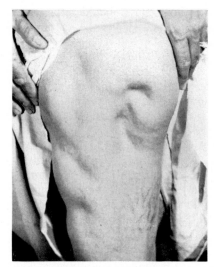

Fig. 32. Fat atrophy in patient receiving insulin injections.

Fig. 31. Fröhlich's syndrome.

One of the most striking types of fat people is seen in patients suffering from diseases of the endocrine glands. The most characteristic, perhaps, is that seen in *Fröhlich's syndrome,* due to disease of the pituitary gland. These patients show an infantilism of the sexual organs associated with a marked deposit of fat, which has a central distribution, occurring mainly upon the lower part of the abdomen and thighs. The face of such patients may be of normal appearance, and the arms, hands, legs and feet normal in size. Such persons are fat centrally, while peripherally they are of normal size (Fig. 31).

Diabetic patients occasionally show a striking atrophy of the subcutaneous fat following continued administration of insulin subcutaneously (Fig. 32).

Closely related to the obesity due to endocrine disorders are the localized deposits of fat forming true *fatty tumors* or *lipomata.* Such fatty tumors are usually located symmetrically upon the neck and arms, also at times over the

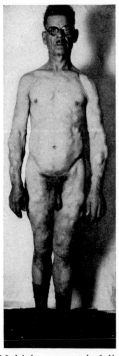

Fig. 33. Multiple symmetrical lipomatosis.

chest, abdomen and legs, and are better known as "multiple symmetrical lipomatosis" (Fig. 33). This condition occurs both in overnourished and normally nourished persons. Hypothyroid obesity is less common. Patients who suffer from it show other signs of hypothyroidism. Another disease closely related is *Dercum's disease,* or *adiposis dolorosa.* This name suggests at once the most striking characteristics of the disease—fatty deposits and pain. These patients, already fat, acquire painful masses of fat.

Fatty people are proverbially the butt of numerous jibes and jokes. But obesity is no joking matter, as the fat man learns when he applies for life insurance and is heavily penalized. Beall has calculated that every pound of fat requires five sixths of a mile of blood vessels to supply it and that a man who is 30 pounds overweight is carrying around 25 miles of excessive blood vessels with a resultant strain upon the circulatory system. He points out that fat is a parasite and that as we lengthen the waistline we shorten the life line.

Edema, or *general anasarca,* may cause a marked increase in weight. This should be suspected when a patient gains weight with phenomenal rapidity. Such edema is commonly the result of heart disease or kidney disease, and more recently is often seen in diabetics taking insulin. We have seen diabetic patients gain as much as 15 pounds a week, the increase being mainly due to retention of fluid with the production of an insulin edema. The student should remember that 10 pounds of edema may be present without being obvious.

Underweight. Underweight, or loss of weight, is most commonly seen in conditions in which there is an excessive destruction of tissue, as in continued fevers, and in wasting diseases such as pulmonary tuberculosis (Fig. 34) and cancer. Pulmonary tuberculosis, however, may be present in a patient whose nutrition is excellent. The patient shown in Figure 252 had advanced pulmonary tuberculosis with cavitation. In Graves' disease, or hyperthyroidism, we see a marked loss in weight just as we see a gain of weight in myxedema or hypothyroidism. Graves' disease shows an increase in the metabolic rate, while myxedema shows a decrease.

In *Simmonds' disease,* a syndrome caused by atrophy of the anterior lobe of the pituitary, there is marked emaciation with a decrease in the metabolic rate (Fig. 35).

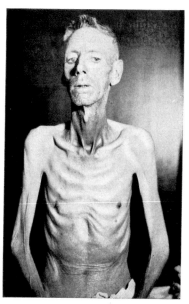

FIG. 34. Extreme emaciation in patient suffering from pulmonary tuberculosis.

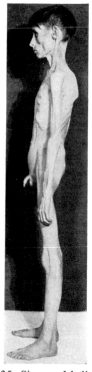

FIG. 35. Simmonds' disease.

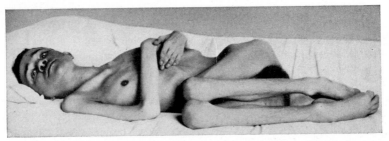

Fig. 36. Extreme emaciation as a result of poliomyelitis.

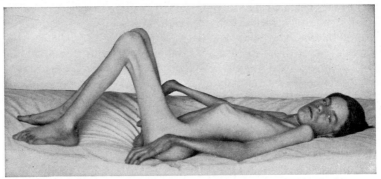

Fig. 37. Extreme emaciation in late stages of muscular dystrophy.

Diabetics lose weight rapidly, loss of fluid being in part responsible. The sudden disappearance of a cardiac or renal edema accompanied by a marked increase in the output of urine produces a rapid and striking loss of weight.

One of the most striking pictures of loss of weight with emaciation is seen in *amyotrophic lateral sclerosis,* fortunately a relatively rare disease, some of the unfortunate victims of which are exhibited in side-shows as "living skeletons." An attack of poliomyelitis in childhood producing an extensive paralysis may lead later to extreme emaciation (Fig. 36). Extreme emaciation is also seen in the late stage of muscular dystrophy (Fig. 37).

Mental diseases or simple "worry" with the common accompaniment of loss of appetite and sleep often result in a marked loss of weight.

STATURE

When the stature of people is increased above normal limits, we class them as giants and, when decreased, as dwarfs. Both these types have loomed large in the mythology, fables and fairy tales of the past, but now lose much of their mystery in the explanation of modern science.

Giants. The legends of giants in past ages probably developed from the occasional discovery of the bones of prehistoric animals. An immense thigh bone of some prehistoric monster, for instance, was discovered by some primitive people, who immediately assumed it to be a human bone and estimated the size of the man to whom it belonged. Thus originated the stories of large monsters who were able to step over houses or ships with the greatest ease.

Many giants, however, of more modest proportions have undoubtedly existed. Goliath's height, according to Scripture, was "six cubits and a span," or about 9 feet 9 inches. One of the most interesting giants in medical history was O'Brien, the famous Irish giant, whom John Hunter saw and coveted. Hunter was determined to have his skeleton, while O'Brien was equally determined that he should not. Finally, O'Brien on his deathbed paid some men to take his body after death, put lead in his coffin and sink it in the Thames. Hunter, getting wind of this arrangement, hurried to the scene, plied the men with drink, and finally secured the body at a cost of 500 pounds. The coffin, filled with lead, was towed out in the Thames and sunk while Hunter hastened away with his treasure, now one of the curiosities of the Museum of the Royal College of Surgeons. O'Brien was 8 feet 4 inches in height. The Russian giant, Machnow, one of the tallest known, measured 9 feet 3 inches in height (Fig. 38). The tallest giantess known was Wassiliko Calliandji, a Greek, who measured 7 feet 6 inches.

Many classifications of giants have been proposed, but that of Launois and Roy is most generally accepted. They recognized two types:

1. ACROMEGALIC GIANTS. These cases of gigantism are the best known and understood, and are produced by a hyperactivity of the anterior lobe of the pituitary gland. Most of the giants who have been autopsied have shown definite evidence of disease of the pituitary. The skull of O'Brien shows a marked enlargement of the sella turcica, indicating a large and hyperactive pituitary gland. "Acromegaly is gigantism of the adult, gigantism is acromegaly of the adolescent" (Brissaud and Meige). This may be expressed by saying that when the pituitary hyperactivity begins during adolescence, gigantism appears; when the hyperactivity begins in the adult, acromegaly results.

2. INFANTILE GIANTS. These giants resemble eunuchs, who, it will be recalled, often attain great stature and in whom castration is performed before puberty. These giants have extremely long legs, marked atrophy of the genitalia and failure of the epiphyses to unite (Fig. 39). They do not show the marked bony overgrowth characteristic of acromegaly such as the hypertrophy of the frontal bone and of the mandible.

Such giants with infantilism, however, often show at autopsy enlarged pituitary glands. Acromegalic giants, conversely, often show infantilism. Frequently both types of giants really merge into each

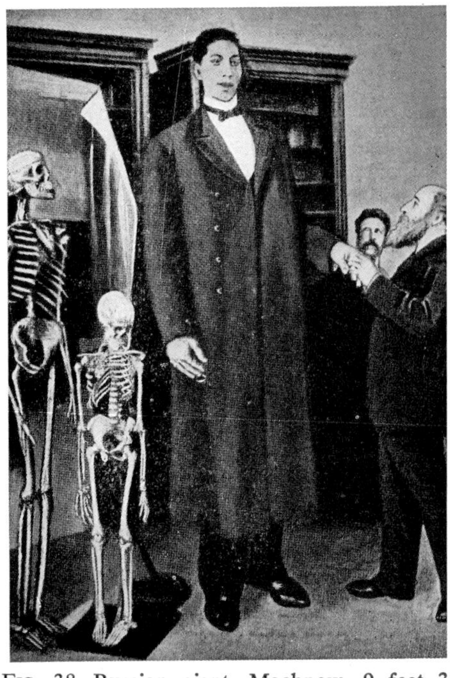

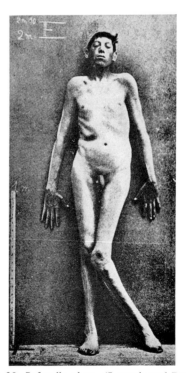

Fig. 38. Russian giant, Machnow, 9 feet 3 inches in height. (Launois and Roy.)

Fig. 39. Infantile giant. (Launois and Roy.)

other. "If all giants are not acromegalic, all those who are not are apt to become so" (Launois and Roy). Gigantism is a disease in which both the pituitary and the gonads may play a role, but the role of the pituitary is by far the more important.

Dwarfs. Dwarfs are persons with stunted growth when compared with persons of the same race and age. The history of dwarfs is no less interesting than that of giants. The Greeks ignored dwarfs in their sculpture, but the Romans have left us many examples. Many painters, including Holbein, Van Dyck and Velasquez, have painted dwarfs with such fidelity that we can look at their pictures and diagnose the type of dwarfism.

Dwarfs have been divided into three groups:

1. ATELEIOTIC DWARFS. These are dwarfs who are perfectly proportioned, but are small in all their parts. They are simply "pocket editions of adults" —"a man seen through a reversed opera-glass." Many famous dwarfs belong to this category, among them Charles G. Stratton, better known to the world after his introduction by P. T. Barnum under the cognomen of General Tom Thumb (Fig. 40). At the age of

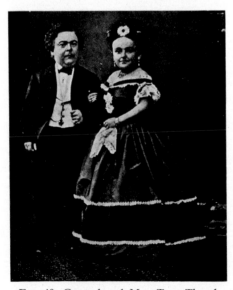

FIG. 40. General and Mrs. Tom Thumb.

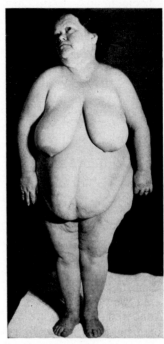

FIG. 41. Ateleiotic dwarf showing scar of cesarean section. (The patient's mother and grandmother were also ateleiotic dwarfs.)

twenty-five Tom Thumb was 31 inches in height.

Ateleiotic dwarfs are clever, intelligent and quite normal except for their stature. They marry and often beget children, although pregnancy is dangerous to the mother because of the small size of her pelvis, and a cesarean section is commonly necessary (Fig. 41).

2. ACHONDROPLASTIC DWARFS. These dwarfs are not perfectly formed like the first group, but have abnormally short legs. The Egyptian dwarf Puoinhetef, who belonged to this group (Fig. 42), had such legs as his portrait on his tomb shows clearly. Puoinhetef was a dancer who lived circa 340 B.C. The entire body of these dwarfs is small, often deformed, the legs are curved and unusually short, the spine is crooked, and the head commonly as large as that of a full-grown adult (Fig. 43). These dwarfs are of normal intelligence, the musculature is well developed, and their genital organs are of normal size and function normally. "This latter characteristic," as Pagniez remarks, "is

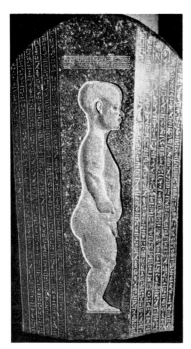

FIG. 42. The Dwarf Puoinhetef. (Cairo Museum.)

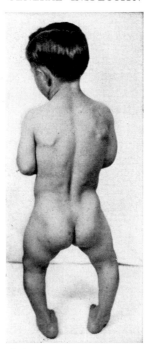

FIG. 43. Achondroplasia in boy aged seven and one-half years. Note extremely short and curved legs.

fortunate for the man but unfortunate for the women, for the pelvis being contracted, the grave complications of dystocia result, which make necessary cesarean sections, embryotomies, etc."

3. CRETINS. Cretins, who are examples of endemic dwarfism, are markedly abnormal in many ways. Short in stature, often being less than 3 feet in height, their extremities are short, and often curved with the spine deviated to either side. The expression is dull, the forehead narrow and low, the eyelids are puffy, the nose is flat, and the jaws are pendulous. The mouth is large, often habitually open, with thick lips constantly dripping saliva. The tongue is usually large and protrudes from the mouth (Fig. 44). The chin is small and the ears seem swollen. The skin is dry, leathery and rough, and the hands and feet are cyanosed, thick and rough. There is little or no axillary and pubic hair. The genitalia are infantile and immature. Cretins are always of low mentality and frequently are idiots.

Other types of dwarfs are also occasionally encountered. A very severe rickets may lead to dwarfism, particularly when the fetus is rachitic, but

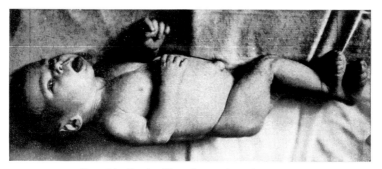

FIG. 44. Cretin. Note large size of tongue.

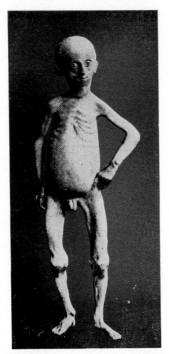

FIG. 45. Progeria. (Hastings Gilford.)

dwarfism may also appear when the rachitis occurs in early infancy. Such dwarfs naturally show other characteristics of rickets: the rickety rosary, chicken breast, scoliosis, natiform skull, olympic forehead and marked deformi-

ties of the legs. Two other types, seen occasionally, are *mitral dwarfism* in children who suffer mitral disease early, and *renal dwarfism* in children with advanced chronic nephritis. A remarkable and rare type of dwarfism is the condition called *progeria* (Fig. 45), which affects youthful persons, producing a marked stunting of growth, underdevelopment of the genitalia and premature senility. These patients resemble little old men both in their appearance and in their facial expression. At autopsy they show marked arteriosclerosis and other signs of advanced age. The cause of this condition is entirely unknown, although some workers think it of pituitary origin. Syphilis may produce a type of dwarfism. Congenital heart disease may lead to a marked shortening in stature.

Rischbieth and Barrington published a photograph of an unusual collection of dwarfs (Fig. 46), showing the achondroplastic dwarfs with short legs, ateleiotic dwarfs perfectly proportioned, and a dull-faced, pot-bellied cretin.

TEMPERATURE

The taking of the temperature is such a commonplace occurrence that it is

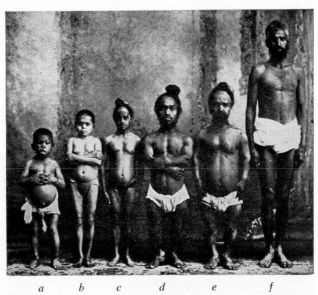

a   b   c   d   e   f

FIG. 46. Various types of dwarfs with normal man for comparison (Rischbieth and Barrington): *a*, cretin; *b*, *c*, ateleiotic dwarfs; *d*, *e*, achondroplasia; *f*, normal.

Inſtrumentum Primum.

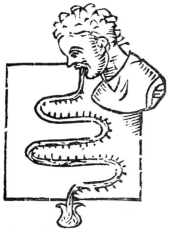

FIG. 47. Santorio's thermometer, (Sanctorii Sanctorii: Commentaria in Primam Feu Primi Libri, Venice, 1646.)

hard to realize that the systematic recording of temperature dates only from 1852. Galileo invented the thermometer, while Santorio (1561–1636), professor at Padua, was the first physician to use a clinical thermometer. He devised several types of instruments. One type was inserted into the mouth (Fig. 47), while another type was described to be held in front of the mouth, so that the hot breath of the patient might strike it. More than two centuries elapsed before his discovery bore fruit.

The first systematic temperature records of patients were begun in the Leipzig Clinic in 1851, and the first published curve was that of Ludwig Traube in 1852 (Fig. 48). This innovation was the source of many jibes, and a prominent French clinician called it an unprofitable subtlety, which could only be carried out in little German hospitals where there were as many physicians as patients. Sir Clifford Allbutt, whose death occurred as late as 1922, recalled as an old man the jibes that he endured while a young practitioner, because he carried a thermometer and used it upon his patients.

The American physician, with a devotion worthier of a better cause, still stands shoulder to shoulder with his British colleague in using the Fahrenheit thermometer, although the rest of the world has long since abandoned it in favor of the Centigrade. Even his own American scientific colleagues now use the Centigrade thermometer.

The normal range of temperature does not usually exceed 98.6° F. by mouth, or 99° F. by rectum. The method of taking the temperature is too well known to need description, although it may be well to call attention to the necessity of "shaking down" a thermometer before using it.

The temperature may be normal, subnormal or increased. A marked fall in temperature in a patient who is quite ill and whose temperature has been normal is of bad prognostic report. Cardiac patients often show a subnormal temperature a few hours or a day or two before death.

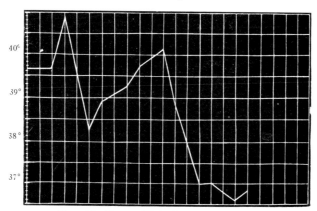

FIG. 48. First published curve of fever.

It is not unusual, however, for normal persons, or those not seriously ill, to show a subnormal temperature, particularly in cold weather. If one examines temperature charts in hospitals, particularly of children, he is often struck with the fact that patients (without fever) show a much higher average in hot weather than in cold.

Fever. An increase in temperature above 98.6° F. by mouth is known as fever. Every degree above normal is spoken of as a degree of fever. When a patient has a temperature of 99.6° F., he has one degree of fever. Patients are often said "to have a temperature," when what is obviously meant is that they have fever or have an increase in temperature, since everybody has a temperature.

Fevers are divided into remittent, intermittent and continuous. A *remittent fever* is one in which there are marked exacerbations in temperature, and marked falls, but not to normal. This type of temperature is often seen in malaria and in sepsis, and may occur in typhoid fever. An *intermittent fever* is one in which the temperature may go high, but some time during the day falls to normal or subnormal. This intermittent fever is seen in malaria, in sepsis, liver abscess and often in cholecystitis (Fig. 49). Some use the term "remittent fever" to include cases where there is a high fever one day and a normal temperature the next, as in tertian malaria (Fig. 50). *Continuous fever* is one in which the temperature remains consistently elevated for many days, showing no greater fluctuations than those seen in normal temperatures. Typhoid fever is the classic example of this type (Fig. 51).

Fevers may disappear either by lysis or by crisis. If the temperature gradually falls to normal in the course of two, three or more days, we speak of the fever falling by *lysis* (Fig. 52); if the temperature falls to normal within thirty-six hours, we speak of a fever falling by *crisis* (Fig. 53). The terms "lysis" and "crisis" are used particularly in lobar pneumonia. When the temperature in lobar pneumonia falls by crisis, the event is so dramatic that it is well remembered by the observer,

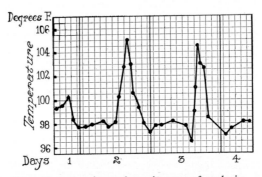

FIG. 49. Intermittent fever in case of malaria.

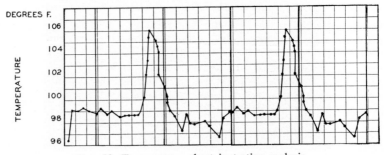

FIG. 50. Temperature chart in tertian malaria.

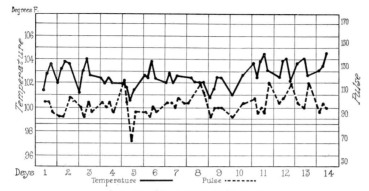

FIG. 51. Chart in typhoid fever.

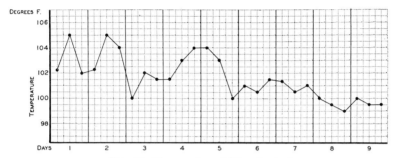

FIG. 52. Temperature falling by lysis.

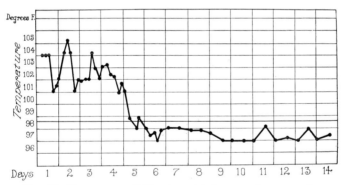

FIG. 53. Temperature falling by crisis in case of pneumonia.

while the less dramatic fall by lysis is soon forgotten. This has led to the popular belief that the temperature in lobar pneumonia usually falls by crisis. Cole found, however, that a true crisis occurred in not more than 15 per cent of his cases.

The most common cause of fever is an infectious disease. The commonest causes of fever of short duration are tonsillitis, acute nasopharyngitis, sinusitis, acute enteritis and pneumonia; the commonest causes of a fever of long duration are typhoid fever, tuberculosis, undulant fever, subacute endocarditis, rheumatic fever and malaria.

There is a small group of diseases in which the temperature is alternately elevated and normal for varying periods of time. In relapsing fever due to the spirillum of Obermeier the temperature is markedly elevated for four or five days, then suddenly falls to normal and remains normal four or five days, then rises again (Fig. 54). In brucellosis (Malta fever), a disease which is com-

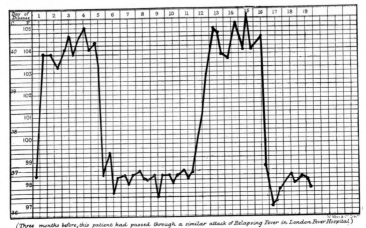

(*Three months before, this patient had passed through a similar attack of Relapsing Fever in London Fever Hospital*)

Fig. 54. Temperature in relapsing fever. (Murchison.)

mon in the United States, the fever is usually of the remittent type and, after lasting for one to three weeks, falls to normal for two or more days and then rises again. This process repeats itself until the disease has lasted three months (the average time), although cases have been known to last two years.

Another interesting fever of this group is the *relapsing pyrexia* occurring in Hodgkin's disease, which is usually referred to as the Pel-Ebstein fever. "Following on a period of low pyrexia, or of normal or subnormal temperatures,

there is a steady rise occupying two or four days to a maximum, which may reach 105° F. For about three days it remains at the high level and then there is a gradual fall by lysis, occupying about three days, and the temperature then becomes sub-normal" (Fig. 55).

Smallpox is commonly ushered in by a chill, or even convulsions in children, followed by an abrupt rise of temperature to 103° or 104° F. With the appearance of the eruption, the fever usually remits, then rises again on the seventh day (Fig. 56).

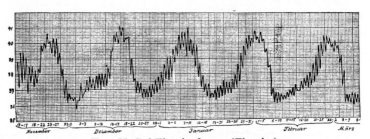

Fig. 55. Pel-Ebstein fever. (Ebstein.)

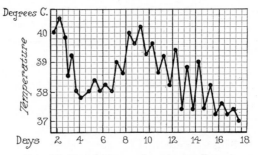

Fig. 56. Temperature chart in smallpox.

Chills commonly mark the onset of certain infectious diseases such as lobar pneumonia, malaria and sometimes typhoid fever. Other diseases such as scarlet fever, cholecystitis, liver abscess and peritonitis may begin with a chill. The phenomena accompanying a chill are striking. The skin is pale, cyanotic and cold. The capillaries are often constricted and the peripheral circulation is slowed. The patient feels cold, and shivers. Although the skin remains cold, the internal temperature of the body rises rapidly. The patient soon breaks out into a profuse perspiration, and the skin becomes warm and moist. The mouth or rectal temperature, which was normal at the onset of the chill, rises rapidly.

Chills following instrumentation, particularly of the bladder, urethra or kidneys, may be accompanied by an elevation of temperature. In hysterical chills the temperature remains normal.

Sweating, particularly at night, is commonly associated with tuberculosis. In such patients the sweating usually occurs while the patient sleeps. If he reverses the order of things, sleeping during the day and remaining awake at night, he has day sweats. Sweating is often an accompaniment of many other infectious diseases, notably pneumonia, influenza, endocarditis, undulant fever, rheumatic fever and typhoid fever. It is commonly present in any infectious disease.

Certain noninfectious diseases, such as leukemia, Hodgkin's disease and Graves' disease, may be accompanied by fever. In Graves' disease, however, the pulse rate is increased out of all proportion to the temperature, while in typhoid fever, particularly early in the disease, the reverse is the rule. The patient's chart in Graves' disease resembles the chart of a typhoid fever patient turned upside down (Fig. 57). Malignant tumors may produce fever. Patients in diabetic coma usually show fever. Many patients with anemia show slight but persistent fever. In cerebral hemorrhage, when the hemorrhage occurs in the basal ganglia, the temperature is frequently elevated.

Sunstrokes, as is well known, may produce a sudden marked rise of temperature, the temperature often reaching 110° F. or higher. In heat exhaustion, by contrast, the temperature becomes subnormal and may fall to 95° F.

Starvation may produce fever. A marked loss of body fluids or a deprivation of water often causes a marked rise in temperature. This type of fever is common in children. Certain drugs such as belladonna, iodides and sulfonamides may cause fever in susceptible persons. Psychogenic fevers have been described. The body temperature may be elevated during a hysterical attack. Genuine habitual hyperthermia is the term given to a condition in which the persons are apparently perfectly well, but show regular elevations of temperature above normal.

Frequent sweating is often observed in pernicious anemia. Many nervous patients sweat, particularly when they are subject to a physical examination. The physician often sees the sweat trickle down from the axillae while examining an apprehensive patient.

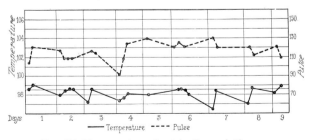

Fig. 57. Temperature chart in Graves' disease.

SKIN

The condition of the patient's skin should always be carefully noted by the physician. Many skin conditions are associated with general systemic disease, while others are skin diseases *per se* and belong entirely within the domain of dermatology. A discussion of skin diseases does not lie within the scope of this book and is treated both exhaustively and completely in textbooks of dermatology. The student of physical diagnosis should be familiar with certain common skin conditions. He may also be reminded with profit that many great clinicians have also been competent dermatologists.

State of Skin. The state of the skin should always be noted. A very loose skin which can be picked up in folds is a good indication that the patient has lost weight. A harsh, greasy skin is often, although not invariably, seen in tuberculosis. A moist skin is frequently observed in hyperthyroidism—particularly on the palms of the hands. In myxedema, by contrast, the skin is dry and harsh. A marked harshness and thickening of the skin is a characteristic finding in scleroderma, a disease which is fortunately relatively rare. In ichthyosis or "fish skin" the condition is admirably described by the name (Fig. 58). The skin is furrowed and scaly, like the scales of a fish. Mild degrees of ichthyosis are common in the Negro race, particularly on the legs. This condition is congenital, and usually most marked in winter. Edema of the skin is seen especially in nephritis, heart disease, diabetes mellitus and inanition.

Color of Skin. The color of the skin is one of the first characteristics that should be studied. An *extreme pallor* is commonly the first abnormality that calls attention to a severe anemia. It should be stressed, however, that many pale persons are so because of a lack of a rich superficial blood supply to the skin. Such persons apparently have an unusual degree of capillary constriction. Pallor of the mucous membranes is of

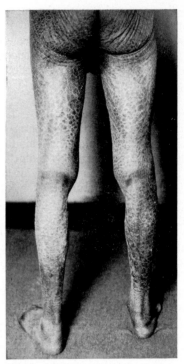

Fig. 58. Ichthyosis.

far more importance in the diagnosis of anemia than pallor of the skin.

An unusual *redness of the skin* is present in a fresh sunburn. It is most marked in the exanthem of scarlet fever. Yet the author once saw a patient with an intense erythema, fever and albuminuria—the whole picture suggesting most strongly an attack of scarlet fever. The absence of the characteristic tongue, together with the history of a prolonged sun bath, established the correct diagnosis.

In *polycythemia vera* the skin, especially of the face and hands, is extremely red, often somewhat purplish. The ruddy, purplish complexion of these patients often permits a tentative diagnosis.

A *lemon-yellow tint* of the skin is commonly seen in pernicious anemia, but may occur also in severe secondary anemia. A peculiar orange color of the skin, especially of the palms of the hands, occurs in diabetes mellitus. This condition, known as *xanthosis,* is sometimes associated with small orange-colored nodules—*xanthomata diabeti-corum*—an unusual skin complication of diabetes mellitus, first described by Thomas Addison and usually associated with a high blood cholesterol. This remarkable diabetic complication bears no special relation to the severity of the disease (Fig. 59).

The best-known cause for a yellowish discoloration of the skin is *icterus* or *jaundice*. In icterus the color of the skin may vary from a light yellow to a greenish or even brownish. This condition is most commonly due to "catarrhal jaundice," usually infectious hepatitis, to gallstones or to malignant disease of the bile ducts, all examples of obstructive jaundice. Very intense jaundice may be the result of fulminant acute hepatitis with massive necrosis of the liver. Jaundice is also seen in some cases of pernicious anemia.

In *hemolytic jaundice* the icterus is distinct but not intense and is not associated with clay-colored stools. This type of jaundice is commonly familial, and the patient shows enlargement of the spleen with a severe anemia.

It must be remembered that jaundice is best diagnosed by daylight and may not be perceptible under artificial light. Patients with jaundice usually suffer from intense itching and scratch a great deal. The presence of scratch marks over the chest or abdomen sometimes gives the clue to the diagnosis when the patient is examined under artificial light and the jaundice is not apparent. Patients with jaundice also show an icteric tint of the sclerae of the eyes and also of the mucous membranes.

A condition sometimes confused with jaundice is *carotinemia*. This condition, most commonly seen in children eating large amounts of carrots, causes an orange tint of the skin rather than a yellow. In our experience the sclera of the eye is not stained in carotinemia as it is in icterus.

Cyanosis, a bluish color of the skin, is associated with anoxemia or a diminution in the oxygen-carrying capacity of the blood. It is noted most commonly

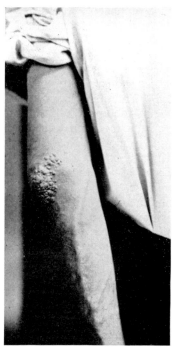

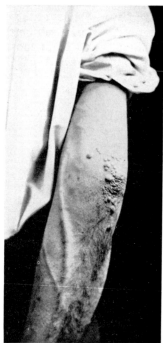

FIG. 59. Xanthomatosis diabeticorum.

in cardiac disease with heart failure and in pneumonia. In these conditions the cyanosis is often observed first in the ears and on the tip of the nose. A chronic cyanosis is seen in congenital heart disease and in polycythemia vera, in both which conditions there is a marked increase in the number of red blood cells. The cyanosis in both is especially marked in the lips. A striking cyanosis is produced by occlusion of the vena cava. When the superior vena cava is occluded, the upper half of the body, including the face and arms, becomes strikingly cyanotic. This is often associated with edema of the neck and upper part of the thorax, a condition referred to as "Stokes collar." When the inferior vena cava is occluded, cyanosis of the lower half of the body appears. A similar picture is present when there is a fistula between the aorta and the vena cava, which occasionally occurs in aneurysm of the aorta. Cyanosis may also be due to poisoning with certain chemicals and to the continued use of certain drugs, notably coal-tar products. Attacks of acute and intense cyanosis have followed the use of certain shoe polishes and dyes. Studies of these cases have shown the toxic substance producing this effect to be in most cases aniline or nitrobenzene. A patient was seen recently who gave this interesting history. Before joining a group of friends at cards he went to a barber shop where his shoes were dyed and polished. A short time later, while in the midst of a poker game, he noticed that all eyes were turned upon him with a look of amazement. On asking the reason, his friends told him to look in the mirror. He did so and was horrified to see that he had turned blue. His cyanosis disappeared in the course of the night. A striking form of cyanosis involving the face and neck, but stopping sharply at the level of the clavicles, has been observed in crushing injuries of the chest. Cyanosis is also seen in fibrosis of the lungs, advanced emphysema and mitral stenosis.

Argyria resembles cyanosis, but need never be confused with it. This grayish-blue discoloration of the skin and mucous membranes is the result of the ingestion of silver. In the days when silver nitrate was extensively used for internal medication, cases of argyria were more common. The staining is permanent and, although its cosmetic effects

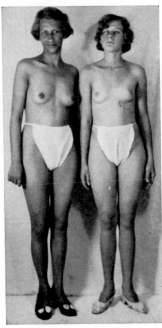

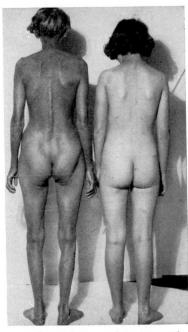

Fig. 60. Addison's disease compared with normal.

Fig. 61. Hemochromatosis compared with normal.

are deplorable, it has no detrimental effect upon the health. In the circus side shows these persons are often demonstrated as examples of a patent foramen ovale.

Two other permanent pigmentations should be mentioned. In Addison's disease there is a striking *brownish* or *bronze-like discoloration* of the skin (Fig. 60), and a similar type of pigmentation is seen in *hemochromatosis* (Fig. 61). Other features in the clinical picture of these two diseases permit a differential diagnosis between the two. Patients suffering from Addison's disease show a low blood pressure and are usually extremely weak. In hemochromatosis, glycosuria is commonly present.

Skin Eruptions. The various types of skin eruptions that may be seen are manifold and are best studied in a textbook of dermatology. A few of the most

common and most characteristic may be considered.

Skin eruptions are frequently caused by drugs, such as bromides (Fig. 62), by sulfonamides, and particularly by antibiotics (Fig. 63).

In typhoid fever the *rose spots* which appear over the abdomen in successive crops are characteristic (Fig. 64).

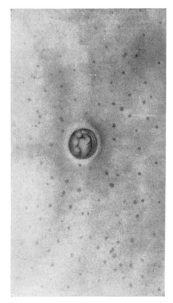

FIG. 64. Rose spots in typhoid fever. (Murchison.)

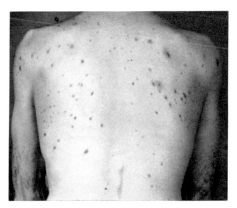

FIG. 62. Skin eruption following bromide therapy.

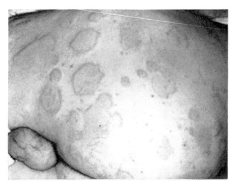

FIG. 63. Skin eruption following penicillin therapy.

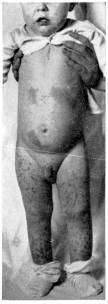

FIG. 65. Purpura haemorrhagica in legs.

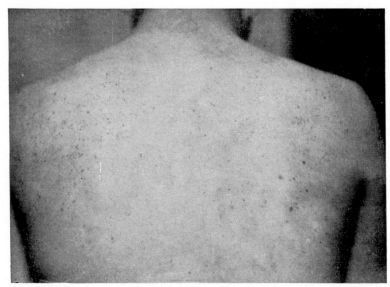

FIG. 66. Petechiae in patient with lymphatic leukemia.

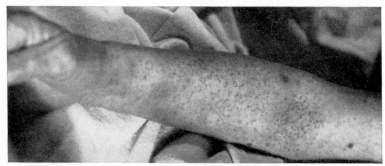

FIG. 67. Petechiae produced by pressure of cuff of sphygmomanometer around the arm.

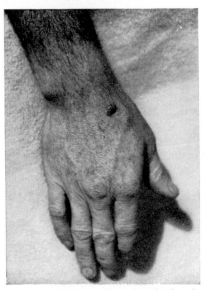

FIG. 68. Melanotic sarcoma of the hand arising from a pigmented mole.

These rose spots are small, slightly elevated reddish papules. On pressure, the color fades completely, since it is due to excessive vascularity and the blood is contained within the blood vessel walls. They are usually most numerous and most obvious over the abdomen, but may appear also over the chest, the back and even the shoulders. In that other classic disease, *typhus fever*—long confused with typhoid fever—small red spots are present which do not disappear on pressure, because the spots are due to small extravasations of blood under the skin. These spots resemble flea-bites, and, indeed, Jerome Cardan, who first described this disease, called it "morbus pulicaris," or flea-bite disease, because of this resemblance. This type of lesion, where there is an extravasation of blood

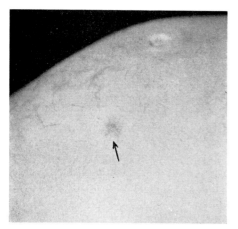

FIG. 69. Spider nevus on abdomen. Patient suffering from cirrhosis of liver.

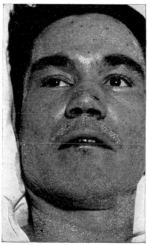

FIG. 70. Urea frost in patient with chronic nephritis.

under the skin, we speak of as *purpura,* and very small spots are called *petechiae.* Petechiae are approximately the size of a pin head. When the extravasations exceed 2 mm. in diameter, they are called *ecchymoses.*

The most striking form of purpura is seen in purpura haemorrhagica, "morbus maculosus Werlhofii"—the spotted disease of Werlhof (Fig. 65). This disease is commonly due to a decrease in the number of blood platelets. It may occur in avitaminosis, especially scurvy, and in the course of certain infectious diseases, especially in typhus fever. It appears often in severe cerebrospinal meningitis; hence the name "spotted fever."

Petechiae are seen in a variety of conditions. They are an important and often pathognomonic sign in subacute infectious endocarditis. They are often seen in leukemia (Fig. 66), in Hodgkin's disease and in aplastic anemia. Less frequently they are seen in nephritis, cancer, chronic tuberculosis and cachexia. In conditions associated with increased capillary fragility such as a deficiency of vitamin K, slight trauma may produce numerous petechiae (Fig. 67).

The skin should be carefully examined for the presence of large pigmented *moles.* These moles sometimes become malignant, giving rise to a melanosarcoma, which is one of the most malignant of all tumors (Fig. 68).

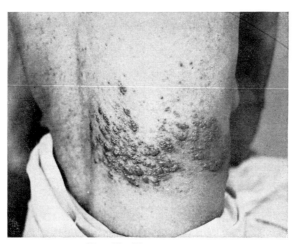

FIG. 71. Herpes zoster.

Spider nevi (Fig. 69), small reddish spots which on close examination prove to be small blood vessels radiating from a center, always suggest liver disease, especially cirrhosis. They are, however, seen occasionally in pregnancy and in deficiency diseases. There is some uncertainty whether these nevi are of arterial or venous origin.

Sudamina are small vesicles the size of millet seeds which contain sweat. An eruption of these vesicles may occur after profuse sweating or in certain febrile diseases. We have recently seen a marked eruption of sudamina in a diabetic patient who had intense perspiration following insulin shock.

A striking phenomenon which occasionally appears in uremia is the *urea frost.* The term is very descriptive. The skin, especially of the face, is covered in places by a fine white glistening crystalline frosting, a thin coating of crystalline urea excreted through the skin (Fig. 70).

Herpes, when it involves the lips (herpes labialis), is readily recognized as the well-known "fever blister" or "cold sore." It frequently involves the nose, and when the conjunctiva of the eye is attacked the condition may be serious. *Herpes zoster* (ζωστήρ—zoster, girdle), called "shingles" by the laity, an acute inflammatory skin lesion similar to herpes labialis, commonly causes severe pain on one side of the trunk before the eruption appears. The unilateral girdle-like location of a crop of vesicles on a red inflamed base usually permits a ready diagnosis (Fig. 71).

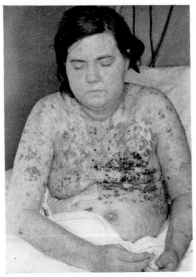

FIG. 72. Pemphigus vulgaris.

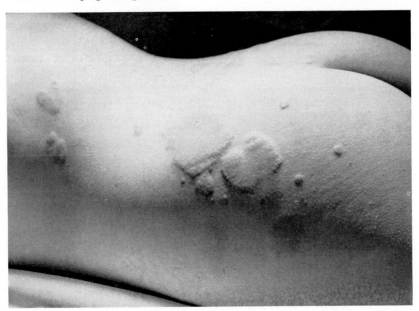

FIG. 73. Urticaria.

Pemphigus, a very distressing and frequently fatal skin disease, begins usually with a crop of bullae which later burst, form scabs and sores with a most disagreeable fetid and nauseating odor (Fig. 72).

Urticaria or *hives,* also known as nettle rash, is "an acute inflammatory affection characterized by the development of whitish, pinkish or reddish wheals which are usually evanescent and are accompanied by itching and stinging sensations" (Sutton). This eruption may occur anywhere on the body and is usually due to sensitization to some foreign substance.

In some persons the skin at times exhibits a striking instability of the cutaneous vascular supply, so that stroking or rubbing the skin produces wheals or welts. This condition, called *dermatographism* or *autographism* (Fig. 74), has played a prominent role in the history of witchcraft. The so-called "witch's marks" were often examples of dermatographism, and the unlucky subjects perished at the stake when this peculiarity was demonstrated.

The striking condition known as *generalized neurofibromatosis,* or von Recklinghausen's disease, is shown in Figure 75. This condition is characterized by the presence of nodules, some sessile, others pedunculated, scattered over the skin in various places.

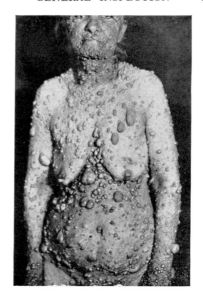

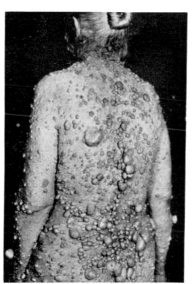

Fig. 75. Von Recklinghausen's disease—multiple neurofibromatosis.

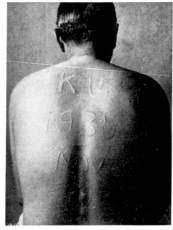

Fig. 74. Dermatographism.

BIBLIOGRAPHY

Barber, Hugh: Renal dwarfism, Quart. J. Med., *16:*205, 1920.

Beall, K. H.: Parasitism of fat. South. M. J. *17:*319, 1924.

Bean, William Bennet: The cutaneous arterial spider, a survey. Medicine *24:*243, 1945.

Blumer, George: The diagnosis of the obscure fevers of the temperate zone, particularly in adults. Med. Rec. *150:*233, 271, 1939.

Büttner, H. E., and Robbers, H.: Schwere Urämie mit Harnstoff und Kochsalzablagerungen auf der Haut. Klin. Wchnschr. *14:* 372, 1935.

Ebstein, E.: Ueber Lage und Lagerung von Kranken in diagnostischer und therapeutischer Beziehung. Ergebn. d. inn. Med. u. Kinderh., Berlin, 8:379, 1912.

Gilford, Hastings: Ateleiosis. Brit. J. Child. Dis. 8:289, 1911.

Gilford, Hastings: Progeria. Brit. J. Child. Dis. 8:292, 1911.

Gilford, Hastings: Progeria. Practitioner *73:* 188, 1904.

Jackson, Chevalier, and Jackson, Chevalier L.: The Larynx and Its Diseases. Philadelphia, W. B. Saunders Co., 1937.

Keefer, Chester S.: The diagnosis of the causes of obscure fever. Texas State J. Med. *35:*203, 1939.

Launois, P. E., and Roy, P.: Études Biologiques sur les Géants. Paris, Masson et Cie, 1904.

Lisser, H., and Escamilla, R. F.: The clinical diagnosis of Simmonds' disease (hypophyseal cachexia). Tr. A. Am. Physicians *53:*210, 1938.

Miller, J. Roscoe: Diagnosis and treatment of fevers of obscure etiology. M. Clin. North America *25:*287, 1941.

Mitchell, S. Weir: The Early History of Instrumental Precision in Medicine. New Haven, Tuttle, Morehouse & Taylor, 1892.

Muehlberger, C. W.: Shoe dye poisoning, J.A.M.A. *84:*1987, 1925.

Pagniez, Ph.: Troubles du Développement Général. In Nouveau Traité de Médécine, Roger, Widal and Teissier. Paris, Masson et Cie, 1925.

Pullen, Roscoe L.: Medical Diagnosis, Applied Physical Diagnosis. 2nd ed. Philadelphia, W. B. Saunders Co., 1950.

Rischbiet, H., and Barrington, Amy: Treasury of Human Inheritance Eugenics Laboratory Memoirs XV. University of London, London, 1912.

Roger, G. H., Widal, F., and Teissier, P. J.: Nouveau Traité de Médécine, Fascicule VIII. Paris, Masson et Cie, 1925.

Ruffer, Sir Marc Armand: Studies in the Paleopathology of Egypt. Chicago, University of Chicago Press, 1921.

Sahli, Hermann: A Treatise on Diagnostic Methods of Examination. 2nd ed. Philadelphia, W. B. Saunders Co., 1911.

Sutton, Richard L., and Sutton, Richard L., Jr.: Diseases of the Skin. 9th ed. St. Louis, C.V. Mosby Co., 1935.

Thayer, W. S.: On fever in tertiary syphilis. Internat. Clin. 22 Ser., IV: 94, 1923.

CHAPTER 5

EXAMINATION OF THE HEAD AND NECK

Head

In a systematic examination of the body we should begin with the head. After the general survey has been completed, we must retrace our steps and examine the head in more detail. In this study we rely almost entirely upon inspection aided at times by palpation. Percussion and auscultation are of little value, although in a few conditions percussion may be used to a limited extent.

The *size and shape* of the head should be noted first. In hydrocephalus the large head with the bulging fore-

head is quite striking (Fig. 76). An equally striking picture is the tower skull or steeple head (Fig. 77)—the "Turmschädel" of the Germans or the "crâne en tour" of the French. This type of head is seen in oxycephaly, a condition due to premature synostosis of the coronal and sagittal sutures, and sometimes in acholuric family jaundice. These patients show a marked exoph-

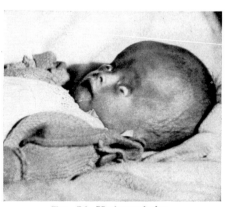

Fig. 76. Hydrocephalus.

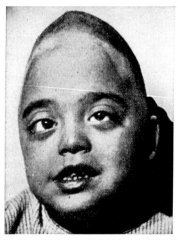

Fig. 77. Steeple head. (Griffith and Mitchell.)

59

thalmos with heavy eyelids, resulting in a dull, vacant expression of the face. The skull in rickets often has a flattened or squared appearance. Paget's disease produces a characteristic deformity in the skull which consists in an enlargement of the cranial vault so that the shape of the head resembles that of an acorn (Fig. 78).

The forehead in congenital syphilis may show bilateral bosses or at times bilateral anterior and posterior bosses. This latter condition gives the skull such a distinctive appearance that it has been described as a *cross-bun skull.*

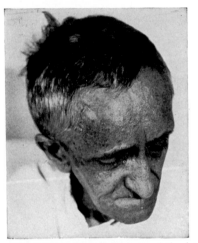

FIG. 78. Head in Paget's disease of the bone.

The bosses are commonly referred to as *Parrot's nodes* (Fig. 79). *Gumma* of the forehead is occasionally seen (Fig. 80). *Tumors* originating in the skin or subcutaneous tissue of the forehead may produce a striking appearance. Figure 81 shows a lipoma of the forehead. Sebaceous cysts of the scalp are common. They may be either singular or multiple (Fig. 82). Tumors of the frontal bone, such as an osteoma (Fig. 83), cause a marked prominence of the forehead. A frontal sinusitis often produces a marked swelling of the forehead accompanied by intense frontal headache and fever. The normal person, in looking up to the ceiling of a room, wrinkles his forehead; the patient with exophthalmic goiter looks upward without wrinkling his forehead. This phenomenon is called *Joffroy's sign.*

FACE

The *color of the face* is characteristic in certain conditions. Pallor, cyanosis, argyria, jaundice are all well seen in the face. In certain *heart lesions* the appearance of the face may be characteristic. The patient with aortic insufficiency is usually pale, the patient with mitral disease is ruddy or flushed. Girls in their teens who have mitral lesions

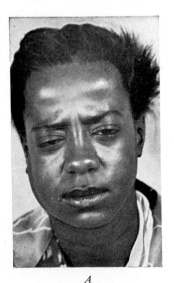

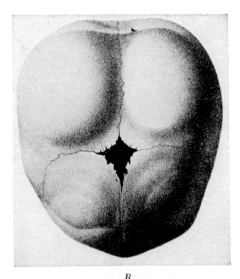

A   *B*

FIG. 79. Parrot's nodes. *A,* Appearance of patient. *B,* Original illustration by Parrot.

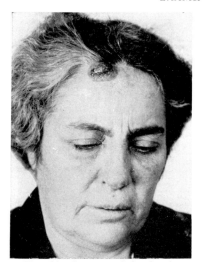

FIG. 80. Gumma of forehead.

often have beautiful complexions with high coloring. In the stage of cardiac failure, patients with both aortic and mitral disease are cyanotic. In congenital heart disease marked cyanosis of the face and lips is common. Marked flushing of the cheeks, "hectic flush," is common in pulmonary *tuberculosis*.

The size and shape of the head as well as the facial features are quite typical in *acromegaly* (Fig. 84). The features of an acromegalic are so striking that any one who has seen and carefully observed a case will immediately recognize a subsequent case, often without being able at first fully to ex-

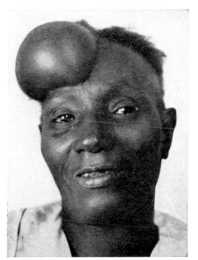

FIG. 81. Lipoma of forehead.

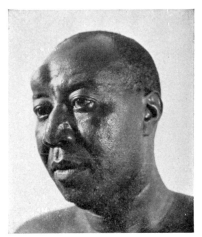

FIG. 83. Osteoma of skull.

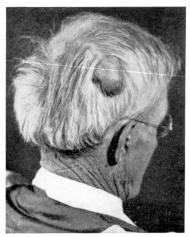

FIG. 82. Sebaceous cyst of the scalp.

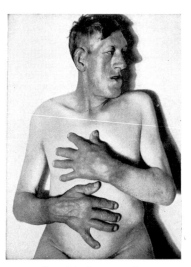

FIG. 84. Acromegaly.

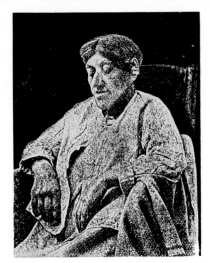

FIG. 85. First illustration of acromegaly. (Pierre Marie.)

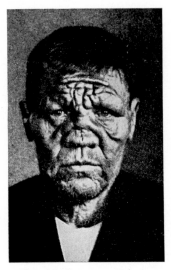

FIG. 86. Leprosy. (Stitt.)

plain his reasons for the diagnosis. Here again, as frequently in medicine, the visual sense seems more acute and more rapid than the processes of reasoning. The massive face with its craggy eyebrows, prominent nose and massive lower jaw forms a characteristic and unforgettable picture. The whole face seems molded on larger lines, with features magnified. Figure 85 is a reproduction of the picture illustrating Marie's description of acromegaly, one of the earliest and indeed the classic description of this disease.

The appearance of the face in *leprosy* is often pathognomonic. Here again the experienced physician makes an instantaneous diagnosis because he has seen the condition before. The characteristic appearance of the leper's face is due to a subcutaneous infiltration over the forehead, the cheeks and chin, combined with a flattening and broadening of the nose (Fig. 86). The resemblance to a lion's face is striking and gave origin to the term *leonine facies*. This change in facial expression is also apparent in the photograph taken of Father Damien after he contracted leprosy on the Island of Molokai (Fig. 87).

The facial expression produced by *adenoids* is characteristic, the mouth hanging open and the chin receding

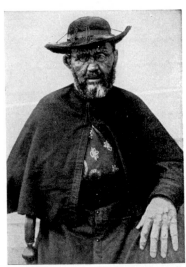

FIG. 87. Father Damien after he became a victim of leprosy. (Morrow.)

somewhat. The impassive, sphinx-like expression of patients suffering from paralysis agitans is so striking that the "Parkinsonian mask" is recognized as one of the cardinal signs of this disease. This expressionless face with the elevated eyebrows and facial immobility, which was not mentioned by Parkinson himself, may be a very early sign of the disease. The *Hippocratic facies* indicative of approaching death remains after more than two thousand years the classic description—"a sharp nose, hol-

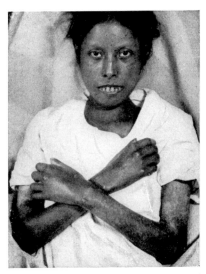

FIG. 88. Scleroderma. The skin is very tight over the hands and also over the face. The patient is trying to smile and show all her teeth.

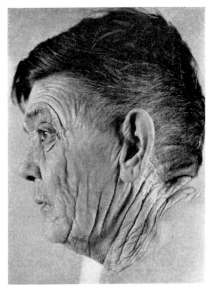

FIG. 89. The face and neck of a eunuch showing marked creases and wrinkles.

low eyes, collapsed temples; the ears cold, contracted, and their lobes turned out; the skin about the forehead being rough, distended, and parched; the color of the whole face being green, black, livid, or lead-colored."

The skin of the face may be markedly thinned and tightened in *scleroderma*. This tightening may be so marked that the patient is unable to close his lips over the teeth or to smile (Fig. 88).

The skin of the face and neck of eunuchs is often deeply creased and wrinkled. In early stages, the wrinkles are particularly noticeable about the eyes (Fig. 89).

In some patients suffering from tonic spasm of the muscles of the face the eyebrows may be raised and the angles of the mouth drawn out, forming the so-called sardonic grin or *risus sardonicus*. This condition is seen most frequently in tetanus.

In *paralysis of the facial nerve* (Bell's palsy), which is almost always unilateral, the muscles on the affected side of the face are paralyzed. When the patient is asked to wrinkle his forehead, the forehead on the affected side remains smooth. He is unable to shut

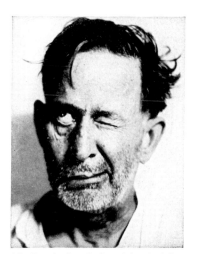

FIG. 90. Paralysis of the right facial nerve, Bell's palsy.

his eye on the affected side, and when he is asked to show his teeth, the affected half of the mouth cannot be moved (Fig. 90). The patient is also unable to whistle.

When the involvement of the facial nerve is supranuclear or nuclear, there is an accompanying hemiplegia or evidence of involvement of other cranial nerves. In most instances, however, only the nerve trunk itself is involved, and the signs are those due to paralysis of the muscles supplied by the nerve. In cases in which the facial nerve is involved after the chorda tympani has joined it, the sense of taste is lost over the anterior two thirds of the tongue on the affected side.

MOVEMENTS OF THE HEAD

The movements of the head are often suggestive of certain diseases. In Parkinson's disease there is a slight though constant tremor of the head. Patients with a *habit spasm* make sudden, unexpected movements of the head often accompanied by facial grimaces. In aortic insufficiency there is commonly present a constant jerking of the head forward and backward synchronous with the heart beat. This sign is called by the French *de Musset's sign,* after the poet, de Musset, who suffered from aortic insufficiency and showed this phenomenon. Sudden jerky movements of the head may be seen in chorea.

HAIR

In syphilitic disease and in diabetes the hair may be scanty or may show small, irregular patches of baldness. Occasionally, there may be a complete loss of hair or a total baldness in these diseases (Fig. 91). In some patients with pituitary insufficiency the hair may be extremely sparse (Fig. 92). This is particularly true in Simmonds' disease. In alopecia areata the patient suddenly

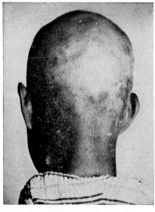

FIG. 91. Alopecia in diabetes.

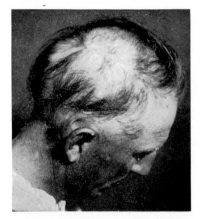

FIG. 92. Alopecia.

loses patches of hair, leaving spots of baldness. Patients suffering from this disease often wake up in the morning to find a handful of hair on the pillow and a bald spot on the scalp where the hair fell out. Loss of hair in typhoid fever is common.

In myxedema the hair is scanty and invariably harsh, dry and lusterless. This harsh, dry hair is a pathognomonic sign in thyroid deficiency. In pediculosis capitis the hair is matted together and covered with nits. Close observation discloses numerous pediculi running about among the hairs. This condition in an exaggerated form is known as "plica polonica."

EYES

The eyes give significant information about a patient. The *expression of the eyes* is often of great importance. The wild expression of the maniac contrasts strikingly with the apathetic appearance of a patient suffering from a marked psychic depression. The experienced physician can often distinguish sanity from mental aberration by the expression of the eyes. The eyes in hyperthyroidism have a bright, interesting expression as contrasted with the cretin, whose eyes are dull and expressionless. In psychoneurotic patients the eyes are commonly bright and alert.

Physical divergences from the normal often indicate particular conditions.

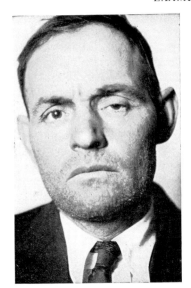

FIG. 93. Ptosis of the left lid.

orbicularis oculi, is unable to close the eye on the affected side, while the eyeball turns up during the attempt (Fig. 90). The eyelids are markedly swollen and the eyes often nearly closed in the *edema* of nephritis, erysipelas and angioneurotic edema (Figs. 94 and 95). Marked edema of the eyelids is commonly present in trichinosis. The appearance produced by this edema of the eyelids is heightened by the edema of subcutaneous tissues of the face.

The lacrimal glands are markedly enlarged in an unusual syndrome called *Mikulicz's disease* (Figs. 96 and 97).

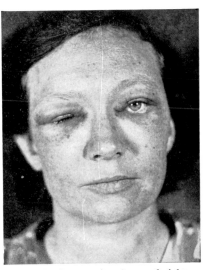

FIG. 95. Angioneurotic edema of right eye.

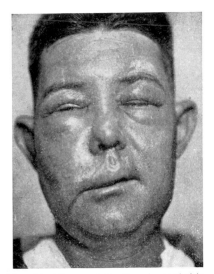

FIG. 94. Edema of the face in nephritis.

Ptosis of the upper lids is the result of paralysis of the oculomotor nerve (Fig. 93). Narrowing of the palpebral fissure occurs in paralysis of the cervical sympathetic. There is marked feebleness of the upper eyelids in myasthenia gravis. The patient often wakes in the morning with his eyes wide open, but as the day wears on his lids droop more and more until at nightfall his eyes are completely closed and he is unable to open them. In facial paralysis the patient, because of paralysis of the

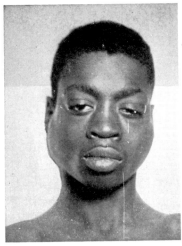

FIG. 96. Mikulicz's syndrome. Enlarged parotid glands.

In this condition there is also a bilateral enlargement of the parotid and submaxillary glands.

The upper eyelid may be the seat of a *chalazion,* a small hard nodule, the result of an obstruction in the sebaceous ducts and glands of the lid. *Xanthomata* are yellowish-orange nodules in the lids, often of diabetic origin, but usually not (Fig. 98). These nodules often occur in the skin just below the lower lid. An infection of the hair follicles of the eyelashes produces a *hordeolum,* the well-known "sty."

There is usually protrusion of the eyeballs, or *exophthalmos,* in Graves' disease. Because of this exophthalmos, which is one of the cardinal signs of this disease, it is also called exophthalmic goiter. This exophthalmos gives the patient a striking appearance, described by Moebius as an expression of "frozen terror" (Figs. 99 and 100). In oxycephaly, a congenital defect with premature union of the cranial sutures (Figs. 101 and 102), the orbits become shallow and the eyeballs are forced forward. Optic atrophy and papilledema are common. A striking picture is produced by the pulsating exophthalmos which is the result of a fistula between the internal carotid artery and the cavernous sinus.

A marked exophthalmos may also be present in cavernous sinus thrombosis (Fig. 103).

Exophthalmos may be unilateral or bilateral. When unilateral, it is usually the result of a local condition, such as a tumor or aneurysm, and when bilateral, the result of a systemic disease. While exophthalmos is commonly associated with hyperthyroidism, in some instances it becomes progressively more marked after thyroidectomy and is apparently associated with a hypothyroidism rather than with a hyperthyroidism. Such exophthalmos is probably caused by an excess of a hormone of the anterior pituitary lobe and resembles the condition described as progressive idiopathic exophthalmos, which is characterized by gradually developing and increasing exophthalmos, but is not associated with hyperthyroidism.

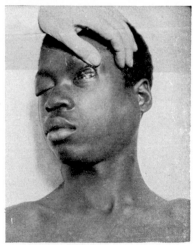

Fig. 97. Mikulicz's syndrome. Enlarged lacrimal glands.

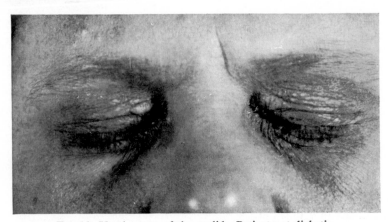

Fig. 98. Xanthomata of the eyelids. Patient not diabetic.

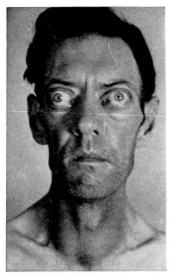

FIG. 99. Exophthalmos in Graves' disease.

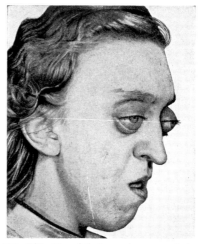

FIG. 102. Exophthalmos in oxycephaly.

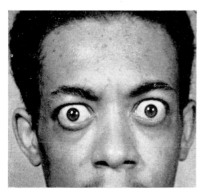

FIG. 100. Extreme exophthalmos in hyperthyroidism.

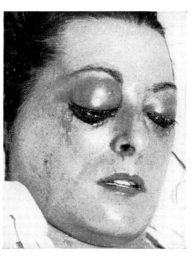

FIG. 103. Exophthalmos in cavernous sinus thrombosis.

Exophthalmos is also frequently seen in arterial hypertension and in nephritis, as pointed out by Barker and Hanes.

Enophthalmos is an abnormal retraction of the eye into the orbit. It may follow loss of orbital tissue or disease of the oculopupillary center in the medulla. Horner's syndrome, which consists of enophthalmos, miosis and ptosis, follows a lesion of the medullary tegmentum.

The eyeballs feel hard to the touch in glaucoma and very soft, often almost mushy, in diabetic coma.

Ectropion ($\epsilon\kappa$ = out + $\tau\rho\epsilon\pi\epsilon\iota\nu$ — trepein = to turn) is an eversion or turning out of the edge of the eyelids; *entro-*

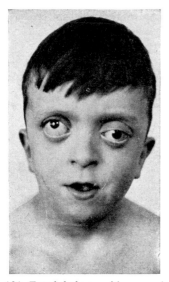

FIG. 101. Exophthalmos with oxycephaly.

pion is an introversion or turning in of the edge of the eyelids. Both processes are usually the result of inflammation or of trauma. Entropion may occur in exophthalmos associated with hyperthyroidism.

The *conjunctiva may be inflamed* in certain infectious diseases, notably influenza and measles. It may be the seat of hemorrhages, particularly in high blood pressure and in whooping cough. In the latter disease the hemorrhages are the result of the paroxysms of coughing. The conjunctivae are stained yellow in jaundice. In subacute infectious endocarditis, small petechiae commonly appear in the conjunctiva of the lower lid. This may be the clinching point in the diagnosis (see Fig. 355). Petechiae in the conjunctiva occur also in leukemia and in aplastic anemia.

The conjunctiva is markedly reddened in conjunctivitis, the reddening usually being more marked at the lid borders. In iritis the inflammatory process is more marked near the iris, and the reddened vessels are most numerous about the margin of the cornea.

The *sclerae of the eyes* have invariably a striking bluish tint in a rare disease—osteogenesis imperfecta. In tuberculosis of children and young adults the sclerae are often bluish.

The *cornea* may show opaque spots as the result of an old injury or a previous infection. Gonorrheal ophthalmia may lead to the production of opaque scars. In interstitial keratitis, or inflammation of the cornea caused by congenital syphilis, the cornea shows a diffuse clouding (Fig. 104). These lesions all interfere markedly with sight. The "arcus senilis" is a whitish opaque circle or part of a circle about the outer margin of the cornea. The presence of a complete circle is the exception. This phenomenon is associated with senility, but may occur in comparatively youthful persons, being fairly common in Negroes. In Wilson's disease there is often an annular brownish green ring of pigmentation of the cornea, the Kayser-Fleischer ring.

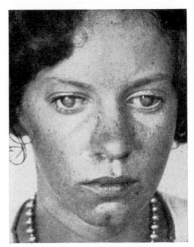

Fig. 104. Interstitial keratitis.

The *pupil of the eye* may be dilated or contracted. The dilatation or contraction is most significant when unilateral. *Mydriasis,* or dilatation of the pupil, occurs in neurasthenia and in lesions of the oculomotor nerve, associated here with a marked ptosis. *Miosis,* or contraction of the pupil, is often seen in tabes dorsalis and after the use of morphine. In tabes the pupils are often not only miotic, but fixed and do not react to light, although they react actively to accommodation. Such a pupil is called an *Argyll Robertson pupil* and is one of the pathognomonic signs in the diagnosis of tabes dorsalis. It has also been described in disseminated sclerosis, epidemic encephalitis, chronic alcoholism and mesencephalic tumors. Miosis occurs in iritis, mydriasis in glaucoma. This distinction is important, since both conditions are accompanied by pain and injection of the cornea. In iritis, mydriatics, such as atropine, are used; in glaucoma, miotics such as eserine.

Irregularities in the contour of the pupil are most commonly the result of adhesions of the iris. Inequality in the size of the two pupils is called *anisocoria* (Fig. 105). It is common in paresis and in tabes dorsalis, and may often be seen in aneurysm of the aorta or in patients with a cervical rib. An aneurysm

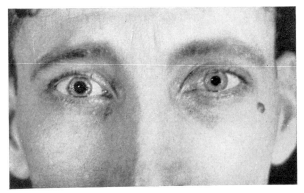

Fig. 105. Anisocoria.

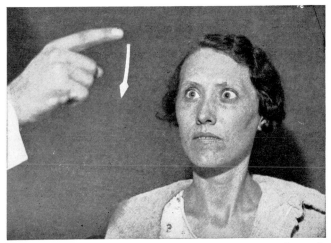

Fig. 106. Von Graefe's sign. The patients' eyes are following the finger downward.

of the aorta pressing on the sympathetic nerves may produce a stimulation and dilatation of the pupil on that side. Later, however, it may produce paralysis of the sympathetic nerve with constriction. In a patient with a cervical rib the dilated pupil is usually on the same side as the cervical rib.

The *movements of the eyes* are important in the diagnosis of many diseases. In meningitis they commonly wander, as it were, from side to side, each eye apparently independent of its fellow. In Graves' disease the eyes converge poorly—"Moebius' sign"—and the upper eyelid fails to follow the eyeball on looking downward—"lid lag" or "von Graefe's sign" (Fig. 106). By *nystagmus* we mean rapid oscillation of the eyeball as the patient looks from side to side, or up and down. The former variety, lateral nystagmus, is by far the more common and is an important sign of multiple sclerosis. It also occurs in myasthenia gravis, Friedreich's ataxia and among miners working in mines which are poorly lighted, the so-called "miners' nystagmus." This condition has become comparatively rare with the improvement in the lighting condition in mines. There is a hereditary type of nystagmus transmitted from generation to generation. Albinos usually show a lateral nystagmus. Vertical nystagmus is relatively uncommon. It is seen most frequently in epidemic encephalitis in which there is involvement of the brain stem.

Corneal Reflex. The corneal reflex is produced by touching the cornea gently with a feather or hair or by blowing a little puff of air on it. This produces normally a contraction of the orbicularis oculi which produces blinking, normally in both eyes. Bilateral loss of corneal reflexes on stimulating the cornea may occur in any type of coma, including general anesthesia. In hemiplegia the corneal reflex is often absent on the paralyzed side. The loss or diminution of the corneal reflex on one side may be an early sign of trigeminal nerve disease. Unilateral or bilateral loss of corneal reflex may be present in hysteria.

The bilateral nature of the corneal reflex is of value in determining whether we have involvement of the trigeminal nerve or the facial nerve. If there is a loss of the reflex on one side, stimulation of the cornea of the affected side will produce no blinking in the opposite eye if the trigeminal nerve is involved. If the facial nerve alone is paralyzed, however, this stimulation will produce blinking in the opposite eye.

Retina. Examination of the retina is now a recognized part of every complete physical examination, thanks to the electric ophthalmoscope (Fig. 107). The most important lesions easily recognized are the following:

1. Retinal hemorrhages, seen commonly in nephritis, arterial hypertension, severe anemias, leukemias, endocarditis, diabetes and purpura.

2. Arteriosclerosis may be more readily recognized in the eyegrounds than elsewhere. The vessels often have an appearance which has been compared to that of a silver wire, and may apparently obliterate a retinal vein in crossing it.

3. Choked disk or papillary edema is a sign of increased intracranial pressure. In this condition the margins of the disk are blurred or obliterated and the normal cupping is replaced by a bulging. It is seen in brain tumors, in meningitis, brain abscess, cerebral hemorrhage and not infrequently in marked arterial hypertension.

4. Optic atrophy is often seen in tabes dorsalis and paresis. The disk is smaller than normal and glistening white in color.

5. Pallor of the temporal side of the disk is common in multiple sclerosis.

In aortic insufficiency marked pulsation of the retinal arteries is usually visible. Visible pulsation of the retinal arteries is a normal physiologic occurrence.

Frequently it is impossible to study the retina satisfactorily without dilating the pupil. Before this is done, however, the tension of the eyeball should be tested and the patient carefully questioned regarding a possible earlier attack of glaucoma. The instillation of mydriatics into the eye may provoke an attack of acute glaucoma.

EARS

The ears should be carefully examined in suspected cases of gout for the presence of *tophi* (Fig. 108), which are hard nodular deposits of sodium biurate upon the cartilages. The deformed, so-called "cauliflower" ears of the professional pugilist are familiar. This deformity is due to the injuries received by the ear in boxing. *Lupus vulgaris* may attack the ears and erode large areas. The ears may show a developmental deformity present at birth (Fig. 109). *Tenderness over the mastoid* process may be elicited by pressure and is an important sign in mastoiditis.

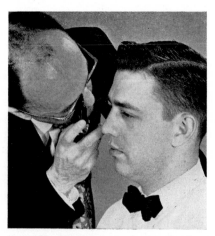

Fig. 107. Ophthalmoscopic examination.

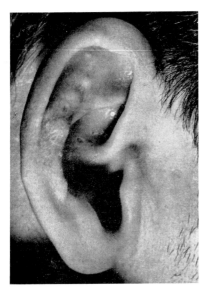

FIG. 108. Multiple tophi of ear. One on helix, five on anthelix. (From Leopold, Physical Diagnosis.)

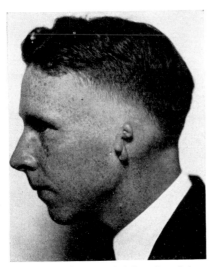

FIG. 109. Developmental deformity of the ear.

Furunculosis and inflammation of the external auditory canal cause pain, tenderness, itching and some diminution in hearing. On inspection the skin of the external meatus is red and swollen. Examination of the auditory canal and the ear drum is best carried out with the otoscope (Fig. 110).

The hearing of the patient may be roughly tested by holding a watch away from the ear while the patient closes

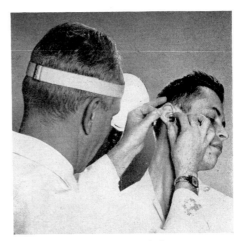

FIG. 110. Employment of the otoscope.

with his finger the ear which is not being tested. The distance at which a watch is heard normally varies with the watch, but averages perhaps 40 to 50 inches. Other tests for hearing are described on page 315.

Chronic otitis media, one of the common causes of deafness, may present a variety of findings. Some patients hear better during clear, dry weather than when it is damp and rainy, or they may hear a watch tick at the normal distance, but cannot hear spoken words distinctly. Thomas Willis, in the seventeenth century, described a woman "who, although she was deaf, whenever a drum was beaten in the room, heard every word clearly," and mentions a deaf man "who, passing close to a bell-tower when one of the numerous bells rang, could hear one's voice very easily, but not otherwise." This phenomenon, frequently observed since, is known as *hyperacusis,* or *paracusis Willisii,* and is often seen in chronic otitis media.

CHEEKS

The cheeks may show characteristic deformities as the result of an involvement of the neighboring structures. *Facial paralysis* produces a characteristic expression when the patient attempts to smile, the paralyzed side refusing to function (Fig. 90). A marked difference in the depth of the nasolabial fold

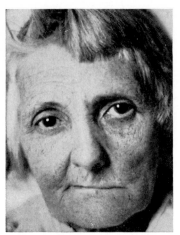

FIG. 111. Deepening of right nasolabial fold in left-sided hemiplegia.

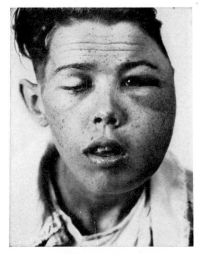

FIG. 113. Lymphosarcoma of face.

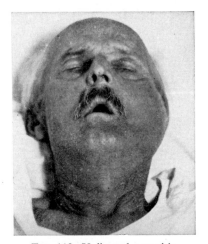

FIG. 112. Unilateral parotitis.

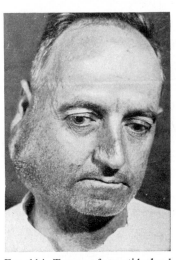

FIG. 114. Tumor of parotid gland.

on the two sides occurs in this condition (Fig. 111). Single or bilateral enlargement of the parotid glands occurs in mumps, in Mikulicz's disease (Fig. 96) and sometimes as a terminal event in severe infections (Fig. 112). The boy shown in Figure 113 has a marked facial deformity due to a lymphosarcoma of the soft tissues. Figure 114 shows a tumor arising in the parotid gland—the so-called "mixed" tumor of the parotid.

Chvostek's sign is a pathognomonic finding in tetany. It is elicited by tapping sharply with the finger just in front of the external auditory meatus over the facial nerve at its point of emergence from the parotid gland. This produces a contraction or spasm of the facial muscles on this side, due to stimulation of the hyperexcitable facial nerve. The most marked examples of tetany are seen after accidental removal of the parathyroid glands, but it is also observed in a milder form after prolonged vomiting and after continued hyperventilation of the lungs.

NOSE

In diseases associated with difficulty in respiration, notably pneumonia and, to a less extent, heart disease, the nostrils dilate with inspiration and contract with expiration.

The nose in syphilis may present the typical "saddle nose" (Fig. 115) caused by erosion of the nasal bones. In rhinophyma the nose is red, large and bulbous. Ghirlandajo and Holbein have immortalized rhinophyma on canvas, (Fig. 116) and Cyrano de Bergerac was a well-known example. Lupus erythematosus produces the characteristic "butterfly" lesion on the nose with the wings extending out over the cheeks. (Fig. 117). This lesion, sometimes called Cazenave's disease, consists of

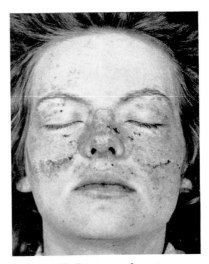

FIG. 117. Lupus erythematosus.

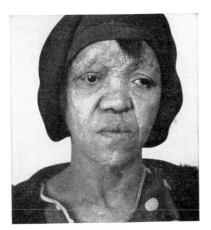

FIG. 115. Saddle nose.

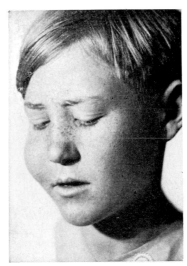

FIG. 118. Sarcoma of maxillary bone.

disk-like patches covered with scales or crusts which fall off leaving dull-white cicatrices.

Acne rosacea produces a marked reddening of the tip of the nose which instantly suggests that the owner of the nose has a weakness for alcoholic beverages. Often, however, these persons are teetotalers, or even rabid prohibitionists, and resent the insinuation.

Tumors originating within the nose, or from the nasal sinuses, may produce marked deformity of the face. Figure 118 shows the marked asymmetry of the face produced by a sarcoma of the

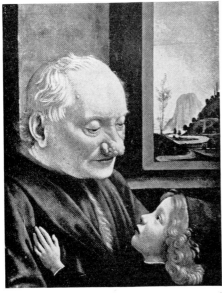

FIG. 116. "The Old Man and His Grandson" by Domenico Ghirlandajo (1449–1494), showing rhinophyma of grandfather.

maxillary bone. The patient shown in Figure 119 has a basal cell carcinoma of the face involving the nose especially and producing marked deformity.

One should never neglect to look into the *nostrils* (Fig. 120). A *perforation of the nasal septum* is due most frequently to syphilis, but may be the result of a nonspecific ulceration or of chrome poisoning. Workers in chrome mines, it is said, after a certain length of service almost invariably suffer a perforation of the nasal septum. Such "seasoned" workers commonly carry a piece of bent wire in their pockets and

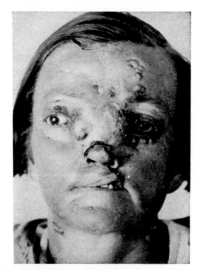

FIG. 119. A basal cell carcinoma of face.

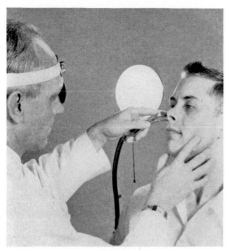

FIG. 120. Inspection of nostrils.

amuse their friends by demonstrating that the wire enters one nostril and emerges from the other.

Nosebleed may be an early symptom in typhoid fever, often occurs in high blood pressure and polycythemia, or may be the result of an erosion of the small vessels in the mucous membrane.

LIPS

The lips may be deformed from birth as in the well-known *harelip* (Fig. 121) due to a failure of union during fetal life. The lips may be markedly swollen from the edema of a nephritis (Fig. 94) or of angioneurotic edema (Fig. 122). Extremely dry lips are often seen in fever and in diabetes mellitus.

The lips show a marked *cyanosis* in pneumonia, in cardiac failure, in congenital heart disease and in polycythemia vera (Vaquez-Osler disease).

One of the commonest lesions on the lips is *herpes labialis,* the well-known "cold sore" or "fever blister" (Fig. 124). This begins as a collection of small painful vesicles rapidly proceeding to scab formation. This eruption is often not limited to the lips, but extends to the nose or cheek.

The lips, particularly the upper lip, may be the seat of a *chancre,* which should always be suspected when a patient shows a large, persistent, firmly indurated, but relatively painless, sore

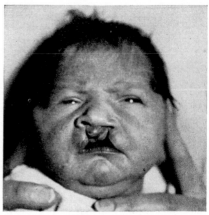

FIG. 121. Harelip.

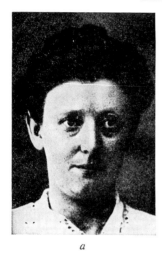

a

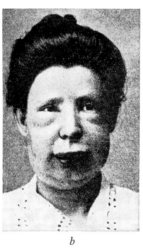

b

FIG. 122. Angioneurotic edema: *a,* before attack; *b,* during attack. (Lewandowsky.)

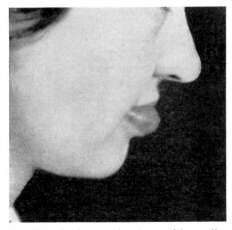

FIG. 123. Angioneurotic edema of lower lip.

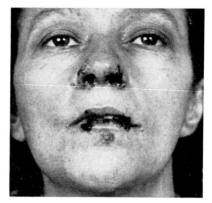

FIG. 124. Herpes labialis et nasalis.

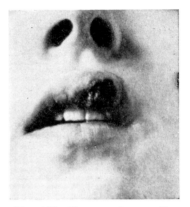

FIG. 125. Chancre of upper lip.

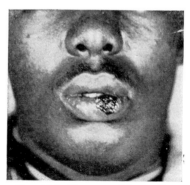

FIG. 126. Chancre of lower lip.

on the lip (Fig. 125). Chancres also occur on the lower lip (Fig. 126). In an old or middle-aged person a firm, painless, slowly growing ulceration with hard borders is usually a *carcinoma* (Fig. 127). Adults who have suffered from congenital syphilis in their youth often show "rhagades" small linear

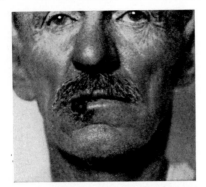

FIG. 127. Epithelioma of lip.

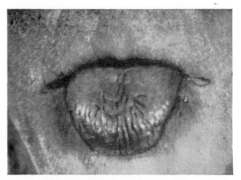

FIG. 130. Fissures in corners of mouth, in riboflavin deficiency. Patient also has glossitis, the result of niacin deficiency.

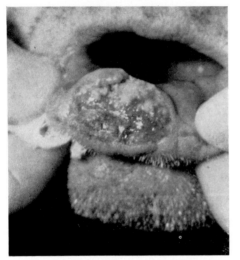

FIG. 128. Epithelioma of lower lip.

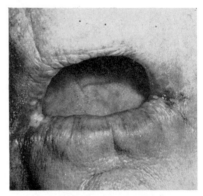

FIG. 131. Perlèche.

missures, particularly of children but also of adults, producing thickening and desquamation of the epithelium at the corners of the mouth, often produces fissures (Fig. 131).

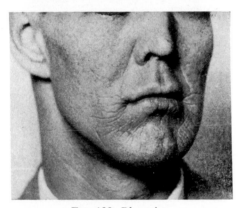

FIG. 129. Rhagades.

TEETH AND GUMS

scars running out from the mouth upon the cheeks (Fig. 129). In riboflavin deficiency, fissures in the corner of the mouth are common (Fig. 130). Perlèche, an infection of the labial com-

The teeth and gums often give important indications of disease. The condition of the teeth and gums often has a profound bearing on health. The presence of *pyorrhea alveolaris* (Riggs' disease) is established by demonstrating retraction of the gums from the roots of the teeth and by pressing out small quantities of pus from the root sockets. In elderly persons pyorrhea leads to marked loosening or loss of teeth. The teeth should be further examined for caries or cavities, and the presence or absence of crowned teeth noted. Perhaps the most striking appearance of the teeth is in *congenital syphilis,* first described by Sir Jonathan Hutchinson and since known as "Hutchinson's teeth" (Fig. 132). His original description was as follows:

The central upper incisors are the test-teeth. . . . The teeth are short and narrow. Instead of becoming wider as they descend from the gum, they are narrower at their free edge than at their crowns, their angles having been, as it were, rounded off. In the centre of their free edge is a deep vertical notch, made by the breaking away or nondevelopment of the middle lobe of the tooth-crown. This notch taken together with the narrowness and shortness of the tooth, is the main peculiarity.

The well-known "Hutchinson's triad," described as characteristic of congenital syphilis, consists of Hutchinson's teeth, interstitial keratitis, and labyrinthine disease causing deafness. Another type of tooth very characteristic of congenital syphilis is the "screw driver tooth" (Fig. 133).

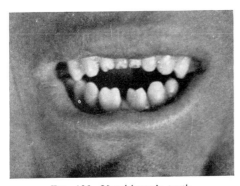

FIG. 132. Hutchinson's teeth.

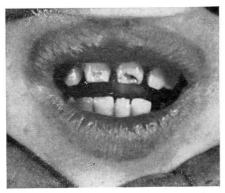

FIG. 133. Screw driver teeth in syphilis.

In disorders of the pituitary gland, patients may show an unusually *wide spacing of the teeth.* The patient shown in Figure 134 is suffering from hypopituitarism.

Imperfect dentition or crumbling, decayed teeth may call attention to dietary faults. In inveterate chewers of tobacco the molars usually show a smooth polished surface and sometimes may be ground down to the level of the gums. A similar condition is often seen in Indians who grind their corn in a primitive stone mortar. During the process of grinding cornmeal a fine stone powder becomes mixed with the meal and is baked in the bread. Constant eating of this bread wears down the molars.

The presence of minute amounts of fluorine in drinking water, more than 1.5 parts per million, produces teeth that are pitted and stained yellow, brown or black (Fig. 135). This condition is called *mottled enamel* or *fluorosis.*

The *lead line* in chronic lead poisoning is an important diagnostic sign and has saved many patients with severe abdominal pain from an unnecessary surgical operation. This lead line consists of a black, finely stippled line oc-

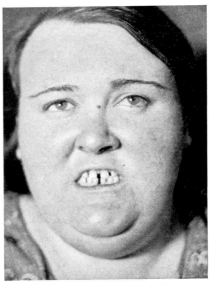

FIG. 134. Wide spacing of teeth in pituitary disease.

curring on the gums just below the point at which the teeth emerge, or at the border of teeth and gums. Henry Burton, who first described this phenomenon, wrote, "The edges of the gums attached to the necks of two or more teeth of either jaw, were distinctly bordered by a narrow leaden-blue line, whilst the substance of the gum apparently retained its ordinary colour and condition." Examination of this line with a hand lens shows it to consist of innumerable dots, placed close together in a row (Fig. 136).

Bismuth produces a similar line. This *bismuth line* is not infrequently seen in patients who have had continued courses of bismuth injections for the treatment of syphilis. These patients also show at times small dark areas on the tongue and on the mucous membranes of the mouth produced by these bismuth deposits (Fig. 137).

In *scurvy* the gums are soft, tender and spongy, the teeth often so loose that they can be plucked out with the fingers.

Hyperplasia of the gums may be the result of various causes, such as acute monocytic *leukemia* (Fig. 138) or the excessive employment of Dilantin (Fig. 139). At times the etiology is obscure.

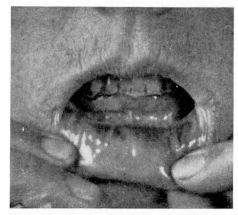

FIG. 137. Bismuth line on gums. Note also the dark deposit of bismuth on the mucous membranes of the lower lip.

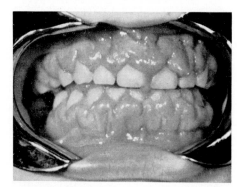

FIG. 138. Hyperplasia of the gums in acute monocytic leukemia.

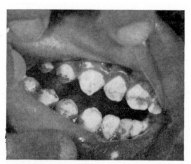

FIG. 135. Mottled enamel due to fluorine in water.

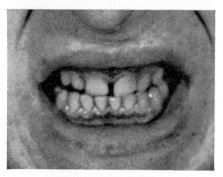

FIG. 136. Lead line.

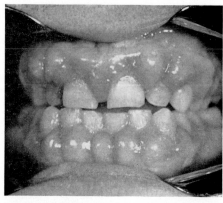

FIG. 139. Hyperplasia of the gums in Dilantin administration.

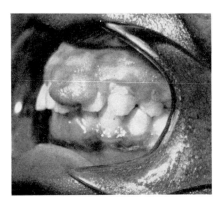

FIG. 140. Fibroma of the gum.

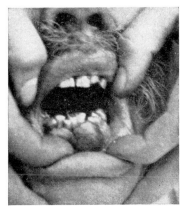

FIG. 141. Epulis. Note tumor of lower gum between two forefingers of examiner.

Fibroma of the gums presents a striking picture (Fig. 140).

Osteomyelitis and tumors of the mandible may produce marked distortion of the gums and the teeth of the lower jaw. The tumor most commonly seen in the lower jaw is the so-called *epulis,* a giant-cell sarcoma of a low grade of malignancy (Fig. 141).

TONGUE

The old-time physician always looked carefully at the patient's tongue, and many stories were told of his uncanny ability in diagnosing diseases from its appearance. His modern successor should never omit this time-honored but simple procedure, for in certain diseases the tongue shows a characteristic appearance.

In scarlet fever we have the so-called *strawberry tongue,* which is very red, covered with a slight fur and showing enlarged reddened papillae. This tongue is especially striking because there is commonly an area of pallor around the mouth. In typhoid fever the tongue is heavily coated, furred and often covered with brownish sordes. The tongue in pernicious anemia and sprue forms one of the striking diagnostic signs—pale, smooth and glossy (Fig. 142). In the early stages of pernicious anemia, however, the tongue, although sore, may appear normal. In sprue the tongue, though commonly pale and smooth, may at times be red, inflamed or fissured. The tongue in pellagra at first is rough and swollen; later it becomes smooth and very red, often showing glossitis (Fig. 130). Excessive smoking may produce mild glossitis.

The tongue in Ludwig's angina may be acutely inflamed, painful and so swollen that it protrudes from the mouth, preventing the patient from closing his mouth. In *leukoplakia* the tongue is covered with firm white indurated lesions, resembling firmly attached crusts. In myxedema and cretinism the tongue may be enlarged and protrude from the mouth, but it is not painful (Fig. 44). In dehydrated patients it is small and dry.

Among the *tumors* of the tongue that

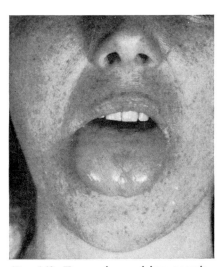

FIG. 142. Tongue in pernicious anemia.

one encounters, carcinomata should be mentioned. These tumors produce a marked induration of the tongue with destruction and ulceration. Hemangiomata of the tongue are occasionally seen (Fig. 143). They produce some local discomfort.

The *geographical tongue* (Fig. 144) presents a striking appearance, may be a cause of great worry to the patient, but is quite harmless of itself. It is commonly seen in nervous persons. The patient shown in the illustration was suffering from a mild hyperthyroidism. The geographical tongue changes its appearance daily, the "map" commonly passing through a certain cycle of changes.

A curious-looking tongue is the so-called *scrotal tongue,* which presents grooves and markings much like those on the surface of the scrotum (Fig. 145). This condition may be caused by vitamin B deficiency and is often relieved by treatment with vitamin B complex. The tongue in Addison's disease shows at times small, irregularly shaped, round or oval areas of black or brown pigmentation.

Marked *furrowing of the tongue* (Fig. 146) is in most instances congenital.

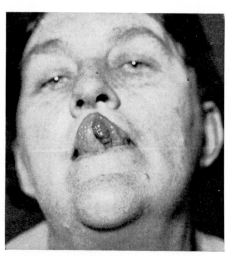

FIG. 143. Hemangiomata of tongue.

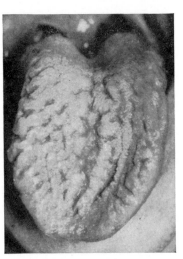

FIG. 145. Scrotal tongue. (Kindness of Dr. Hayes Martin)

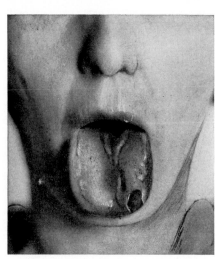

FIG. 144. Geographical tongue.

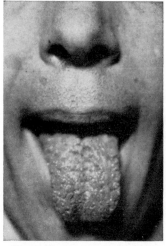

FIG. 146. Furrowed tongue.

Food particles often collect in the deep furrows, undergo fermentation and produce tenderness.

Ulcers under the tongue, on the frenum, are often seen in children with whooping cough. The paroxysms of coughing cause protrusion of the tongue, and the frenum is constantly forced against the sharp edges of the lower incisor teeth, producing an erosion. Scarring of the tongue is often seen in epileptics who commonly bite their tongues during convulsions.

The veins on the under surface of the tongue give us a good indication of the venous blood pressure, according to May. When a person is erect or sitting, the veins are collapsed unless the venous pressure is abnormally high, more than 200 mm.

Clusters of small dilated and varicose veins along the undersurface of the tongue may reach a large size and occupy about the whole under surface of the tongue. Their round shape and black color has suggested a resemblance to caviar. These caviar lesions have been recently studied by Bean, who concludes that they are without any pathologic significance (Fig. 147).

In lesions of the central nervous system in which the nucleus of the hypoglossal nerve is involved, the tongue is not protruded in the midline, but *deviates* away from the normal side and toward the side on which the lesion is located.

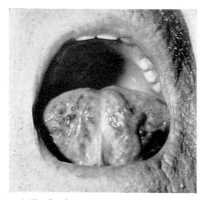

Fig. 147. Caviar tongue. (Kindness of Dr. William Bean.)

In myasthenia gravis the tongue may show an *abnormal fatigability* like that of the eyelids and of other voluntary muscles. Thomas Willis, who first described myasthenia gravis, has left a classic description. "I have now a prudent and honest Woman in cure, who for many years has been obnoxious to this kind of bastard Palsey not only in the Limbs but likewise in her Tongue; This person for some time speaks freely and readily enough, but after long, hasty or laborous speaking, presently she becomes as mute as a fish, and cannot bring forth a word, nay, and does not recover the use of her Voice till after an hour or two."

BREATH

The breath may give important clues in diagnosis. The breath in *alcoholic intoxication* has a characteristic odor. In uremia the breath may have a urinous odor. The breath in diabetes mellitus, particularly when there is a marked acidosis, has a *sweetish "fruity" odor* due to the odor of acetone. Anyone unfamiliar with the odor of acetone should go to the chemical laboratory and become familiar with it. Many patients with severe diabetes breathe out so much acetone that the atmosphere becomes saturated with it and the odor is noted by the physician the moment he enters the room. This acetone breath occurs also in acidosis not of diabetic origin. It is common in infants and in young children who, as the result of illness, have not eaten for twenty-four hours or longer. It is present in professional fasters during their tests. In these conditions the acetone breath is the result of starvation acidosis. The amine odor noted on the breath of patients with severe parenchymal liver disease is quite characteristic. Sometimes referred to as *fetor hepaticus,* it is often described as "a musty smell." Methyl mercaptan has been isolated from the urine in such patients. An oxidation product of this substance eliminated in the breath may be the cause for the odor. It is a highly significant finding and often associated with a grave prognosis.

In oral sepsis the breath may have a disagreeable odor, the condition being known as *halitosis,* a term now quite as well known to the general public as to the physician.

The most disagreeable breath of all is that present in lung abscess with *gangrene of the lungs.* The infection in such cases is largely due to putrefactive organisms, so that the patient's breath has the odor of decaying vegetable or animal matter. Such patients announce their presence to their neighbors and also their diagnosis to an alert physician. The author once saw a patient with gangrene of the lung sit down in a street car. A half dozen passengers sat down beside him in rapid succession and, after sitting by his side for a few moments, moved on to other seats.

The odor of patients with certain diseases was stressed by an earlier generation of physicians. Many of these odors are fairly characteristic, but difficult to describe. The odor in diphtheria may be characteristic. In smallpox the odor is extremely disagreeable. A "mousy" odor has been described in typhus fever, a slight sweetish, fetid odor in measles and an acid sweat smell in rheumatic fever.

BUCCAL CAVITY

The appearance of the buccal cavity aids greatly in the diagnosis of many diseases (Fig. 148). In severe anemias the mucous membrane of the mouth is pale. *Koplik's spots,* which are small bluish-white spots surrounded by a small red margin, appear on the mucous membrane of the cheek opposite the molars and near the parotid duct, and are pathognomonic of measles. They appear before the eruption, and thus permit an early diagnosis of this disease.

Mucous patches, white, sharply circumscribed areas 0.5 to 1 cm. in diameter, a characteristic sign of secondary syphilis, are seen on the mucous membranes of the mouth near the bases of

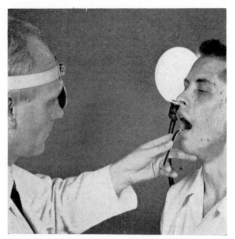

Fig. 148. Inspection of the buccal cavity.

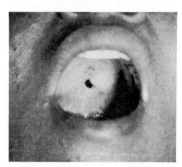

Fig. 149. Perforation of the palate in syphilis.

the gums. They may be present on the palate or anywhere on the mucous membrane of the buccal cavity.

General *redness of the throat* or pharynx may indicate a pharyngitis or the early stage of diphtheria or scarlet fever.

Paralysis of the soft palate is seen occasionally as a sequel of diphtheria. In the days before the use of diphtheria antitoxin it was common. This complication was described by Aretaeus the Cappadocian, who noted that many patients with diphtheria feared to drink water because it would "return by the nostrils."

Perforation of the palate is usually, but not invariably, of syphilitic origin (Fig. 149).

The *tonsils* may be the seat of an acute follicular tonsillitis or of diphtheria. In the former condition the process begins as numerous small abscesses in the tonsillar crypts, the abscesses coalescing later to form a large grayish patch on the surface of the tonsils. In diphtheria there is a dirty grayish membrane which spreads over the surface of the tonsils and frequently spreads to the fauces and uvula. This membrane on removal leaves a bloody surface beneath. The careful physician has learned by experience that a streptococcic sore throat may closely resemble diphtheria and always takes a throat culture in doubtful cases.

Vincent's angina is an infection of the tonsil, usually unilateral, causing necrosis with a dirty yellow exudate which leaves a bleeding surface when removed. It has been mistaken for both diphtheria and syphilis.

A peritonsillar abscess may follow acute tonsillitis. The patient commonly has a high fever, dysphagia, rigidity of the neck which, combined with spasm of the buccal muscles producing "locked jaws," has led to the false diagnosis of tetanus. In such cases the physician may be unable to see the abscess, since the patient cannot open his mouth wide enough, but may feel the swelling by inserting a finger into the mouth.

A *retropharyngeal abscess* may be seen on inspection in children suffering from tuberculosis of the cervical vertebrae. This swelling may produce a peculiar barklike cough which the French have called "cri de canard" (cry of a duck). The swelling can often be better felt than seen.

In inflammation of the pharynx or fauces the *uvula is enlarged,* pendulous and semitranslucent. Such an enlarged uvula frequently produces a shallow, irritating cough, worse at night when the patient lies down, allowing the uvula to fall down on the base of the tongue. The *uvular pulsation,* described by F. Müller in aortic insufficiency, is an interesting diagnostic sign. With each heart beat there is pulsation of the uvula.

Neck

Examination of the neck should always be done in an unhurried and careful manner. Familiarity with the landmarks of the muscles, vessels and bony or cartilaginous structures as illustrated in Figure 150 will facilitate the examination.

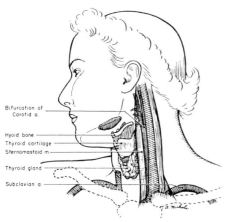

Bifurcation of Carotid a.

Hyoid bone
Thyroid cartilage
Sternomastoid m.

Thyroid gland

Subclavian a.

FIG. 150. Anatomic structures of neck.

As always, the first maneuver is that of inspection of the neck for asymmetry, unusual pulsations, tumors or limitation of motion. By simple extension and lateral deviation of the neck, tension of the sternocleidomastoid brings into view the boundary of the anterior and posterior triangles. Enlargement of the thyroid, unusual swelling of the lymph nodes, or abnormality of the vascular structures may immediately become apparent.

Both normal and abnormal structures should then be further studied by palpation. First, attention should be given to identification of the thyroid cartilage, the thyroid, the sternocleidomastoid muscle and the carotid arteries. Palpation of the lymph nodes should be carried out as indicated in Figure 151 using the tips of the fingers and gentle pressure. Fixation and positioning of the patient's head can be accomplished

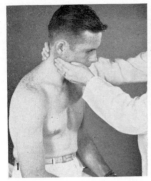 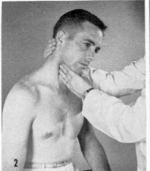 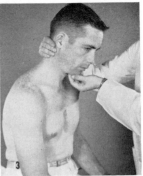

FIG. 151. Palpation of neck.

by placing one hand behind the occiput, while palpating with the other hand. Slow, gentle, sliding, or rotary motions with the palpating fingers, first in the anterior triangle, and then in the posterior triangle, and finally in the submental region will more likely reveal slightly enlarged lymph nodes than heavy palpation.

Palpation of the thyroid deserves individual consideration. Usually the normal thyroid is palpable as a firm, smooth mass, which moves upward with swallowing. In the patient with a short obese neck, it is extremely difficult or impossible to identify.

When enlargement or nodularity of the thyroid is noted, careful outlining of the structures, with the palpating fingers is required. This is most easily and accurately done with the examiner standing behind the patient, with the finger tips of both hands resting firmly on the structures of the thyroid with the trachea separating the fingers of the hands of the examiner as indicated in Figure 152. The patient is then asked to swallow. As he does so the thyroid slips between the fingers permitting evaluation of the two sides for size, contour, firmness or tenderness. More exact evaluation of each lobe and poles of the thyroid can be carried out as indicated in Figure 152, 2, while the examiner retracts the sternocleidomastoid and palpates the lobe or nodule with the other hand. If the lower pole is not palpated, it probably is beneath

the sternum as will be revealed by percussion.

If the examiner now returns to the front of the patient he may gather further information by displacing the trachea as shown in 152, 3. It may be helpful to palpate the upper pole of the thyroid between the thumb and forefinger as indicated in 152, 4.

In aortic disease of the heart the carotid arteries often beat with unusual force and violence. These *throbbing carotids* are an important diagnostic sign in aortic insufficiency. Indeed, the diagnosis is frequently suggested by this sign alone. Throbbing carotids are, however, occasionally seen in other conditions, notably severe anemia, hyperthyroidism and arteriosclerosis, especially when the latter is associated with arterial hypertension. Careful inspection of the carotids may show clearly an irregularity of the heart beat, such as that due to premature contractions or to auricular fibrillation. Indeed, these two conditions may often be diagnosed by simple inspection of the carotid pulse without palpating the radial pulse or listening to the heart.

Dunning has pointed out that occlusion of the internal carotid artery can be diagnosed by pharyngeal palpation. The examiner, wearing a rubber glove which has been moistened with water to minimize the friction that initiates the gag reflex, gently palpates the posterior wall of the pharynx with the forefinger and slowly draws the finger later-

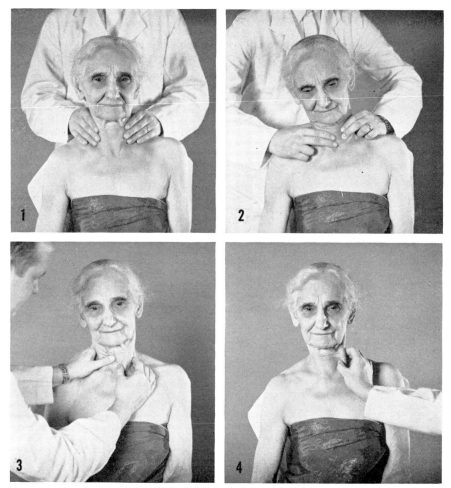

Fig. 152. Palpation of thyroid gland.

ally as far as the pharyngopalatine muscle. When this muscle is relaxed, the pulsations of the internal carotid can be felt particularly if the thumb of the other hand is pressed firmly externally in the carotid fossa. Absence of pulsation indicates occlusion of the internal carotid artery.

Pulsation above the right clavicle may be due to elongation of the aorta with buckling of the innominate artery. It is seen especially in hypertensive and arteriosclerotic patients and may be falsely diagnosed as an aneurysm of the innominate artery.

An aneurysm of the carotid artery may produce a striking *enlargement on one side of the neck* (Fig. 153). Such an enlargement pulsates with the heart beat and also shows an expansile pulsation.

The *venous pulse in the jugular veins* should be studied carefully. When there is obstruction to the flow of blood into the large thoracic veins, the jugular veins are markedly distended. This is seen particularly in intrathoracic tumors. In cardiac failure the veins of the neck are usually engorged.

The venous pulse consists of three waves designated by Mackenzie as *a, c,* and *v.* Mackenzie used this terminology in the belief that the *a* wave was due to auricular contraction, the *c* wave to a transmitted carotid pulsation, and the *v* wave to ventricular contraction,

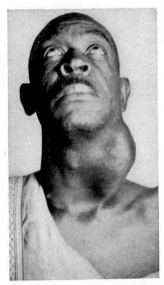

FIG. 153. Aneurysm of left carotid artery.

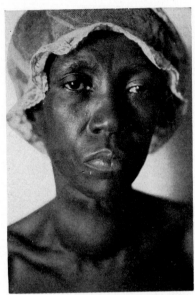

FIG. 155. Thyroid cyst.

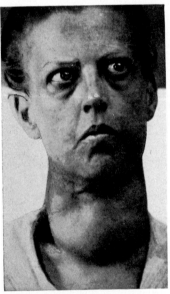

FIG. 154. Graves' disease. Note diffuse enlargement of thyroid gland.

and that the *v* wave is produced during the diastolic filling of the heart. If one examines the jugular vein of a healthy person, these three waves can often be seen. In tricuspid insufficiency, instead of the normal three waves, one large wave is seen—the so-called *positive venous pulse.* In auricular fibrillation, when the auricles are not beating, but are fibrillating, the venous wave caused by auricular systole, the *a* wave, is absent and there are only two waves present in the venous pulse. In this condition there is also a striking irregularity of the heart rate which can be readily detected by careful observation of the venous pulse. In auricular flutter the flutter waves are often visible in the veins of the neck.

A generalized *enlargement of the thyroid gland* is a striking feature of Graves' disease (Fig. 154). An enlarged thyroid gland rises when the patient swallows because of its attachment to the larynx. This is a differential point of great value. Cysts of the thyroid gland, unaccompanied by any marked generalized enlargement, are common (Fig. 155). On auscultation over the thyroid gland, a systolic bruit is commonly heard in Graves' disease. This systolic *thyroid bruit* must not be confused with a cardiac murmur transmitted along the carotid artery. It should also be remembered that a bruit may be heard over the carotid artery if the bell of the stethoscope is applied with too much pressure. A systolic thrill, synchronous with the bruit, is felt in some patients.

A thyroid bruit or thrill is almost pathognomonic of Graves' disease and

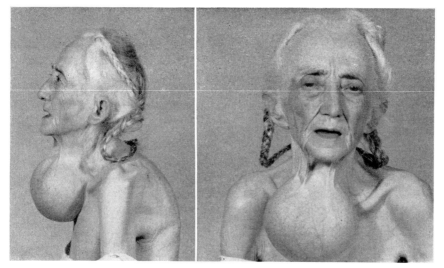

FIG. 156. Enormous cyst of thyroid gland.

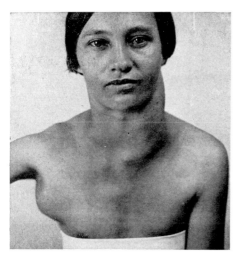

FIG. 157. Hodgkin's disease. Note collar-like enlargement of cervical glands and enlarged glands in the right axilla.

mass about the neck resembling a horse-collar. Frequently this marked enlargement is unilateral (Fig. 157). The lymph nodes in Hodgkin's disease in the early stages are usually firm and discrete and show little tendency to mat together. In tuberculous lymphadenitis they are often matted together, and, by the time they reach the size of the large glands seen in Hodgkin's disease, the tuberculous glands fluctuate or rupture. In their earlier stages, however, the lymph glands in tuberculous cervical adenitis may be discrete (Fig. 158). It

occurs only rarely in colloid goiters and other thyroid abnormalities.

Branchial cleft cysts may produce marked swellings in the neck. Branchial fistulae may open along the anterior margin of the sternocleidomastoid muscle near the episternal notch. They secrete a thin, watery mucoid substance.

Enlargement of the cervical lymph nodes may produce striking *swellings in the neck*. Hodgkin's disease often produces a marked bilateral enlargement of the cervical lymph nodes forming a

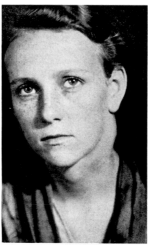

FIG. 158. Tuberculosis of cervical lymph glands.

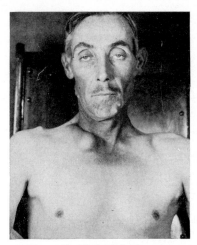

FIG. 159. Hodgkin's disease.

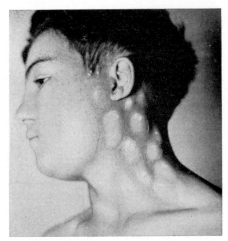

FIG. 160. Enlarged cervical lymph glands in lymphatic leukemia.

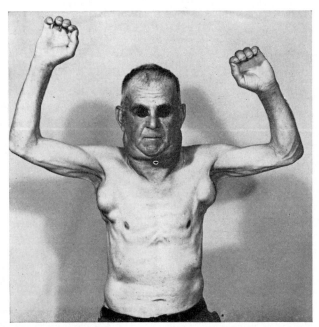

FIG. 161. Enlargement of cervical and axillary glands in lymphatic leukemia.

is commonly impossible to differentiate between Hodgkin's disease of the neck and tuberculous lymphadenitis except by a pathologic study of the tissue. Hodgkin described seven cases in his original paper, but reanalysis of his paper and restudy of the tissue with the aid of the microscope have revealed that one patient had tuberculosis, one syphilis, one acute leukemia and one lymphomatosis, leaving only three cases of

what we understand today as Hodgkin's disease.

Though the enlarged cervical lymph glands in Hodgkin's disease have a tendency to produce the "horsecollar" effect, they may at times present the appearance of scattered smaller groups of discrete glands (Fig. 159).

In lymphatic leukemia the cervical lymph glands are markedly enlarged and discrete (Fig. 160). In this disease we usually find also a generalized enlargement of the lymph glands, the axillary and inguinal lymph glands showing marked enlargement (Fig. 161). The cervical lymph glands, especially the posterior, are often enlarged in pediculosis capitis. This condition is rarely seen in hospital or private practice in America, but is not infrequent among the lower classes in some countries. At one time it seemed to have been frequent among all classes of society, the famous Samuel Pepys recording in his Diary that his wife found "I am lousy, having found in my head and body about twenty-five, little and great, which I wonder at being more than I have had I believe these 20 years."

A *lipoma* of the neck may produce a striking enlargement, usually unilateral (Figs. 162, 163). In multiple symmetrical lipomatosis there may be numerous symmetrically enlarged cervical lymph glands (Fig. 33, p. 38). Certain unusual tumors arising from structures in the neck are seen occasionally. Examples of such tumors are branchial cyst tumors, tumors of the carotid body (Fig. 164) and sarcomata arising from the cervical lymph glands.

An interesting type of enlargement of the cervical glands is seen in the so-called *indurative headache* in which

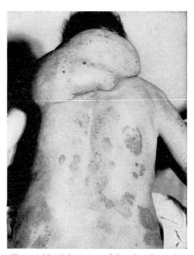

FIG. 163. Lipoma of back of neck.

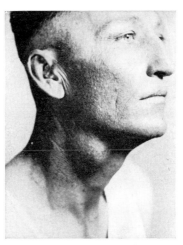

FIG. 164. Tumor of carotid body.

there is a row of small nodules along the outer margin of the trapezius muscle in the back of the neck.

A *torticollis* or *wryneck* causes a characteristic deviation of the head toward the affected side (Fig. 165). Commonly such wryneck is due to rigidity and tenderness of the sternomastoid and trapezius muscles, probably of infectious origin. Other forms of torticollis are encountered at times. A dislocation of the upper cervical vertebrae may produce torticollis with marked pain, at times extending down into the arm. Tuberculosis of the cervical vertebrae may produce a similar picture. Congenital torticollis is also seen occasion-

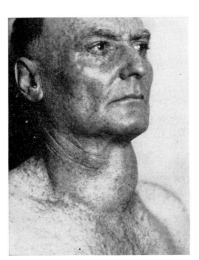

FIG. 162. Lipoma of neck.

ally. This is due to shortness of the muscle and is usually on the right side.

Poliomyelitis may produce atrophy of the trapezius muscle on one side, causing a marked asymmetry of the posterior surface of the neck (Fig. 166).

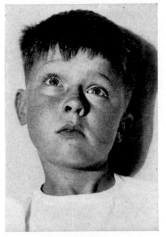

FIG. 165. Torticollis.

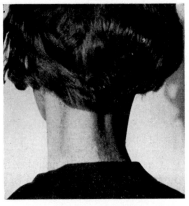

FIG. 166. Atrophy of right trapezius muscle following poliomyelitis.

Marked *rigidity of the neck* is seen in meningitis (Fig. 167). The child shown in this illustration had a boardlike rigidity of the neck and could be raised nearly to the sitting position by holding the hand back of the head.

A cervical rib can at times be palpated in the neck. More commonly, however, it is an accidental x-ray finding.

A very important finding in aortic aneurysm is the well-known *Oliver's sign* or *tracheal tug*. No one has described this sign more accurately or in fewer words than Oliver himself. "Place the patient in the erect position, and direct him to close his mouth, and elevate his chin to the fullest extent, then grasp the cricoid cartilage between the finger and thumb, and use gentle upward pressure on it, when if dilatation or aneurysm exist, the pulsation of the aorta will be distinctly felt transmitted through the trachea to the hand."

BIBLIOGRAPHY

Barker, Lewellys F., and Hanes, Frederick M: Exophthalmos and other eye signs in chronic nephritis. Am. J. M. Sc. *138:*469, 1909.

Bean, William Bennett: The caviar lesion under the tongue. Tr. Am. Clin. & Climat. A. *64:*40, 1953.

Brown, G. E., and Rountree, L. G.: Right sided carotid pulsations in cases of severe hypertension. J.A.M.A. *84:*1016, 1925.

Challenger, F., and Walshe, J. M.: Fetor hepaticus. The Lancet *268:*1239, 1955.

Davis, Loyal, and Martin, John: The pathogenesis and treatment of unilateral exophthalmos. Surg., Gynec. & Obst. *72:*557, 1941.

Dickinson, W. Howship: The Tongue as an Indication in Disease. London, Longmans Green, 1888.

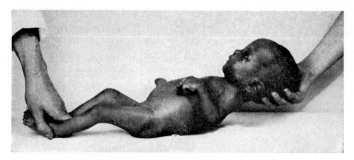

FIG. 167. Rigidity of neck in meningitis.

Dunning, Henry S.: Detection of occlusion of the internal carotid artery by pharyngeal palpation. J.A.M.A. *152:*321, 1953.

Dunphy, J. Englebert, and Botsford, Thomas W.: Physical Examination of the Surgical Patient. Philadelphia, W. B. Saunders Co., 1953.

Fox, Herbert: Remarks on the presentation of microscopical preparations made from some of the original tissue described by Thomas Hodgkin, 1832. Ann. Med. Hist. *8:*370, 1926.

Griffith, J. P. Crozer, and Mitchell, A. Graeme: The Diseases of Infants and Children. 2d ed. Philadelphia, W. B. Saunders Co., 1937.

Hale-White, Sir William: Thomas Hodgkins. Guy's Hosp. Rep. *74:*117, 1924.

Hertzler, Arthur E.: A Treatise on Tumors. Philadelphia, Lea & Febiger, 1912.

Keyes, John E. L., and Hatcher, William F.: The interpretation of visible pulsation in the retinal arteries. J.A.M.A. *114:*2089, 1940.

Lewandowsky, M.: Handbuch der Neurologie. Berlin, Julius Springer, 1910.

Locke, C. E.: Intracranial arterio-venous aneurism or pulsating exophthalmos. Ann. Surg. *80:*1, 1924.

Marie, Pierre: Two cases of acromegaly, transl. by Proctor S. Hutchinson, M.R.C.S. London, New Sydenham Society, 1891.

Martin, Hayes, and Koop, C. Everett: The precancerous mouth lesions of avitaminosis. Am. J. Surg. n.s. *57:*195, 1942.

Martin, J. D., Jr., and Mabon, Robert F.: Pulsating exophthalmos, review of all reported cases. J.A.M.A. *121:*330, 1943.

May, Angelo: The tongue sign for high venous pressure. Am. Heart J. *26:*685, 1943.

Morgan, Winfield S.: Mikulicz's disease and Sjörgrens syndrome. New England. J. Med. *251:*5, 1954.

Morrow, Prince: A System of Genito-urinary Diseases, Syphilology and Dermatology. New York, D. Appleton & Co., 1893–1894.

Naffziger, Howard C.: Progressive exophthalmos associated with disorders of the thyroid gland. Ann. Surg. *108:*529, 1938.

Oliver, W. S.: Physical diagnosis of thoracic aneurism. Lancet *2:*406, 1878.

Parrott, J.: La Syphilis Hereditaire et le Rachitis. Paris, G. Masson, 1886.

Pullen, Roscoe L.: Medical Diagnosis, Applied Physical Diagnosis. 2nd ed., Philadelphia, W. B. Saunders Co., 1950.

Squires, B. T.: Pattern of the human tongue. Lancet *268:*647, 1955.

Stitt, E. R.: The Diagnosis and Treatment of Tropical Diseases. Philadelphia, P. Blakiston's Sons & Co., 1929.

Sydenstricker, V. P., Geeslin, L. E., Templeton, C. W., and Weaver, J. W.: Riboflavin deficiency, J.A.M.A. *113:*1697, 1939.

CHAPTER 6

INSPECTION, PALPATION AND PERCUSSION OF THE CHEST

FOR CONVENIENCE in describing and locating certain points on the surface of the chest it is customary to draw imaginary lines. The first line drawn through the center of the sternum and extending down through the xiphoid is called the *midsternal line*. Two lines drawn along the border of the sternum on either side are called the *sternal lines*. Two lines drawn through the nipple on either side are called the *mammillary lines* (mammilla = nipple). Since, however, the location of the nipple varies with the size of the breast, a more constant line is the mid-clavicular line drawn through the middle of the clavicle (Fig. 168). On the sides of the chest we distinguish three lines, the *anterior axillary line* drawn downward from the origin of the anterior axillary fold, the *midaxillary line,* and the *posterior axillary line* descending from the termination of the posterior axillary fold (Fig. 169). On the back we speak of the *midspinal line,* the *scapular areas* over the scapulae, the *interscapular areas* between the scapulae and the *infrascapular areas* below the scapulae (Fig. 170).

INSPECTION OF THE CHEST

The Skin. The first feature of the chest which attracts our attention is the skin. In certain skin diseases and in the exanthemata the appearance of the skin

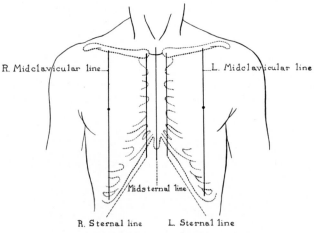

FIG. 168. Sternal lines and midclavicular lines.

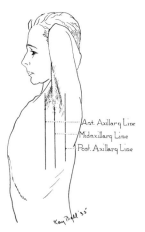

FIG. 169. Axillary lines.

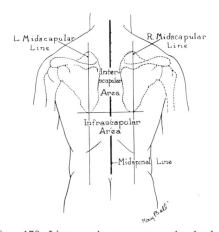

FIG. 170. Lines and areas over the back.

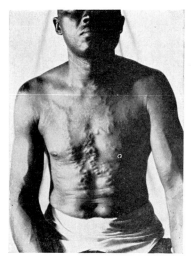

FIG. 171. Dilated veins of chest in mediastinal tumor.

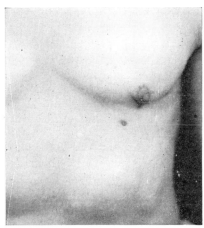

FIG. 172. Supernumerary nipple, seen just below the nipple and slightly toward the midline.

may be so characteristic as to establish the diagnosis. The petechiae, or small pinpoint hemorrhages of infectious endocarditis, aplastic anemia, benzol poisoning and lymphatic leukemia, as well as the larger purpuric spots of purpura haemorrhagica and of Hodgkin's disease, are often seen on the chest. Scratch marks on the chest may give important clues of disease. In jaundice and in Hodgkin's disease an intense itching of the skin often provokes continued scratching, the marks of which may be obvious.

Marked dilatation of the superficial veins of the chest is often seen in mediastinal tumors (Fig. 171).

Supernumerary nipples are often seen (Fig. 172). They are of no pathologic importance. In the sixteenth and seventeenth centuries they were often regarded as witch marks.

The character of the skin itself is often of importance. In tuberculosis we often find the skin of the chest oily and of coarse texture with the pores apparently further apart than in normal skin, but this is not pathognomonic, and also is frequently absent. In this disease the skin of the chest is often atrophied. The presence of scars resulting from old injuries or operations is apparent, and the possible relationship between them and the present condition should be considered.

Shape of the Chest. The shape of the chest may give us important information. The so-called *phthisic chest* is a flat chest in which the scapulae stand forth prominently—the *winged* or *alar scapulae*. This type of chest was once thought to be pathognomonic of pulmonary tuberculosis. Hippocrates noted that consumptives often had chests "with the scapulae having the appearance of wings." Though it is frequently seen in tuberculosis, it does not always accompany this disease (Fig. 253).

The *barrel chest* has been described as pathognomonic of emphysema of the lungs, but may be seen in elderly persons with no obvious emphysema (Fig. 247).

The *funnel chest,* an appearance produced by a deep funnel-like depression of the lower part of the sternum, is readily recognized (Fig. 173). This deformity, the "Trichterbrust" of the Germans, has been described as the result of rickets in childhood and as the result of the continued pressure of the last against the chest in shoemakers. In many patients, however, its cause is unknown.

The *chicken breast,* the "thorax en bâteau" of the French, presents a striking deformity in which the sternum bulges forward like the keel of a ship, while the ribs slope away on either side. This deformity results commonly from early rickets (Fig. 174).

A striking deformity of the chest is produced by *Harrison's grooves,* which result from the pull of the diaphragm on the ribs already softened by rickets or from a softening of the bones. The marked depression or groove occurs along the line of the diaphragmatic attachment.

The *rickety rosary* occasionally visible in young children is produced by a beadlike enlargement of the ribs at their junction with their cartilages (Fig. 175). Certain abnormalities within the

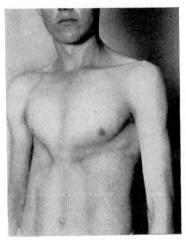

FIG. 174. Chicken breast.

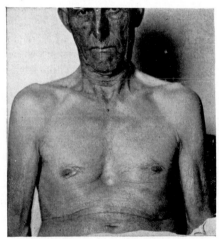

FIG. 173. Funnel breast.

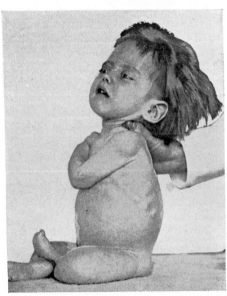

FIG. 175. Rickets showing "rosary" (Foster).

chest may produce marked deformities of the thorax. Figure 363 shows a large aneurysm of the aorta which produced a *bulging,* pulsating mass, so characteristic that inspection alone was sufficient for diagnosis. A tumor of the thymus or a new growth in the anterior mediastinum may cause a marked localized *bulging* of the thorax. Atelectasis of the lobe of one lung often causes a marked *unilateral depression* of that side of the chest (Fig. 252).

In women, breast tumors cause obvious abnormalities. Such a patient is seen in Figure 176. A carcinoma of the breast has produced the characteristic distortion with a *retraction of the nipple.* The nipple itself may be the seat of a primary carcinoma (Fig. 177) (Paget's disease of the nipple). Occasionally a chancre may develop on the nipple (Fig. 178). Carcinoma of the breast is also occasionally seen in the male. Figure 179 shows a *lactating male breast* in a patient with a chorioma of the testis.

Enlargement of the axillary lymph glands is seen in carcinoma of the breast, in Hodgkin's disease (Fig. 157), in tuberculous lymphadenitis, in lymphatic leukemia (Fig. 161), and in patients with infections of the hand or arm on the corresponding side. In tularemia there is usually enlargement of the axillary glands which drain the in-

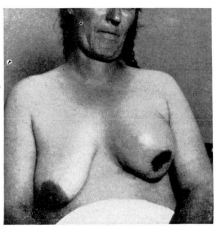

FIG. 176. Carcinoma of the left breast.

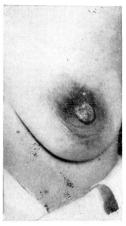

FIG. 178. Chancre of breast.

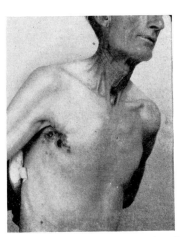

FIG. 177. Paget's disease of the right nipple.

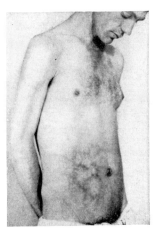

FIG. 179. Lactation of male breast. Patient suffering from syncytioma of testis.

fected wound (Fig. 180). The same is true when there is a chancre of the hand or finger.

The Back. The patient's back should always be examined most minutely. Lesions of the back usually produce symptoms in the back, but at times the pain may be referred elsewhere. *Kyphosis* is produced by an abnormal curvature of the spine with a dorsal prominence (Fig. 181). The term "kyphosis" is derived from the Greek word κυφός (kyphos) meaning humpbacked. The patient with this deformity, shown in Figure 182, suffered from Paget's disease of the bone. It may also be present in marked spondylitis of the spine. It is frequently due to tuberculosis of the spine (Pott's disease) (Fig. 183). Tu-

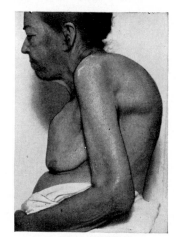

FIG. 182. Kyphosis in Paget's disease.

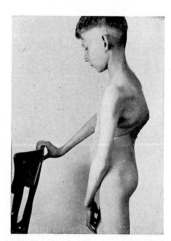

FIG. 183. Kyphosis due to tuberculosis of spine.

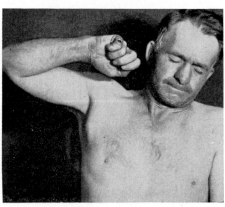

FIG. 180. Tularemia. Enlarged right axillary glands. Sore on right little finger.

berculous disease of the spine may at times produce a local prominence or "gibbus" (Figs. 184, 185).

The association of kyphosis with tuberculosis was recognized by Hippocrates. "In most instances patients with kyphosis have hard cheesy nodules in the lungs and also collections of pus in the flanks and in the lumbar region."

Scoliosis, or lateral curvature of the spine (σκολίωσις—skoliosis = curvation), is seen in Figures 186 and 187. This condition often produces marked deformity and distortion of the chest. It is frequently the result of poliomyelitis, but may appear in persons who are otherwise in perfect health and give no history of any antecedent serious illness.

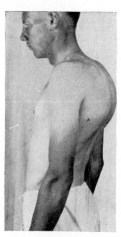

FIG. 181. Kyphosis.

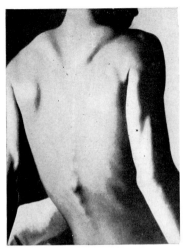

FIG. 184. Gibbus in tuberculous disease of spine.

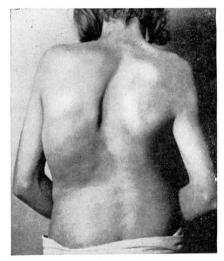

FIG. 186. Scoliosis.

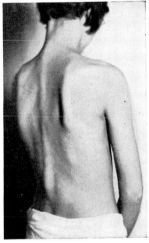

FIG. 185. Gibbus in tuberculous disease of spine.

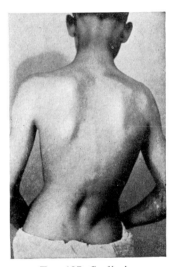

FIG. 187. Scoliosis.

Scoliosis is especially evident if the observer makes a dot with a skin pencil just over the tip of the spinous process.

Lordosis (λορδοῦν—lordoun = to bend) is a curvature of the spinal column with a forward convexity (Fig. 188). Lordosis occurs in pregnancy, with large abdominal tumors, in marked obesity, in bilateral congenital dislocation of the hip, tuberculous disease of the hip, or compensatory to kyphosis in another part of the spine. Marked lordosis is also common in syringomyelia.

The *movements of the spine* forward, backward and laterally should always be carefully tested. In marked spondylitis of the spine we may see complete fixation of the thoracic and lumbar spine. In this condition, known as "poker spine" or "poker-back," the back is as rigid as the proverbial poker. The patient, in attempting to pick up an object from the floor, can only do so by bending his knees until his hands touch the floor (Fig. 189).

In Figure 190 the patient showed a large, bulging, fluctuating mass which proved to be a tuberculous abscess originating from a tuberculous process in the ribs.

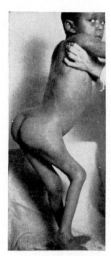

FIG. 188. Lordosis—tuberculosis of the hip.

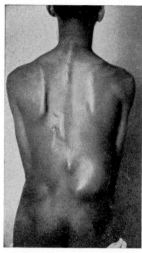

FIG. 190. Tuberculous abscess in right lumbar region. Note two small sinuses in left lower interscapular region.

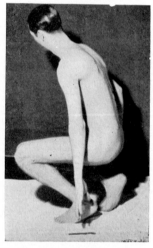

FIG. 189. Characteristic attitude assumed by patient with poker spine when picking a pencil from the floor.

In *perinephritic abscess* a slight but definite bulging may be noted in the back just below the costal margin. This slight bulging may be sufficient to establish the diagnosis in a patient showing fever, chills and pain in the lumbar region.

At the lower end of the spine there occurs occasionally a *pilonidal cyst.* This is a small cyst or sinus of embryonic origin in the sacrococcygeal region, which may discharge from time to time a mucoid secretion and may become infected.

Respiration. Since breathing is one of the most important functions of the chest and certainly the most obvious, the next observations are those concerning the rate, depth and type of respiration, and equality on the two sides.

In health two types of respiration are observed, *costal or thoracic,* and *diaphragmatic or abdominal.* In men respiration is mainly diaphragmatic, in women costal. The costal type of respiration in women was thought at one time to be produced by tight lacing, the staves about the waist interfering with the movements of the diaphragm. This explanation is obviously incorrect, since the era of tight lacing has passed, but the respiration in women continues to be the thoracic type. This type of breathing is also present in young girls and seems to be a characteristic of the sex, not influenced by any mode of dress or type of activity.

An increase in the respiratory rate is called *tachypnea,* while a slowing of the respiratory rate is known as *bradypnea.*

The respiratory rate is increased in cardiac failure, in lobar pneumonia, in bronchopneumonia, in cerebrospinal meningitis and often in chronic nephritis. In fever, especially in children, it is also increased. A child with fever may have such a marked and obvious increase in the rate of respiration that pneumonia is suspected where it does not exist. In pulmonary tuberculosis an increase in the respiratory rate is often as significant in arriving at a diagnosis as the evening elevation in temperature. In diabetes mellitus with an impending or established coma, the respirations are both increased in rate and depth—the air hunger of Kussmaul. The patient in this condition may be conscious and much alarmed at this deep breathing which he is unable to control.

The *respiratory rate is slowed* in some cases of brain tumor, in obstruction to the bronchus and in opium poisoning.

In health a careful examination of the respiration shows that the two sides of the chest move synchronously and equally. A comparison of the movements of the two sides of the chest should always be made, since certain diseases may modify most profoundly the movements on one side of the chest.

Amplitude of Respiratory Movement. In lobar pneumonia the affected side of the chest may show a marked decrease in the amplitude of the respiratory movements, while the healthy side shows a great increase in amplitude. A similar picture is seen in pneumothorax, the chest on the side of the collapsed lung moving slightly or not at all during respiration, while the healthy side moves with a greatly increased amplitude.

Lesser differences in the excursion of the two sides of the chest may be of great importance in diagnosis. In pulmonary tuberculosis the respiratory movements on the affected side often show a characteristic lagging. In children or adults who have aspirated a foreign body into the bronchus, the respiratory movements on the affected side are shallow when compared with the healthy side. Dr. Thomas McCrae, who studied many such patients, stated that this phenomenon appears immediately after aspiration of the foreign body and may be the only physical sign present. In

pleural effusion the excursions of the chest are less on the affected side if the effusion be large.

The *movements of the diaphragm* are profoundly affected by disease in the thorax and abdomen. The diaphragmatic excursions on that side may be abolished by the presence of fluid on that side.

Hoover's sign, movement of the costal margins toward the midline in inspiration, is often easily seen and of important diagnostic significance. It appears bilaterally in pulmonary emphysema and unilaterally in conditions causing a flattening of the diaphragm such as pleural effusion and pneumothorax. They may also be absent on the one side when there is a subdiaphragmatic abscess.

The excursions of the diaphragm may be studied by noting the well-known *Litten's sign,* which Litten described as follows: "The phenomenon takes the form of a wave motion, which begins on both sides at approximately the height of the sixth intercostal space, travels downward with maximum inspiration in the form of a straight line or shallow furrow at an acute angle with the ribs, over several intercostal spaces, at times as far as the costal margin. With expiration, it rises again over the same area." This sign is best elicited by placing the patient on a bed or examination table, placing his head toward a well-lighted window while the observer stands at his feet first on one side and then on the other. As the patient inspires, a small linear vertical shadow travels down the lower part of the thorax below the axilla; on expiration the shadow passes upward. This shadow, due to the "peeling off" of the diaphragm from the costal pleura, is normally present on both sides during inspiration. It is best seen in thin subjects (Fig. 191). When the movements of the diaphragm are diminished or abolished on one side because of fluid in the chest, a subdiaphragmatic abscess or lesions of the phrenic nerve, the shadow is either absent or shows a much diminished excursion on the affected side.

One of the most striking types of

respiratory irregularity is the *Cheyne-Stokes respiration*. Hippocrates was familiar with this phenomenon and described the case of "Philiscus, who lived by the Wall," whose "respiration was like that of a person recollecting himself." A tracing from a patient with Cheyne-Stokes respiration is shown in Figure 192. No one has described this type of respiration better than Cheyne

himself, who, in describing his patient, wrote, "His breathing was irregular; it would entirely cease for a quarter of a minute, then it would become perceptible, though very low, then by degrees heaving and quick, and then it would gradually cease again." This type of respiration is seen in patients who have a disturbance in the respiratory center in the medulla. The most commonly accepted explanation is that during the period of apnea, or cessation of respiration, the carbon dioxide accumulates in the blood and gradually stimulates the respiratory center until it reaches a height of activity and produces deep and heavy breathing. This forced respiration drives the carbon dioxide out through the lungs, the carbon dioxide content of the blood is lowered, stimulation of the respiratory center is removed, and the respiration again ceases until the reaccumulation of the carbon dioxide stimulates it anew. This type of respiration is seen in brain tumors, in cardiac disease, in chronic nephritis, in hypertensive cardiovascular disease, in epidemic and tuberculous meningitis, in pneumonia and in diseases accompanied by profound intoxication. Though a sign of grave prognostic import, it does not always signify a fatal termination.

Another striking type of respiration, most commonly seen in meningitis, was first accurately studied by Biot and has since been known as *Biot's respiration*.

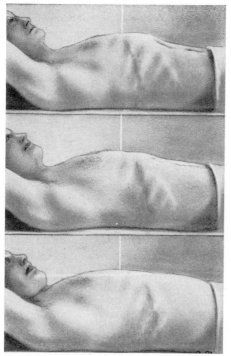

FIG. 191. Litten's sign. (After Sahli.)

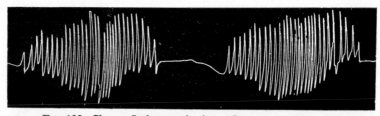

FIG. 192. Cheyne-Stokes respiration. (Conner and Stillman.)

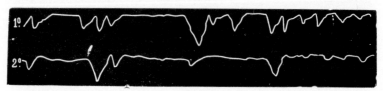

FIG. 193. Biot's respiration. Original tracing published by Biot.

"This irregularity of the respiratory movements is not periodic, sometimes slow, sometimes rapid, sometimes superficial, sometimes deep, but without any constant relation of succession between the two types, with pauses following irregular intervals, preceded and often followed by a sigh more or less prolonged" (Fig. 193). This respiratory irregularity is reminiscent of the total cardiac irregularity in auricular fibrillation.

PALPATION OF THE CHEST

The first use for which palpation should be employed is to confirm the findings of inspection. The condition or texture of the skin, which on inspection appears harsh, dry or oily, may feel definitely so on palpation. The differences in excursion of the two sides of the chest which were noted on inspection may become more striking when the hands are placed upon the chest and the differences in their movements are both seen and felt.

Vocal Fremitus. Testing of the vocal fremitus is one of the most important palpatory procedures in examining the chest. The vocal fremitus is elicited by placing both hands upon the chest, one on either side, symmetrically placed, and then asking the patient to repeat the words "one, two, three" or "ninety-nine." Both hands are then moved to various parts of the chest, keeping them symmetrically placed and comparing the vibrations of the chest wall produced by the sounds uttered (Fig. 194).

The vocal fremitus is produced by the vibrations caused in the larynx passing down the bronchi so that the lungs as well as the chest walls vibrate in sympathy whenever the spoken tone corresponds with their fundamental tones. This phenomenon is similar to that produced when a certain note struck on a piano causes the vibration of some small object nearby which has the same fundamental tone. The fundamental tone of the female voice is often higher than that of the lungs, and in such women the vocal fremitus may be markedly di-

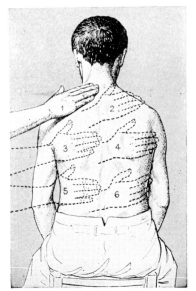

FIG. 194. Method of testing vocal fremitus. (Letulle.)

minished or even absent. In children, however, the voice, although higher in pitch, corresponds to the fundamental tone of the smaller lung, and for this reason the vocal fremitus is usually easily felt in children.

Normally, the intensity of the vibrations varies in different parts of the chest, being felt more strongly upon the right side. Their intensity varies according to the distance from the source of the sound, i.e., the larynx. It is stronger on the right side of the chest because of the shorter length of the right bronchus.

The vocal fremitus is increased when the lung is consolidated. Thus, if we have a lobe of the lung consolidated by a pneumonic process, the vocal fremitus is much stronger over the consolidated area than over other parts of the chest.

The vocal fremitus is decreased when a pathologic condition interferes with the transmission of sound waves from the lungs to the surface of the chest. Any condition producing a decrease in vocal fremitus may, if marked enough, cause a disappearance of the fremitus. The two conditions which most commonly cause decreased vocal fremitus are an effusion of fluid into the pleural cavity between the lung and the chest wall and thickening of the pleura. Figure 195 is a tracing of a normal fremitus and of a diminished vocal fremitus on the side of a pleural effusion. Figure 196 illustrates the inability of the sound causing vocal fremitus to penetrate through a thickened pleura. An infiltrating tumor mass lying between the lung and the chest wall may diminish or abolish the vocal fremitus. The vocal fremitus is absent or markedly diminished on the affected side in atelectasis of the entire lung due to bronchial obstruction or in a unilateral pneumothorax with resulting collapse of the lung.

The vocal fremitus may be localized and increased by applying an Erlenmeyer flask to the chest, placing the mouth of the flask against the skin, and holding the base of the flask in the palm of the examiner's hand. Reich introduced and recommended this procedure.

Some authors distinguish between vocal fremitus as a thrill perceived by the ear and tactile fremitus as a thrill felt by the hand. Most authorities, however, consider vocal fremitus and tactile fremitus as synonymous terms and follow the lead of Austin Flint, who noted that "if the palmar surfaces of the hands be lightly applied over the healthy chest in certain situations, the vibrations of the vocal cords, propagated along the bronchial tubes, and communicated to the thoracic parties, give rise to a thrilling sensation, called the vocal fremitus."

PERCUSSION OF THE CHEST

Physics of Sound. Before proceeding to a discussion of percussion and auscultation of the chest, it is necessary to consider briefly the physical basis of these two methods of examination. Since both percussion and auscultation are intimately associated with the production of sound, an understanding of the physics of sound is necessary. Skoda, it will be recalled was the first physician to

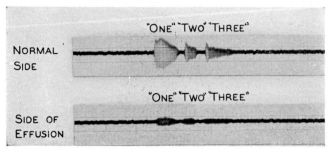

FIG. 195. Phonogram showing differences in intensity of vocal sounds on the normal side of the chest and the side of pleural effusion in the same person.

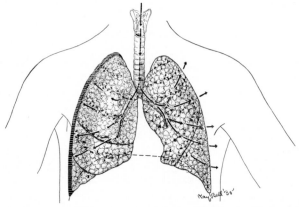

FIG. 196. The voice sounds producing fremitus pass readily through the chest wall on the normal left side, while on the right, transmission is interfered with by the thickened pleura.

apply the laws of physics to the explanation of percussion and auscultation. Helmholtz, the physicist, added greatly to our knowledge of the physics of sound, and Friedrich Müller and his school have made further advances by applying the methods of Helmholtz to a study of the sound phenomena observed in percussion and auscultation.

The source of every sound is a vibrating body which produces a series of waves in the surrounding medium, usually the air. These waves, which vibrate at the same rate as the vibrating body, reach the ear, cause a vibration of the

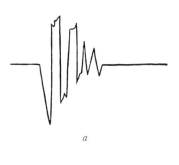

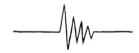

FIG. 197. a, Resonance (lung); b, flat note (liver).

ear drums and middle ear, so that the sensation of sound is produced. When we tap on the chest, the lung is set in vibration and the waves passing from the vibrating lung through the air produce a characteristic sound.

Sounds are divided into tones and noises. Sounds produced by regular oscillations, causing a uniform series of waves, are called *tones*. The simplest example of this is the tone produced by a tuning fork vibrating at a regular rate. Tones have a generally recognized musical quality and have three well-defined characteristics:

1. *Intensity.* The intensity of a tone depends upon the amplitude of the vibrations. A loud tone has a wider amplitude of vibrations than a soft tone. Figure 197 shows the difference in the amplitude of the waves produced when one percusses with the same intensity over the normal lung and over the liver. The tone over the lung is louder than that over the liver, since the lung is a more elastic tissue and vibrates more readily when struck.

2. *Pitch.* Pitch or tonality depends upon the number of vibrations produced. When the vibrations are rapid, the pitch is higher than when they are slower. If one walks inside a pipe organ while the organist is playing, he feels the vibrations produced when the pipes are playing and notes readily that the vibrations of the larger pipes producing deep tones are much slower than those of the smaller pipes which have a higher pitch. Figure 198 shows the difference

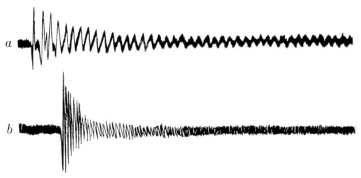

FIG. 198. a, Normal lung note; b, loud high tympanitic note over abdomen. (Seifert and Müller.)

in the number of the vibrations produced when the normal lung and the abdomen are percussed. The sound produced by percussion of the abdomen (tympany) shows more rapid oscillations and is in consequence higher in pitch.

3. *Quality*. The quality or timbre of a tone is a characteristic that escapes every attempt at a precise definition. The most ingenious descriptions that have been proposed are utterly inadequate to describe, for example, the difference in quality of the same note when played on the violin and on the violoncello. When one, however, has heard and recognized the difference, he can, without necessarily having a very musical ear, always recognize the difference between the two instruments. This difficulty of description, however, has led to much confusion, as shown by the varieties of accounts which different observers have given of the same acoustic phenomenon heard on percussion and auscultation. The timbre of a note is an elusive thing to describe precisely, something like the flavor of a certain kind of tobacco or the taste of a certain wine.

When, however, we study the physics of the timbre, we are treading upon much firmer ground. A simple note like that produced when a tuning fork is struck emits a single fundamental tone, produced by the vibrations of the fork (Fig. 199). When a violin string, however, is plucked, a more complicated phenomenon results, for we have not only an intense fundamental tone, but a series of faint overtones as well, superimposed upon the fundamental tone (Fig. 200). It is these overtones that give the violin string its characteristic quality or timbre. The differences in rate and amplitude of these overtones determine the timbre of different musical instruments. The human voice (Fig.

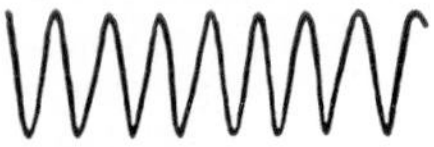

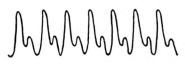

FIG. 200. Vibration waves of fundamental note with faint overtones in violin (recorded with cathode-ray apparatus).

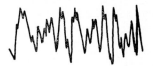

FIG. 201. Human voice (recorded with cathode-ray apparatus).

201) produces a fundamental tone with numerous overtones. These physical observations, it may be remarked, explain the timbre of a note even though we must admit that the terms describing timbre are usually inadequate.

TONES AND NOISES. A noise, in contrast to a tone, has no regular vibratory rate. A tone has a definite vibratory rate which gives it a certain pitch, while a noise, which has no regular rhythmic vibrations, but is a series of sound waves all vibrating at different vibratory rates, produces no pitch.

Gilbert, Tzanek and Gutmann have demonstrated the difference between tones and noises by an ingenious experiment. These observers constructed an apparatus consisting of a bellows attached to a large tube pierced by a single hole. Over this tube ran a cinematographic film which was turned by two cylinders on either side. The rate of turning could be increased by increasing the speed of the motor attached to one of the cylinders. They inserted into this apparatus, first, a film pierced by small holes placed at uniform intervals, and started the motor. As the small holes passed regularly before the steady current of air coming from the bellows, a musical note of a definite pitch was produced; as the speed of the motor was increased, the pitch of the note was raised. They then inserted a film pierced with small holes placed at irregular intervals and started the motor. This produced no tone, but a noise, and as

FIG. 199. Vibrations of tuning fork (recorded with cathode-ray apparatus).

the speed of the motor was increased there was no elevation in pitch. This experiment and similar ones prove convincingly that a noise has no true pitch, and the explanation as to how they produced a tone and a noise is obvious. The rotating film with regularly spaced holes set up a rhythmic uniform series of vibrations and a definite tone, while the film with irregularly placed holes set up no uniform series of vibrations and the result was a noise.

Resonators and Consonance. Musical tones, both fundamental tones and overtones, are much intensified by the presence of sonorous bodies or accumulations of air which vibrate in unison with the original tone and increase their intensity. This is well illustrated when we strike a tuning fork and note that another tuning fork, string or bell, having the same pitch, will vibrate in unison. In the construction of violins and pianos care is taken by the maker to produce a violin body or piano sounding board that will vibrate with the strings when they are set in motion. Helmholtz made use of this principle in the construction of his resonators which enabled him to carry out his analyses of sound; it is also important in the construction of the stethoscope, since certain types of stethoscope bells intensify the sounds more than others. It should also be kept in mind that different sounds require different types of resonators to intensify the sound and that the bell of a stethoscope may intensify certain sounds, while other sounds may be diminished. It is a well-known fact that the soft murmur of aortic insufficiency may often be better heard by the unaided ear than through a stethoscope. Indeed, at times it may be inaudible with the stethoscope.

This sympathetic vibration or consonance (*con* + *sonare* = to sound with) is of great importance in percussion and auscultation. Its importance was first stressed by Skoda, whose observations upon its role in physical diagnosis remain classic. Skoda emphasized the intensification of various sounds in the lungs through consonation, and compared it with the well-known observation that the sound of a vibrating tuning fork is increased by placing its handle upon a table or box.

A well-known example of consonation is the vibration of some object in a room when a certain note is struck on the piano. This "sympathetic vibration" or consonation is due to the fact that the object which vibrates, a pin tray for instance, has the same fundamental note as that struck on the piano. Pierce states, "It is a pretty well authenticated feat, performed by persons of a clear and powerful voice, to break a drinking-glass by singing its proper fundamental note close to it. Looking-glasses are said to have been broken by music; the excursions of their molecules in the vibrations into which they are thrown being so great as to strain them beyond the limits of their cohesion."

This principle of consonation must always be kept in mind when percussing the chest. When we percuss the chest we not only set the lungs into vibration, but cause the chest walls and thoracic contents to vibrate in unison. Soft organs, not containing air, like the liver, heart and muscles, and substances like fluid, are not set into vibration by the ordinary percussion stroke and thus act as damping bodies. When they interfere with vibrations of the chest wall, changes in the percussion note are produced. The percussion note, as Martini has shown, is determined by three factors: first, the vibratory ability of the chest wall; second, the vibratory response of the lung; and third, the damping effect of nonvibrating solid organs or pathological masses.

The Transmission of Sounds. Sounds are carried from the point of their production to the human ear through an elastic medium. Some sounds are better transmitted through one medium than through another. The ease with which sounds are transmitted depends upon the elasticity, mass and density of the medium through which they pass. The lungs, when removed from the body and inflated, transmit the percussion note extremely well. Bone transmits sound very well, and, as a rule, better than soft tissues. It is a well-known fact that the breath sounds in the trachea are well conducted by the clavicle to its acromial end and that the ribs conduct much of the sound heard when the chest is percussed.

Sound is much better transmitted through a uniform medium than through one which is not. Laennec obtained his inspiration for the invention of the stethoscope by observing that the sound produced by children scratching on a long beam was heard better by other children at the far end, when they applied their ears directly to it. Every boy knows that if he strikes two stones together under the water, the sound is better heard by his fellow if he puts his head under the water. The sound is produced under the water and is better propagated under the water than through the air, since it passes through a uniform medium in reaching the ear. For the same reason, when a stethoscope is applied to the chest, the normal breath sounds are better heard through the healthy lung than through the chest which contains an accumulation of fluid in the pleural cavity. This latter condition produces a medium of transmission which is not uniform (Fig. 202). Simi-

larly, the bronchial breathing, which is produced in the bronchi, is better heard through a consolidated lung than through a normal air-containing lung, since the density of the consolidated lung more nearly approaches that of the bronchus where the sound is produced and consequently transmits the sound better (Fig. 203). Here, however, dispersion also plays a role.

This factor of dispersion plays an important role in the transmission of sound. When the sound waves, after passing through a uniform medium, strike a medium of different density, some of the waves are reflected backward with a consequent diminution in tone. Sound waves spread themselves out much as ripples produced by dropping a stone in a pool, with a consequent diminution in intensity. When such dispersion is prevented by directing the sound within enclosed walls, as a speaking tube or a stethoscope, the intensity of the sound diminishes slightly or may actually be increased. Another closely allied factor is that of absorption. The ability of certain substances to absorb sound is made use of by architects and builders. Similar conditions occur in the human body.

Physics of Percussion. In percussion of the chest, as previously mentioned, *mediate percussion* is universally used.

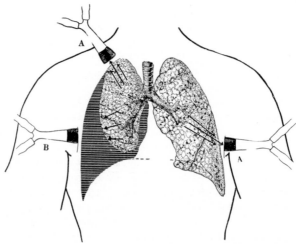

FIG. 202. The normal breath sounds are well heard at A and A', but not at B, since the effusion of fluid in the right chest has interfered with their transmission.

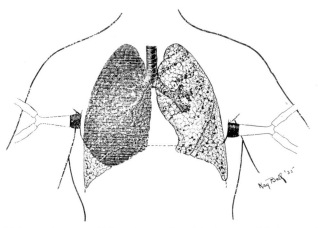

FIG. 203. Bronchial sounds are well heard over the right lung, which is consolidated, but are not heard over the left lung.

For this purpose either the finger striking upon the finger may be used, or a rubber hammer striking upon a piece of ivory (plessimeter). For most purposes the finger is preferable. The rubber hammer striking upon an ivory plessimeter produces of itself an additional tone which may be confusing. Figure 204 shows the difference in the sound waves produced by the two methods and demonstrates the clearer and sharper sound waves produced by finger percussion on the chest, as compared with percussion carried out by the instrumental method.

The *correct method of percussion* is better demonstrated than described. Three essentials for accurate percussion must be emphasized: first, the plessimeter finger must be placed flatly and firmly upon the chest wall. The percussion note can be radically altered by curving the finger instead of keeping it flat, a fact of which every beginner can easily convince himself. Second, a much clearer note is obtained if the hand at the moment of striking is moved at the wrist and the forearm is kept fixed. Third, the percussion stroke must be sharp, clear and decisive, and the percussing finger after striking the blow must be immediately raised. This is the same principle employed in producing a clear tone on a gong. If the hammer, after striking the gong, is not instantly

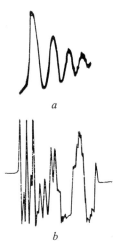

FIG. 204. *a*, Sound waves produced by finger percussion; *b*, sound waves produced by percussion with a hammer and an ivory plessimeter. (Recorded with cathode-ray apparatus.)

withdrawn, a muffled sound results. The same result appears in percussion if the percussing finger is not immediately withdrawn.

When percussing the chest of certain patients, the observer notes that each time he strikes the chest, a small lump of muscle rises and persists for several seconds. This phenomenon is called *myo-edema* and is usually best elicited over the pectoral, platysma and biceps muscles (Fig. 205). Myo-edema was formerly thought to be characteristic of pulmonary tuberculosis, but it occurs

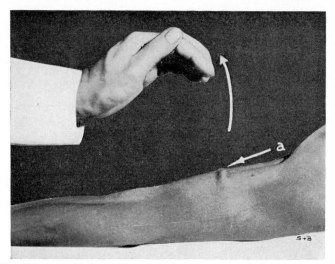

Fig. 205. Myo-edema—the welt is shown at the tip of the arrow (*a*).

commonly in emaciated or poorly nourished persons. It is also seen in persons apparently quite normal.

Before attempting to percuss the chest, the novice as well as the more experienced physician should remember the advice of Friedrich Müller: "We must not explore the chest by percussing our ideas into it; we must rather give our attention to listening to what comes out. The principal task in the course in percussion is to encourage the beginner in an honest method of investigation, and to guard him against the intrusion of previously formed judgments."

When we strike the chest, we set into vibration, not only the lungs, but the chest walls with their curved surfaces as well. These vibrations produce waves which are carried to our ear drums as sound. Anything interfering with these vibrations, such as a pleural effusion or an infiltration of the lungs, causes a damping of the vibrations, with a consequent change in percussion note. Such a damping can also be produced by pressure from without upon the chest wall. Other factors which are less obvious may also modify this vibration of the chest wall and influence the percussion note.

The limits of percussion must be clearly understood to avoid pitfalls of an overrefined technique, which usually means that the examiner percusses his own ideas into the chest. In percussing the chest, it must be borne in mind that we cannot percuss deeper than 5 cm. We cannot demonstrate any pathologic lesion in the chest which is covered by a layer of air-containing lung thicker than 5 cm. While we can demonstrate by percussion a consolidation of the lung which extends to the surface of the lung, a deeper area of consolidation, such as occurs in a central pneumonia, cannot be shown in this way (Fig. 206). Similarly, an aneurysm of the transverse or descending parts of the aortic arch often cannot be made out by percussion, although it can be readily seen in the roentgenogram. Likewise, a tumor in the chest lying deeper than 5 cm. from the surface produces no change in percussion note.

A pathological lesion in the lungs smaller than 2 to 3 cm. in diameter will not cause any change in the percussion note. Free fluid in the pleural cavity may not be detected by percussion unless it exceeds 200 to 250 cc. in amount.

Some observers obtain good results with heavy percussion, while others use minimal or light percussion. In general, light percussion is preferable to heavy percussion, although at times heavy percussion is advantageous. The physician should be able to use either.

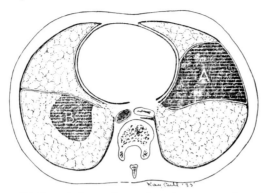

FIG. 206. Area of consolidation at A can be made out on percussion. Area of consolidation at B cannot be demonstrated by percussion, since it is covered by a layer of air-containing lung thicker than 5 cm.

Nomenclature of Percussion Sounds. Since the days of Auenbrugger there has been much confusion in the nomenclature of percussion sounds. Auenbrugger described the percussion sounds as *sonus clarior* and *sonus obtusior,* which Skoda translated by "resonant" and "dull." These terms have since come into universal use, although Friedrich Müller pointed out that, by *clarior,* Auenbrugger meant, not more resonant, but more distinct, and by *obtusior,* less distinct. Skoda found these two terms insufficient to describe the percussion note and introduced two additional terms, a "full or sonorous" sound when "the sound appears more persistent" and "a less full or empty percussion sound." The exact significance of the terms "full" and "empty" has been the matter of much dispute, although it seems clear from Skoda's own words that he referred to the duration of the tone vibrations. Felix Hoppe, later known as Hoppe-Seyler, the great physiological chemist, in 1854 classified the percussion note according to physical characteristics. His classification has been shown to be correct by the work of recent observers studying the problem by means of resonators and string galvanometers. Hoppe-Seyler classified the percussion note according to (1) intensity, amplitude of vibrations; (2) pitch, frequency of vibrations; (3) duration of vibrations; (4) timbre, in which he emphasized the purity of the tone, the absence of bytones and overtones.

According to Friedrich Müller, the qualities of the percussion note consist of first, loud and soft, commonly called clear and dull; second, high and deep; third, full and empty (referring to the duration of the sound); and fourth tympanitic.

Though this classification is unquestionably accurate, such a simple division does not fully describe all the qualities of the percussion sounds obtained. For this reason, and because other terms have been universally used to designate the common findings of percussion, it seems advisable to use the following terms:

1. *Resonant.* A resonant tone is that obtained by percussion over the normal lung. Such a note is loud in comparison to the note obtained over a pleural exudate (Fig. 207). It is higher in pitch than that of an emphysema, and full in comparison to that of a pleural exudate, since it has a longer duration (Fig. 208). But it has also something which is more characteristic, a definite timbre. No other sound precisely resembles the normal lung resonance. The curve shows that it is not a pure tone, but contains numerous overtones which determine its quality or timbre.

It should be emphasized that the term "resonant" is to a certain extent relative. There is no absolute standard of resonance. What is a normal lung

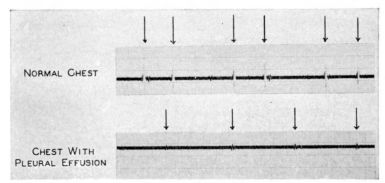

FIG. 207. The normal, loud, low note of the lung contrasted with a very soft, short, dull note over a large pleural exudate. Both records taken from same person. Arrows indicate the moment of percussion.

RESONANT NOTE
OVER
NORMAL LUNG

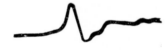

DULL NOTE
OVER
PLEURAL EFFUSION

FIG. 208. Contrast of resonant and dull notes. Resonant note much louder and of longer duration. (Recorded with cathode-ray apparatus.)

resonance for one person may be abnormal for another. A person with a thick muscular chest, or with much subcutaneous fat, shows less resonance than one with a thin, poorly muscled chest wall. Differences in resonance are often obtained in different parts of the same chest.

2. *Dull.* A dull percussion note is frequently called an impairment of resonance, and the degree of this impairment may vary. When all resonance is absent, the percussion note is referred to as flat.

A dull note is sometimes called a soft note, emphasizing that it is not so loud as a resonant tone. When a patient is percussed before a group in an amphitheater, the resonant note is well heard by all present, while a dull note is audible only to those who sit in the first few rows.

A dull note is higher in pitch than a resonant note; it vibrates at a higher rate of frequency (Fig. 209). It is also shorter in duration than a resonant note.

3. *Tympanitic.* A tympanitic percussion note is distinguished from a resonant or dull note by the fact that it has a more distinguishable pitch and apparently is a much purer tone. Its vibrations are simpler and more regular, and it closely approaches a musical tone (Fig. 210). In contrast to a resonant note, it shows an almost complete absence of overtones. Its pitch is usually higher than that of a resonant note.

Normally, a tympanitic note is obtained on percussion over the stomach

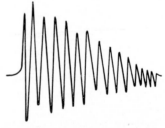

FIG. 209. Tracing of dull note showing pitch higher than that of resonant note. This note has been greatly amplified for purpose of recording. (Recorded with cathode-ray apparatus.)

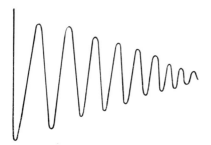

FIG. 210. Tympanitic percussion note. (Recorded with cathode-ray apparatus.)

and intestines. It is a simpler tone than that obtained on percussion over the chest, since percussion of the chest sets into vibration the chest wall and all the organs within with the production of numerous overtones.

4. *Cracked-Pot Resonance*. Cracked-pot resonance is a peculiar type of resonance described as "chinking" which is produced by vigorous percussion which forces air out of a cavity through a narrow orifice. It can be imitated by clasping the hands loosely together, enclosing air between the palms and then striking the under hand sharply against the knee. It was first described by Laennec, who noted that in percussing the chest of consumptives he occasionally "produced a sound like that a cracked pot gives when one percusses it lightly." He added, "This sign indicates the existence of tuberculous cavities." This sound may also be obtained by percussing the chest of a crying child. It is best heard when the patient keeps his mouth open during percussion.

5. *Amphoric Resonance*. Amphoric resonance resembles tympany except that the note is more clanging and echoing, and has a distinctly metallic quality—"a resonance resembling that of an empty cask with a metallic tinkle" (Laennec). The Germans call it "Metallklang," which has been rendered into English as "a metallic ringing" percussion note. Studies of this note show it to consist of high overtones with a low fundamental tone. Its duration is longer than that of tympany.

Amphoric resonance is heard over smooth-walled cavities not less than 4

cm. in diameter. It may be imitated by percussing gently over the cheek markedly distended with air or by holding a small rubber ball against the ear and percussing it with the fingernail.

Auenbrugger, as previously mentioned, used the direct or immediate method of percussion, striking "slowly and softly with the tips of the fingers drawn close together and extended." Experience, however, soon proved the superiority of the indirect or mediate method, that of striking the finger applied to the organ to be percussed, and this method is now so universally employed that we usually understand by the term "percussion," mediate percussion. Two other methods of percussion are used from time to time and are worthy of mention.

Auscultatory Percussion. This method of percussion, mentioned by Laennec in 1826, consists in placing the bell of the stethoscope on the chest, or having an assistant hold it there, and then percussing lightly. Either mediate or immediate percussion may be used.

This method was first carefully studied by Camman and Clark in 1840 and later modified by Bianchi, Runeberg and Smith who, instead of striking the chest, scratched lightly over the surface of the skin. In outlining the heart, the stethoscope is placed over the lower part of the sternum, and the observer scratches lightly over the surface of the skin, beginning in the left axilla and gradually moving toward the sternum. When the left border of the heart is reached—relative cardiac dulness—the sound suddenly increases in intensity. This method is easy to apply and, for outlining the heart, appears as accurate as mediate percussion.

Auscultatory percussion has also been used to outline the area of the liver, the spleen and the lower border of the stomach. To outline the lower border of the stomach by this method, the stethoscope is placed over the xiphoid and the observer scratches upward from the lower parts of the abdomen. This method of outlining the stomach gives information of doubtful value except in cases of marked dilatation of the stomach.

Palpatory Percussion. This method is carried out by what may be termed a series of finger pressures upon the chest. It is not widely used, but in the hands of skilled examiners may yield good results. The heart may be outlined by this method, as well as areas of consolidation in the chest. Pottenger has brought this method of examination to a high degree of perfection in his clinic.

Every physician who examines the chest should pay attention to the tactile sensation which the plessimeter finger experiences. This sensation is produced by the vibrations beneath. In palpatory percussion, however, no blow is struck. It is really a method of palpation and not of percussion.

Tactile Sensation. This phenomenon of tactile sensation, or resistance to percussion, was first stressed by Piorry, and is of great importance. It is commonly designated the sense of resistance felt by the plessimeter finger during percussion, and this sense of resistance is described as greater in areas that are dull and greatest when there is flatness. This sense of resistance refers to waves set in motion by percussion and to the ability of the fingers to perceive differences in the frequencies of these waves. Over areas of dulness the wavelengths are shorter and of greater frequency than over resonant areas. This difference is readily perceived by the sense of touch. The experienced examiner usually depends more upon tactile sensation than upon the actual sound produced by percussion.

Warren Coleman has pointed out that it is quite probable that the so-called "sensation of resistance" is transmitted by the vibratory sense. The vibratory sense is highly developed in certain animals, notably fishes, but less so in man. Helen Keller makes use of this vibratory sense in orienting herself. She states that "There are tactual vibrations which do not belong to skin touch.

They penetrate the skin, the nerves, the bones, like pain, heat and cold. The beat of a drum smites me through from the chest to the shoulder blades . . . every atom of my body is a vibroscope." Percussion of resonant and dull areas sets up different types of vibrations which are perceived by the vibratory sense, some of which, according to Coleman, the ear is incapable of perceiving.

PERCUSSION OF THE NORMAL CHEST

Position of the Patient. If possible, the patient should be examined in the sitting position. Occasionally, however, this is not advisable because of the patient's condition, and percussion of the chest must be carried out with the patient lying in bed. Under these conditions serious errors may be made unless we remember that the position of the patient may influence the percussion note. This is especially true when we examine the patient's chest while he is lying on the side.

When the patient lies on one side with the head propped up on a pillow, a temporary scoliosis may develop because of the spine's sagging downward. The ribs are crowded together on the upper side, thus producing an impairment of tone of the percussion note in this region. There is also an area of impaired resonance on the lower side next to the bed, probably due to the pressure of the bed which interferes with the vibrations produced by percussion. In certain patients less resonance appears throughout the lower side because of compression of the chest by the weight of the body.

These *areas of dulness* shown in Figure 211 vary greatly in different patients, and may shift completely when the patient is percussed lying first on one side and then on the other. The advice of Norris should be followed— "No examination of the lungs, however carefully performed, should be considered entirely satisfactory or final, if made in the recumbent position." Gross

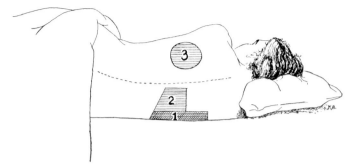

FIG. 211. Zone of dulness produced by position of patient: *1*, zone of dulness due to deadening effect of mattress; *2*, zone of dulness due to compression of chest by weight of body; *3*, zone of dulness due to crowding of ribs. (After Tasker Howard.)

changes, such as complete consolidation of a lobe in pneumonia, can usually be demonstrated in the recumbent position. In such cases, however, it may be safer to change the patient, if possible, from one side to the other in the procedure of percussion.

The upper border of the lungs, the pulmonary apices, extend anteriorly 3 to 4 cm. above the upper margins of the clavicles and posteriorly to the level of the spine of the seventh cervical vertebra. Normally, the percussion note is resonant up to these limits.

Krönig's Isthmus. On percussing the apices posteriorly we find normally an area of resonance over the trapezius muscle on either side, bounded medially by the dulness of the neck and laterally by the dulness of the shoulder.

Normally, this area of resonance is approximately the same at the two apices, measuring 4 to 6 cm. in width (Figs. 212, 254). This area of resonance is markedly diminished in a tuberculous process which has produced a retraction of lung apex. In tuberculosis of one apex the strip of resonance on the affected side may measure only 2 or 3 cm. in width, while the strip of resonance on the normal side is 4 to 6 cm. in width. A retraction of the isthmus of Krönig is a diagnostic sign of great importance.

In percussing the chest it is a good plan to begin by outlining the isthmus of Krönig on either side, and then to percuss downward from the apices, at

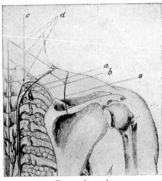

Posterior view

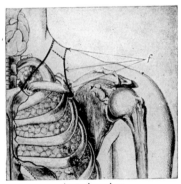

Anterior view

FIG. 212. Krönig's isthmus. (Krönig's original illustrations.)

first over the front of the chest and then over the back. We should always compare symmetrical points on the chest, percussing first on one side and then the corresponding point on the other side.

One should always strike with equal force over the two sides of the chest.

A heavy stroke over the diseased side of the chest may set enough normal tissue vibrating to mask the diseased area and actually produce more resonance than that obtained with a light stroke over the normal side. In the detection of diseased areas in the lung, light percussion is better than heavy. Resonance, as previously mentioned, is a relative term and, in a patient, is judged by comparing the two sides of the chest. It is also dependent in a large measure upon the resonating quality of the thoracic wall. The chest of a thin person with poor muscular development is more resonant than that of a muscular person with much subcutaneous tissue. Auenbrugger recognized this clearly. "The tone," he wrote, "is clearer in thin persons, more indistinct in fleshy individuals; indeed in obese individuals the sound is almost suppressed because of the mass of fat. It is especially the anterior portion of the thorax which is the most resonant; indeed from the clavicle to the fourth true rib. For there the breasts and the pectoral muscles increase the mass and a more indistinct sound results."

Normally, the percussion note of both apices is somewhat higher pitched than the note obtained in lower parts of the lungs. The percussion note of the right apex is often shorter and higher pitched than that of the left apex. This fact often insufficiently emphasized, should always be kept in mind, for, if forgotten, it may lead the examiner to erroneous conclusions. This "normal dulness" of the right apex is probably due to the fact that the right apex of the lung lies directly against the trachea (Fig. 213).

The generally accepted statement that there is a relative dulness of the right apex is disputed by Coleman, who has found the percussion note more often high pitched at the left apex than at the right apex. Coleman, in a study of 223 normal persons, found that the left apex gave a percussion note of higher pitch in 70 per cent of the cases examined. He suggests that the anatomic relationships are the cause of the lower pitch on the right side. These differences in opinion emphasize the differences between the percussion note at the apices of normal lungs and should serve as a warning against sweeping conclusions made from differences in percussion note at the apices. Buck states that "the inventors and early careful observers of the art of percussion did not recognize the existence of physiologic dulness of the right apex, that physiologic dulness is a concept of American clinicians not based upon or justified by objective experimental results and that one must seriously doubt that it exists." At any rate, slight dulness at either apex should be stressed only when rales are present at the apex.

The upper part of the lung lying beneath the infraclavicular fossae is not so resonant as the remainder of the lung anteriorly, since it is covered by a deeper layer of muscle.

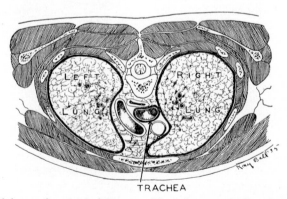

TRACHEA

FIG. 213. Slight dulness of normal right apex. Note close proximity of trachea to right lung at apex. (Viewed from below upward.)

As we pass down the right side of the chest the lung is quite resonant until the fourth costal interspace is reached, when the note becomes impaired by the mass of the liver underneath. At the sixth costal interspace the percussion note becomes flat, since the lung no longer covers the liver. This *liver flatness* ordinarily extends to the costal margin. The percussion note of the right lower border changes with respiration. During inspiration the impaired resonance at the border becomes louder and longer (i.e., more resonant) as the lung descends over the surface of the liver (Fig. 214).

As we percuss downward on the left side of the chest the *percussion note is altered by the heart*. At first there is an impaired resonance over the part of the heart covered by the lungs, this impairment changing gradually to flatness over that part of the heart which is not covered by the lung. These changes in resonance are shown in Figure 215. The lower border of the left lung cannot be percussed accurately, since there is a gradual transition from the softer resonant note of the lung to the loud tympanitic note of the stomach.

At the lower border of the lung on the left we encounter an area of tympany produced by the stomach. The upper part of the stomach tympany is called the *semilunar space of Traube*. It is bounded above by the lung border, on the right by the left margin of the liver, on the left by the splenic dulness and below by the costal border. Traube described the space as follows: "It has an approximately semilunar form, that is, it is bounded below by the costal margin, above by a curved line whose concavity is directed downwards. The semilunar space formed in this manner begins in front below the fifth or sixth costal cartilage and stretches along the costal margin backwards to the upper end of the ninth or tenth rib. Its greatest width is three to three and one-half inches.

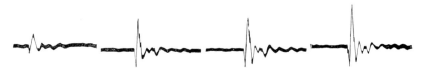

Fig. 214. Phonogram at base of right lung during inspiration. (Kindness of Friedrich Müller.)

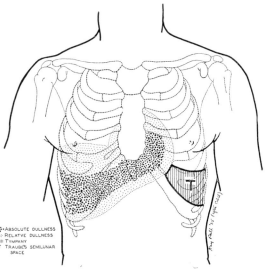

:::•ABSOLUTE DULLNESS
RELATVE DULLNESS
IIIII TYMPANY
T TRAUBE'S SEMILUNAR
SPACE

Fig. 215. Percussion outlines of normal chest. The areas of dulness are due to the heart and liver. (Redrawn after Cabot.)

With deep inspiration, when the lung descends, the semilunar space is markedly diminished in size and this circumstance aids in proving a normal mobility of the lung border. A marked increase in size or widening, usually accompanied by immobility of the lower border of the left lung, is one of the most important signs of its contraction. In a pleural exudate the semilunar space may disappear completely, the beginning of resorption may be demonstrated by its reappearance, and the progress of resorption may be clearly shown by its increasing size. In a pneumonic infiltration of the entire left lobe of the lung the semilunar space is either unchanged

or only a very little narrowed" (Figs. 216, 217).

The *posterior aspect of the chest* is less resonant than the anterior because of a greater muscular development. The percussion note is more resonant in the interscapular area than over the scapulae themselves. It is more resonant on either side in the midaxillary line than in the midscapular line.

It is important to percuss the lower limits of lung resonance on the back, since the mobility of the lung bases on either side may give information of value. The mobility is determined by instructing the patient to take a deep breath and then noting the level to

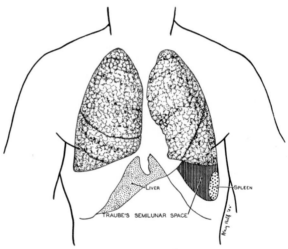

FIG. 216. Traube's semilunar space.

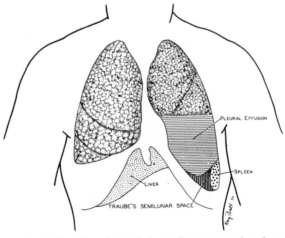

FIG. 217. Partial obliteration of Traube's semilunar space by pleural effusion.

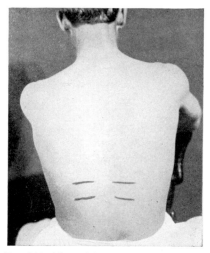

FIG. 218. Normal lung expansion at base.

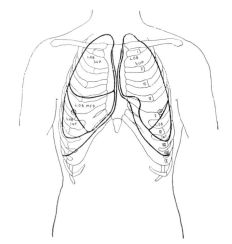

FIG. 219. Topography of lungs, anterior view. (Corning.)

which the lung resonance extends. The patient next makes a forced expiration and the lower limit of lung resonance is noted. Normally, the difference between the lung resonance on forced inspiration and forced expiration is from 4 to 6 cm., and is equal on the two sides (Fig. 218). If the excursion of the lung on one side is prevented or interfered with by adhesions, or by a pleural effusion, this change in resonance during deep inspiration and deep expiration is abolished or diminished, while on the normal side we note the customary difference.

Topography of the Lobes of the Lungs. The outlines of the lobes of the lungs cannot, of course, be made out on percussion. It is important to keep the outlines in mind, however, when locating pathologic processes in the lungs.

The outlines of the lungs when viewed anteriorly are shown in Figure 219. On the right side the lower margin of the upper lobe corresponds to the fourth rib. The middle lobe begins at the fifth rib in the posterior axillary line and extends forward and downward, passing under the nipple and terminating at the costal cartilage of the sixth rib (Fig. 220). Below this lies the inferior lobe, which anteriorly is but a small part of the lung mass. The upper lobe of the left lung extends anteriorly to the fifth

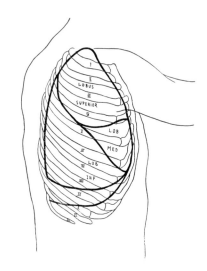

FIG. 220. Topography of lungs, right view. (Corning.)

rib, below which lies the inferior lobe. The upper margin of the inferior lobe begins posteriorly at the fourth rib and crosses the fifth rib in the midaxillary line (Fig. 221). The upper lobe of the left lung shows a notch at the level of the fourth rib which is produced by the heart, here in contact with the anterior wall of the thorax.

The topography of the lobes posteriorly is shown in Figure 222. We note that the line of division between the right upper and lower lobes at first follows the fourth rib, but soon descends

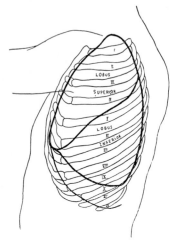

FIG. 221. Topography of lungs, left view. (Corning.)

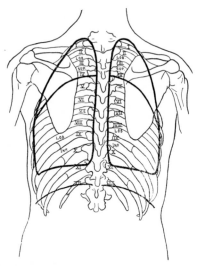

FIG. 222. Topography of lungs, posterior view. (Corning.)

abruptly, crossing the level of the fifth rib under the scapula and reaching the level of the sixth rib in the right posterior axillary line. The line of division between the left upper and lower lobe is approximately the same. Posteriorly, the lower lobes occupy approximately two-thirds of the mass of the lungs, while anteriorly the right upper lobe represents two-thirds of the mass and the left upper lobe approximately five-sixths of the mass. The middle lobe does not extend beyond the right poste-

rior axillary line and cannot be percussed from the back.

Recent studies of the finer gross anatomy of the lungs have shown that the lobes of the lungs can be further subdivided into smaller lobes, on the basis of their bronchial supply. This is shown in Figures 223 and 224. Such a subdivision is of great importance in surgery of the lungs but cannot of course be determined by either percussion or roentgenology.

PERCUSSION OF THE CHEST IN DISEASE

In the preceding paragraphs we have discussed the physical findings in the normal chest on percussion. The dominant note is that of resonance, which varies slightly in various parts of the chest. The areas of impaired resonance and dulness produced by the encroachments of the heart and liver upon the pulmonary resonance form exceptions to the otherwise dominant resonance. These conditions are all normal. The following variations are abnormal:

1. **Hyperresonance.** Normally the percussion note over both sides of the chest is resonant. At times one entire side or a part of the chest may give a hyperresonant or an almost tympanitic note. Vesicular resonance, which is produced by air in the parenchyma of the lung, becomes hyperresonant when the amount of air is greatly increased.

The percussion note is hyperresonant in pulmonary emphysema. The boundaries of the lungs in this condition are increased because the volume of the lung is greater, owing to distention of the alveoli.

In lobar pneumonia the normal lung tissue which is carrying on the entire burden of respiration is hyperresonant. In patients in whom one entire lung is consolidated the other lung may show an extreme degree of hyperresonance.

In pneumothorax the percussion note is usually hyperresonant over the affected side. Here the lung is collapsed and the hyperresonance is due to free air in the thoracic cavity and is pro-

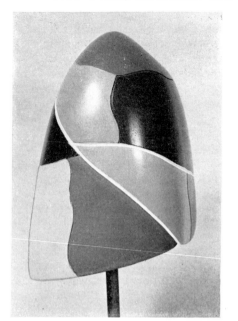 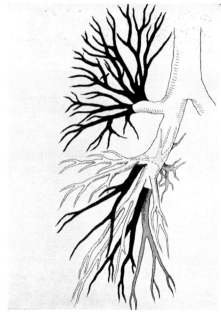

FIG. 223. Model of small lobes of right lung with bronchial supply.
Anatomical Model Research Co. after Jackson & Huber.
Chart of bronchial tree after J. Stauffer Lehman & J. Antrim Crellin. (Courtesy of Eastman Kodak Co.)

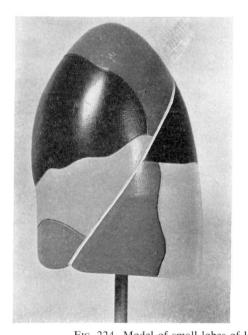 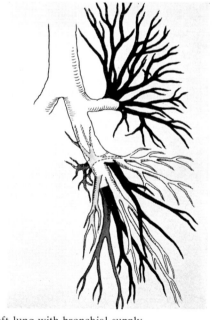

FIG. 224. Model of small lobes of left lung with bronchial supply.
Anatomical Model Research Co. after Jackson & Huber.
Chart of bronchial tree after J. Stauffer Lehman & J. Antrim Crellin. (Courtesy of Eastman Kodak Co.)

duced by the vibrations of the chest wall. At times in pneumothorax the percussion note may be tympanitic, particularly when the chest wall is thin and of poor musculature. This is readily understood when we remember that a tympanitic percussion note is produced when we percuss over a large hollow body containing air, such as the stomach. In pneumothorax the chest, containing a large amount of free air, presents physical conditions similar to those in the stomach.

2. **Dulness and Flatness.** Dulness or impaired resonance is produced by any condition which interferes with the production of normal resonance within the lung or interferes with the transmission of normal resonance outward.

Any consolidation of the lung parenchyma which interferes with the vibrations of that part of the lung when the chest wall is struck, produces dulness. The most common causes of such consolidation are tuberculosis, pneumonia and neoplasms. Any inflammatory disease involving the lung such as syphilis, actinomycosis, and so on, may produce the same signs.

Any pathologic process which interferes with the transmission of the percussion stroke from the chest wall to the lung parenchyma causes dulness. It also interferes with the transmission of the normal resonance outward. The most common examples of this type of disease causing dulness are pleural thickening and pleural effusion. When the pleural effusion is large and replaces a large part of the lung, the percussion note is flat. The lung immediately above the level of flatness may be dull or impaired in resonance. In contradistinction to the flatness which is due to the vibrations set up in the fluid, the area of impaired resonance has its percussion note modified by the air-containing lung beneath the fluid. Above the area of dulness the lung on percussion may be resonant or actually tympanitic. This hyperresonance is due to a local emphysema of that portion of the lung not compressed by the fluid. This finding is called *Skodaic resonance,* after Josef Skoda, who noted "that when the lower portion of the lung is entirely compressed by any pleuritic effusion, and its upper portion reduced in volume, the percussion sound at the upper part of the thorax is distinctly tympanitic" (Fig. 225). This phenomenon was, however, familiar to Auenbrugger, who discovered that when the chest was half filled with fluid, "an increased resonance is obtained in that part which is not occupied by fluid."

Skodaic resonance may also be obtained over normal lung tissue just above an area of consolidation in lobar pneumonia.

Shifting dulness or *movable dulness,* or a change in the area of dulness with

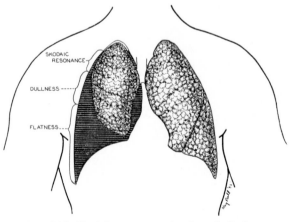

FIG. 225. Skodaic resonance in pleural effusion.

change in position, is considered by many to be the crucial test of free fluid within the pleural cavity. The test is usually carried out by determining the level of the dulness in the mammillary line with the patient first lying down and then sitting up. Several minutes usually elapse before the fluid settles down and the change in the level is demonstrable. When present, this is the surest sign of pleural effusion. It is, however, of limited value, and some observers go so far as to deny its occurrence.

Pitfield has described the "diaphragm sign," which he considers a diagnostic sign for pleural fluid. The patient leans forward a little, while the examiner percusses the suspected area with the finger tips of one hand and palpates with the other hand the quadratus lumborum muscle on the same side. "This will cause the collected fluid to vibrate, and the vibrations are felt by the palpating hand on the muscle."

The resonance over one side of the chest may be impaired in patients showing marked deformities of the chest associated with scoliosis. When a patient has a marked curvature of the spine with convexity to the right, the ribs on the opposite side are pressed closely together and the percussion note over the left side is commonly higher pitched and shows a definite impairment.

In mitral stenosis there is frequently dulness on percussion at the left apex. This dulness is found anteriorly, usually above the third rib, and extends to the clavicle or occasionally above. It extends a variable distance to the left, at times as far as the outer third of the clavicle. This dulness is probably due to enlargement of the left auricle which interferes with the normal percussion note of the left lung.

Grocco's Sign. This sign, commonly present in pleurisy with effusion, was first observed by Korányi in 1897, but was independently and more fully described by Grocco in 1902. The following year Rauchfuss described the same sign, so that it is also known as *Rauchfuss' triangle*. Grocco's original observation is as follows: "When the pleural effusion is sufficiently large, on percussing over the spinal processes from above downward with the patient in the sitting position, there appears at the level of the effusion, a dulness, which is at first relative and then absolute. . . . On percussing from above downward along a horizontal line drawn from the spinous processes on the normal side one succeeds in marking out, opposite the dulness in the median line, a paravertebral area of dulness, triangular in form." This paravertebral triangle of dulness, *on the normal side,* is shown in Figure 226.

The cause of Grocco's triangle was at first believed to be due to the effusion pushing the posterior mediastinum over to the opposite side, thus producing an area of dulness on the normal side. Such displacement of the posterior mediastinum has, however, rarely been demonstrated. A much more probable explanation is that given by Turban. This observer has stressed that vibration of the bony structure of the thorax plays an important role in the production of normal chest resonance and has shown that when the vibrations of the

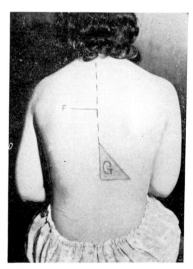

FIG. 226. Grocco's sign. *F* indicates the level to which the fluid can be made out on the left side. *G* is the paravertebral triangle of dulness.

chest wall are interfered with by pressure on the lower posterior surface near the vertebral column, a paravertebral area of dulness appears on the opposite side. Fluid in the chest interferes with vibrations of the chest wall, greater on the side of the effusion but also present on the healthy side. This area of dulness assumes a triangular shape according to Walker because the lung at the base is wedge-shaped, increasing in thickness as one passes upward and outward, this increase occurring abruptly along the line of the lateral border of Grocco's triangle, where it increases suddenly from approximately 5 cm. to 20 cm. in thickness. Normally, there is often a slightly higher pitched percussion note over a triangular-shaped area, and this area is presumably due to the fact that the thin wedge of lung gives a higher note on percussion than the rest of the lung. In a pleural effusion this difference is exaggerated.

Some authors attach little importance to Grocco's sign. In our experience it is a valuable confirmatory sign and is usually present in pleural effusion. It may occasionally be present in a massive consolidation of the lower lobe in lobar pneumonia and in malignant disease of the lung or mediastinum. It may rarely be present in bronchogenic carcinoma with atelectasis of the lower lobe of the lung. Its presence in such varied conditions as pleural effusion, pulmonary consolidation and pulmonary atelectasis suggests strongly that Grocco's sign is produced by an interference with the normal vibratory resonance produced by percussion. In our experience pleural effusion is the cause of Grocco's sign in 90 to 95 per cent of the cases.

Special Percussion Signs. *Wintrich's Change of Tone.* This sign consists in a higher, clearer and louder percussion note over an area during inspiration with the mouth open than closed. It can be closely imitated by percussing over the trachea with the mouth open and then closed, and this experiment closely simulates the conditions under which Wintrich's change of tone is produced.

The change in the percussion note is heard best by listening over the mouth of the patient.

Wintrich's change in tone was first described in pulmonary cavities. It has also been observed in pneumothorax, pneumonia, aneurysm and mediastinal tumors. According to most observers it is of little practical value.

Gerhardt's Change of Tone. The percussion note over an oblong cavity half filled with fluid varies with the position of the patient. If the longest axis of the cavity is parallel to the spine, the percussion note will be lower in pitch when the patient is lying down, since the resonating cavity is longer. This phenomenon is known as Gerhardt's change of tone, or Gerhardt's sign.

Biermer's sign is practically the same except that he describes a metallic resonance over hydropneumothorax which varied with change in position.

Friedreich's Sign. The pitch of the percussion note over a cavity is higher during inspiration than during expiration.

The value of these special percussion signs is limited. They cannot as a rule be demonstrated, but occasionally they may be of some aid. Hoover found Wintrich's change of tone of considerable value in the diagnosis of mediastinal tumors. Fishberg finds that "Wintrich's, Friedreich's and Gerhardt's phenomena are of assistance in the diagnosis of vomicae, but not so frequently as some textbooks would lead us to believe." Cabot thinks these special percussion signs of "no practical importance and should be forgotten." In our experience these special percussion signs have been of little assistance, possibly because the x-ray does so accurately what these signs at best do with such uncertainty.

BIBLIOGRAPHY

Biot, M. C.: Contribution a l'étude de phénomène respiratoire de Cheyne-Stokes. Lyon Méd. 23:517, 561, 1876.

Buck, Robert W.: Physiologic dullness of the right apex. New England J. Med. 219:615, 1938.

Cammann, G. P., and Clark, A.: A new mode of ascertaining the dimension, form and condition of internal organs by percussion. New York. J. Med. & Surg. *3:*62, 1840.

Chapman, Earle M., and Goldstein, Arram: The physics of sound with particular relation to examination of the patient. J. Lab. & Clin. Med. *28:*1535, 1943.

Coleman, Warren: The alleged dulness over the apex of the normal right lung. Tr. A. Am. Physicians *44:*322, 1929.

Coleman, Warren: The alleged dulness over the apex of the normal right lung. Am. J. M. Sc. *197:*141, 1939.

Coleman, Warren: The role of the vibration sense in percussion. Am. J. M. Sc. *197:*145, 1939.

Conner, Lewis A., and Stillman, Ralph G.: A pneumographic study of respiratory irregularities in meningitis. Arch. Int. Med. *9:*203, 1912.

Corning, H. K.: Lehrbuch der topographischen Anatomie. 5th ed. Wiesbaden, J. F. Bergmann, 1914.

Edens, Ernst, and von Ewald, Fritz: Ueber den Perkussionsschall. Deutsches Arch. f. klin. Med. *123:*275, 1917.

Fahr, George, and Brandi, Bruno: Weitere Studien über Perkussion und Auskultation. Deutsch Arch. f. klin. Med. *164:*1, 1929.

Fishberg, Maurice: Pulmonary Tuberculosis. Philadelphia, Lea & Febiger, 1922.

Gilbert, A., Gutmann, R. A., and Tzorck, A.: La percussion. Paris Méd. *16:*37, 1926.

Gilbert, A., Gutmann, R. A., and Tzorck, A.: Les étapes historiques de la percussion. Paris Méd. *16:*193, 1926.

Goodman, Edward H.: Left apical impairment in mitral stenosis. Am. J. M. Sc. *157:*652, 1919.

Grocco, Pietro: Brevi note di semiiotica fisica. Rev. crit. di clin. med., Firenze *3:*274, 1902.

Hoover, C. F.: The diagnostic value of the Wintrich tracheal sound. Am. J. M. Sc. *118:*423, 1899.

Hoppe, Felix: Zur Theorie der Percussion. Virchows Arch. f. path. Anat. *6:*143, 1854.

Howard, Tasker: Percussion note of the back in the lateral position. J.A.M.A. *76:*1229, 1921.

Krönig, G.: Zur Topographie der Lungenspitzen und ihre Perkussion. Berl. klin. Wchnschr. *26:*809, 1889.

Litten, M.: Ueber die normalen bei jeder Respiration am Thorax sichtbaren Zwerchfellsbewegungen. Deutsche med. Wchnschr. *18:*273, 1892.

Martini, Paul: Studien über Perkussion und Auskultation. Deutsches Arch. f. klin. Med. *139-140:*65, 1922.

Müller, Fr.: Aus dem perkussionskurs. München. med. Wchnschr. *75:*6, 1928.

Peirce, Benjamin: An Elementary Treatise on Sound. Boston, James Munroe, 1836.

Pitfield, Robert L.: New methods for detecting fluid in the serous cavities. Lancet *2:*983, 1936.

Pullen, Roscoe L.: Medical Diagnosis, Applied Physical Diagnosis. 2nd ed., Philadelphia, W. B. Saunders Co., 1950.

Reich, Nathaniel: Use of flask as a simple aid to tactile fremitus. New York State J. Med. *39:*1654, 1939.

Rist, E.: L'analyse acoustique des sons de percussion. Ann. de Méd. *21:*19, 1927.

Runeberg, J. S.: Ueber percussorische Transsonanz. Ztschr. f. Klin. Med. *42:*81, 1901.

Smith, A.: Ueber einige neue Methoden zur Bestimmung der Herzgrenzen. Verhandl. d. Congr. f. inn. p. 264, 1900.

Traube, Ludwig: Halbmondförmiger Raum. Berl. klin. Wchnschr. *5:*509, 1868.

Turban, K.: Paralipomena der Tuberkuloseforschung. München. med. Wchnschr. *47:*652, 1927.

Walker, George: Personal communication.

CHAPTER 7

AUSCULTATION OF THE LUNGS

IN LISTENING TO THE LUNGS we have two methods at our disposal; *immediate auscultation,* which consists in placing the ear directly against the chest wall, and *mediate auscultation,* which consists in listening through a stethoscope. The mediate method is the method universally employed, but the student should become familiar with the immediate method as well. The occasion may arise when the physician through unforeseen circumstances does not have his stethoscope with him. In examining babies or children the appearance of the stethoscope may excite the fear of the patient who does not object to the examiner placing his ear against the chest. Again, just as the examiner always has his fingers with him for percussion, so he always has his ears for auscultation.

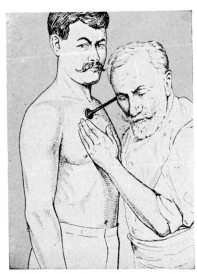

FIG. 227. Application of monaural stethoscope. (Letulle.)

STETHOSCOPES

The earliest type of stethoscope was the *monaural stethoscope,* devised by Laennec. Its modern counterpart, usually made of wood, is 1 foot in length, has a funnel-shaped enlargement on the end which is placed on the chest, and a flat flange on the end which is applied to the ear (Fig. 227). This type of stethoscope, though something of a curiosity in this country, is still extensively used in European clinics, where physicians still champion its superiority and point to its use for more than a century (Fig. 228). There is no question of its value in the hands of those familiar with it. Most, if not all, of the great discoveries in auscultation have been made with this instrument. Yet it

124

is certainly less convenient to use than the binaural type. Thoroughly to explore various regions of the chest with this stethoscope sometimes requires an almost acrobatic agility on the part of the examiner. The American physician usually complains that with the monaural stethoscope he hears too little, to

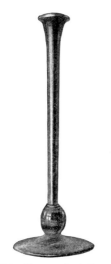

Fig. 228. Monaural stethoscope.

which his Continental colleague retorts that with a binaural stethoscope he hears too much.

The *binaural stethoscope,* which is universally employed in this country, and also in many Continental clinics, is sold in a variety of models. The two most popular models are the Ford type (Fig. 229) and the Bowles stethoscope (Fig. 230). The Ford model has a bell or chest piece shaped somewhat like a funnel, made of hard rubber or metal with a diameter of approximately $\frac{7}{8}$ inch. A metal chest piece is more durable than one of hard rubber, but has the disadvantage of causing some discomfort to a sensitive patient because of its coldness. The Bowles stethoscope, the advantages of which are highly praised by Richard Cabot, has a distinctive chest piece which consists of a shallow steel cup over the mouth of which a thin metal plate is attached. The Bowles stethoscope allows the examiner to listen to the patient's back

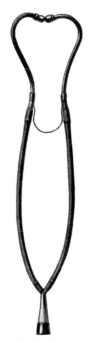

Fig. 229. Ford stethoscope.

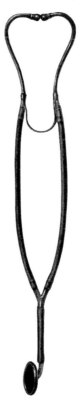

Fig. 230. Bowles stethoscope.

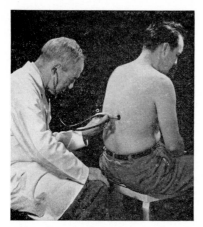

FIG. 231. Auscultation of the lungs. Note comfortable position of examiner and patient.

and axillary regions with a minimum of discomfort. Each type of stethoscope has its champions. In our clinic the Ford model appears to be more popular. One ingenious model avoids any controversy by having two chest pieces, one of the Ford type and the other of the Bowles type, so that by moving a small lever either chest piece may be used.

Another type of stethoscope widely advertised has a large, deep bell-shaped chest piece like a crucible with a tense membrane of rubber drawn over the mouth. Such an instrument produces a great magnification of all auscultatory phenomena, and it is asserted that with it one can hear the breath sounds through the patient's overcoat. The occasion, however, to listen to a patient's breath sounds through his overcoat seldom arises.

The exhaustive investigations of Rappaport and Sprague should be read by everyone interested in physical diagnosis. Their studies have brought out many interesting facts, some of which are mentioned here.

The larger the diameter of the open stethoscopic chest piece, the better the low-pitched sounds are heard but at the expense of the high-pitched sounds. Stethoscopic bells, with the interior shaped like a parabola, have been very popular because of the impression that they collect sounds. Such bells decrease the efficiency of the chest piece because they increase its internal volume. The Bowles stethoscope is especially useful in detecting faint high-pitched sounds, such as the diastolic murmur of aortic insufficiency.

Studies of the transmission of sound waves between 60 and 400 cycles, the auscultatory region for heart sounds and heart murmurs, have shown that the binaural method of auscultation through rubber tubes is, on an average, 20 decibels better than the monaural method with the ear applied directly to the stethoscope. It should be mentioned, however, that a decibel is a unit of the intensity of sound, not of its quality, transmission or of its faithful reproduction.

The tubing employed for the stethoscope should be thick walled, have a small bore the same diameter as that of the chest and ear pieces, and be as short as possible. A bore of $\frac{3}{16}$ inch with a length of 6 to 8 inches should be satisfactory.

The most important point in the use of a stethoscope is the observer's familiarity with the instrument he uses. Familiarity with a certain type of stethoscope invariably gives rise to a certain partisanship on the part of its user. The purchaser of a stethoscope, after deciding upon the model he prefers, must take care that the ear pieces fit his ears.

SOUNDS HEARD ON AUSCULTATION OF THE NORMAL CHEST

It is often said that the beginner in auscultation hears too much rather than too little. This is due to the fact that the beginner has not yet learned to disregard certain sounds that are of no diagnostic importance, or to concentrate his attention upon sounds that are pathologic as well as pathognomonic. The ability to distinguish between important and unimportant sounds is acquired only by practice.

The ideal conditions for auscultation are found in a sound-proof room which shuts out all extraneous noises. Such ideal conditions are rarely present, and the observer must first learn to concentrate his attention upon what he hears through the ear pieces of his stethoscope and to be oblivious of the sounds within the room or in the street.

After excluding all extraneous sounds and making sure that the sounds he hears are coming through the rubber tubes of the stethoscope, the observer must next assure himself that the sounds he hears come from the interior of the chest, the lung and pleura, and not from the exterior, the skin or muscles. The following are the most important sources of error:

1. The observer may breathe heavily on the rubber tubing of the stethoscope, producing a soft roaring sound as he expires. This source of error can be detected and prevented by changing the position of the tubing.

2. Errors may result from an improper application of the bell of the stethoscope. The bell must be firmly and flatly applied. If one side is slightly tilted and air is not excluded, we may hear a soft muffled roaring like that heard when a conch shell is applied to the ear. A similar sound may be heard if the ear pieces of the stethoscope do not fit the observer's ears or if the stethoscope is used upside down. A more common error is produced by allowing the bell of the stethoscope to rub upon the skin of the chest. This may produce sounds which resemble closely a pleural or pericardial friction rub. The student can familiarize himself with these sounds by rubbing the bell of the stethoscope over the skin. Such experimentation will aid him in avoiding this source of error.

3. Sounds produced by friction of the stethoscope on hairs are a frequent source of error. A single hair under the bell of the stethoscope may, during respiration, produce crackling sounds almost indistinguishable from dry rales. The frequency and intensity of these sounds may be increased by rubbing the chest piece over the hairs. In some patients with extremely hairy chests

the difficulty of avoiding these sounds is great. The time-honored method to avoid sounds produced by hairs is to wet them with water or petrolatum and press them down flat against the skin. At times it may be advisable to shave the skin in certain areas.

4. Sounds produced by the muscles, tendons and joints may at times lead to confusion and error. Muscle sounds particularly are a frequent source of error. Patients who are chilled or nervous, or who hold their muscles tense, may produce in these muscles a characteristic set of soft sounds. In patients who are chilled these sounds are of minimal intensity, are of great frequency, and disappear when the patient becomes warm. They are frequently present when the patient ceases breathing for a few moments. The deeper, louder muscle sounds, which are heard particularly over the pectoral and trapezius muscles, are more intense when the patient breathes and may have a loud, creaking, leathery quality. The location of these sounds over the pectoral or trapezius muscles may stamp them as muscle sounds, but occasionally they may be heard over all parts of the chest. Muscle sounds may be confused with rales, but sound more crumpling, muffled and indistinct, and are not affected by coughing, which commonly changes the character and intensity of rales. Muscle sounds are usually more evanescent and transitory than true rales. In doubtful cases it may be necessary to withhold judgment until a second or third examination is made. Sounds produced by joints and fasciae usually disappear when the patient relaxes completely.

NORMAL BREATH SOUNDS

1. **Normal Vesicular Breathing.** This type of respiration was first heard by Laennec, who wrote, "One hears during inspiration and expiration a soft murmur, but extremely distinct, which indicates the penetration of the air into the pulmonary tissue and its expulsion." This description of vesicular breathing and its explanation have not been im-

proved upon by a century of experience. Many new descriptive phrases have since been coined. It has been described as the soughing of the wind, or the swish of a breeze through a distant grove of trees. It is better recognized by hearing the actual sound than by reading a description of it. The student has only to place the bell of his stethoscope on his own chest to obtain a clear impression of this sound. The normal breath sounds, and abnormal as well, can usually be well heard by placing the bell of the stethoscope over the masseter muscle on either side of the face.

Laennec's explanation that vesicular breathing is due to a penetration of the air into the lungs and to its expulsion is still generally accepted. Skoda said, "I explain vesicular breathing, as Laennec did, by the friction of the air against the walls of the fine bronchi and air cells." Some observers have claimed that vesicular breathing has its origin in the larynx, but this explanation is incorrect, since it is still heard after severing the trachea from the larynx. Pottenger believes that not only the air current, the bronchi and alveoli, but also the respiratory muscles and the bony cage are intimately involved in respiration, and that the respiratory sounds are vibrations set up by the entire respiratory mechanism.

According to Pottenger there is little or no difference between the length of inspiration and that of expiration. Indeed, often the expiratory phase of respiration is longer than the inspiratory phase.

Records of vesicular breathing show that it is a complex sound consisting of a dominant tone with a frequency of 100 to 200 vibrations per second, mixed with tones showing a frequency as high as 1000 per second (Friedrich Müller). The pitch of vesicular breathing is relatively low like that of the dominant tone (Fig. 232).

Vesicular breathing is louder during inspiration than during expiration. Figure 233 emphasizes this characteristic.

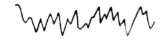

FIG. 232. Tracing of vesicular breath sounds. (Recorded with cathode-ray apparatus.)

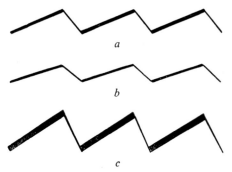

FIG. 233. *a,* Vesicular breathing; *b,* distant vesicular breathing; *c,* exaggerated vesicular breathing.

Vesicular breathing is heard over air-containing and normally functioning lung tissue. When heard over certain areas of the chest it is conclusive evidence that there is air-containing pulmonary tissue beneath the bell of the stethoscope. It is heard over the greater part of the normal lung, but is modified in certain areas where the trachea or larger bronchi are situated near the surface of the chest wall. It is increased in intensity by deep breathing. When the lung on one side is partially or totally thrown out of use by pneumothorax, pleural effusion or by a consolidation due to lobar pneumonia, tuberculosis or a tumor, the lung on the healthy side carries on most of or the entire function of respiration, and vesicular breathing is exaggerated on this side. This exaggeration of vesicular breathing in a normal lung is particularly striking when the other lung is collapsed by pneumothorax. Vesicular breathing is often greatly exaggerated in acidosis.

Vesicular breathing is diminished in emphysema, since the alternate distention and contraction of the lung are diminished. Vesicular breathing is also diminished by a thickened pleura which interferes with the passage of sound to the surface of the chest (Fig. 234). In pleural effusion the vesicular breathing is diminished or absent on the affected side, since the sounds produced in the air vesicles are not well transmitted through the fluid (Fig. 202, p. 106). When a bronchus or bronchiole is completely plugged by exudate or a foreign body, vesicular breathing disappears over the area supplied by the bronchus, since no air can enter this area (Fig. 235). In lobar pneumonia, particularly in the earlier stages, the breath sounds may be markedly diminished or even suppressed over the involved area. This phenomenon is probably due to exudate within the lung alveoli or possibly to an occlusion of the bronchioles.

2. Bronchial or Tubular Breathing.

This type of breathing was also first described by Laennec as "the sound which inspiration and expiration make audible in the larynx, the trachea and the large bronchial trunks situated at the hilus of the lungs. This sound, heard on applying the stethoscope over the larynx or the cervical portion of the trachea, has a character quite distinctive. The respiratory murmur, especially during inspiration, lacks the soft crepitation which accompanies the aeration of the air cells; it is more dry in a certain measure, and one perceives distinctly that the air passes into an empty and rather wide space."

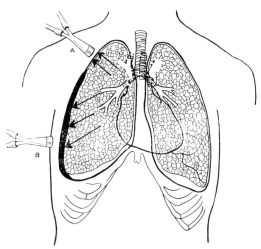

Fig. 234. Thickened pleura interferes with transmission of vesicular breathing. Vesicular breathing heard at *A*, but not at *B*.

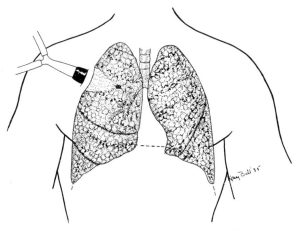

Fig. 235. Obstruction of bronchus abolishes vesicular breathing over area of atelectasis.

Bronchial breathing and tracheal breathing are produced, as Laennec described, by the air passing over the walls of the bronchi and the trachea. Later studies have shown the tracheal breathing and bronchial breathing are similar, but not identical. Tracheal breathing is louder and of a lower pitch than bronchial breathing because the diameter of the trachea is greater than that of the bronchi (Figs. 236, 237). Indeed, the tone in the smaller bronchi is softer and higher in pitch than that in the larger bronchi. This subject has been investigated by Fahr, and the differences in the vibratory rate at different parts of the bronchial tree are shown in Figure 238. The fundamental character of the breath sounds produced in the larynx, trachea, primary bronchi and smaller bronchi is, however, similar.

Expiration is louder and longer than inspiration in contrast to vesicular breathing, in which the opposite is true. Both inspiration and expiration are

usually louder in bronchial breathing than in vesicular breathing (Fig. 239).

3. **Bronchovesicular Breathing.** This type of breathing, as the name indicates, is a mixture of bronchial and vesicular breathing. Austin Flint, who introduced this name, says it denotes "the combination, in varying proportions, of the characters of the bronchial or tubular, and of the normal vesicular respiration. The name expresses such a combination." A tracing of this respiration (Fig. 240) shows its fundamental tones (200 to 500 vibrations per second) to be more rapid than vesicular breathing (120 vibrations) and to be slower than bronchial breath sounds (1000 vibra-

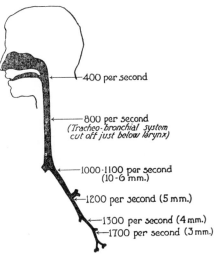

FIG. 238. Difference in vibratory rate at different parts of bronchial tree. (Fahr.)

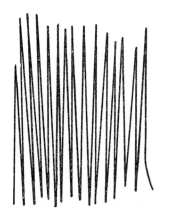

FIG. 236. Tracheal breath sounds. (Recorded with cathode-ray apparatus.)

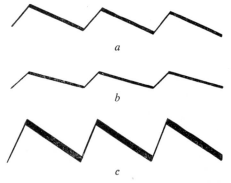

FIG. 239. Bronchial breathing: *a*, bronchial breathing, moderate intensity; *b*, distant bronchial breathing; *c*, loud bronchial breathing.

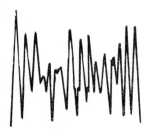

FIG. 237. Bronchial breath sounds. (Recorded with cathode-ray apparatus.)

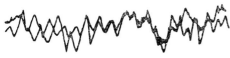

FIG. 240. Bronchovesicular breath sounds. (Recorded with cathode-ray apparatus.)

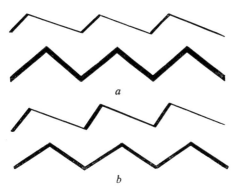

FIG. 241. Bronchovesicular breathing: *a*, bronchovesicular breathing; *b*, distant bronchovesicular breathing.

tions). Its auditory character is illustrated in Figure 241.

Though bronchovesicular breathing is heard particularly over areas of early and incomplete consolidation of the lung, it is also heard normally at the apex of the right lung and over the primary bronchi.

Bronchial and Bronchovesicular Breathing in Disease. Vesicular, bronchial and bronchovesicular breathing are all heard over the normal chest, but it must be emphasized that vesicular breathing alone is heard over almost the entire area of the lungs. Bronchial or bronchovesicular breathing is heard only over the trachea, primary bronchi, over a limited area at the right apex and over the right interscapular area. When it is heard elsewhere, it is pathologic.

The most common causes of bronchial breathing over areas where normally vesicular breathing alone is heard are tuberculosis and lobar pneumonia. In pleurisy with effusion, distant bronchial breathing may be heard above the fluid. Here the tubular breathing is often so faint that it may be missed. Cabot states that bronchial breathing is present in "about one-third of the cases of pleuritic effusion."

In empyema of children, bronchial breathing is often present. During the last pandemic of influenza, patients with empyema often showed loud bronchial breathing over the empyema. In many of these patients the seropurulent exudate accumulated so rapidly in the chest and the bronchial breathing was so intense that the diagnosis of empyema was established only by resort to the exploratory needle.

Any disease process producing consolidation of the lung parenchyma may give rise to bronchial breathing over the diseased area, if the bronchial tree is open.

ABNORMAL BREATH SOUNDS

Amphoric Breathing. Laennec describes this type of breathing as "exactly analogous to that which one produces by blowing into a carafe or into a jar." He designated it as "amphoric" from the Latin *amphora* = a jar. It is never heard in health, but may be heard over large tuberculous cavities and at times in pneumothorax. It is most commonly produced by the air passing in and out of a large cavity, although it may be heard over a closed pneumothorax. Amphoric breathing is almost invariably heard over areas where amphoric resonance is obtained on percussion.

Amphoric breathing is also called cavernous breathing. This type of respiration is pathognomonic of a cavity in the chest, but is sometimes absent, when the entrance from the bronchus into the cavity is filled with exudate or a mucous plug.

Metamorphosing Breathing. In this type of breathing, respiration may begin as a feeble indistinct inspiration and change suddenly into breathing of the bronchial or amphoric type. This sudden change may be due to a bronchial plug being loosened by the force of the inspiration. The characteristics of this type of breathing are shown in Figure 242.

Asthmatic Breathing. This type of breathing is heard during paroxysms of asthma. Inspiration and expiration

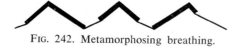

FIG. 242. Metamorphosing breathing.

RÂLES

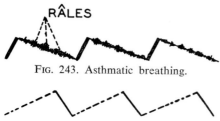

FIG. 243. Asthmatic breathing.

FIG. 244. Cog-wheel respiration.

both show an increase in intensity. Expiration is prolonged, high-pitched and wheezing, and is accompanied by musical rales (Fig. 243). Asthmatic breathing is often audible at some distance from the patient.

Cog-Wheel Respiration. In this form of breathing, inspiration, instead of being heard as a soft, steady, continuous sound, consists of a series of short jerks, puffs and pauses (Fig. 244). At one time it was considered pathognomonic of pulmonary tuberculosis, but it also occurs when pleural adhesions are present, in nervous persons or as the result of chilliness, pain or fatigue. It is caused by irregular inflation and expansion of the pulmonary tissue.

RALES

"Râle is the name commonly given to the noisy murmur caused, in those who are dying, by the air forcing its way with difficulty through the sputum which the lungs are no longer able to expel. For the lack of a more generic term, I take the word in a wider sense and designate as rales, all noises produced during respiration by the passage of air through all such liquids, as may happen to be present in the bronchi or lung tissue. These noises also accompany coughing when it is present; but it is always more convenient to investigate them by means of respiration" (Laennec).

Hippocrates heard rales and mentioned them in several passages describing pneumonia and empyema. Laennec,

more than two thousand years later, first heard them through a stethoscope, studied them and classified them. Laennec recognized four main species: (1) moist or crepitant rales; (2) mucous or gurgling rales; (3) dry, sonorous or snoring rales; (4) dry, sibilant or whistling rales. Laennec's example was emulated by his successors. Each introduced new terms to describe rales, each a new classification. This has caused confusion which persists today. Much of it is unnecessary. Many of the terms which have been introduced are entirely descriptive, describing rales as they appear to the more or less imaginative listener, and presenting characteristics too vague and uncertain to form any basis for classification.

The following classification of rales has been of great assistance to many observers:

1. **Dry Rales.** Dry rales are heard throughout respiration—on both inspiration and expiration. They vary in pitch from a shrill whistle to a deep hum. When high pitched, they are called "sibilant;" when low pitched, "sonorous." Dry rales are also known as rhonchi ($\rho\acute{o}\gamma\chi\circ s$—rogchos = snore) or musical rales and commonly produce vibrations of the chest wall that are easily felt on palpation. Various descriptive terms are also applied to this type of rales, such as wheezing, piping, whistling, snoring, squeaking, groaning, and the like. Here the imagination of the auditor has full play.

Dry rales are heard in inflammation of the mucous membranes of the bronchi, when the tenacious mucus partially occludes the bronchus, but does not entirely close it. These masses of sticky mucus are set into vibration by the currents of air in the bronchi during respiration and produce the rales. This process has suggested to some observers an analogy with the sound of an Eolian harp and has caused some authors to suggest that these rales be called musical rales and the term "dry" be dropped.

Dry rales are heard particularly in bronchial asthma. Here their musical quality is especially striking. The chest of the patient suffering from an attack of bronchial asthma sounds much like a music box.

2. **Moist or Bubbling Rales.** Moist rales, unlike dry rales, are not continuous noises, but are short, discontinuous crackling sounds produced by bubbles in the bronchi. When a bubble formed in the bronchial secretion bursts during respiration, this type of rale is produced. It is designated as coarse, medium or fine, depending upon the size of the bubble which bursts. Coarse bubbling rales arise in the larger bronchi, in bronchiectatic dilatations or in cavities, while fine moist rales originate in small bronchi or in the alveoli. The fine moist rales are usually much more numerous in the same lung than the large bubbling rales.

Moist rales indicate the presence of fluid, transudate, mucus, pus or blood in the bronchi and alveoli, and, when numerous, we assume that the amount of fluid is considerable. They are heard most commonly in lobar pneumonia, bronchitis, tuberculosis and cardiac failure.

Fine moist rales at the apices of the lungs are important diagnostic signs in early pulmonary tuberculosis. Their importance depends not so much on their number as on their persistence. A few moist rales, if persistent, are significant. They may be heard, however, only after coughing and after deep inspiration.

Fine moist rales are often heard at the bases of lungs posteriorly in influenza and in the early stages of typhoid fever.

3. **Crepitant Rales.** Crepitant rales are classified by some authors as a variety of moist rales, while others regard them as a distinct type. These rales are small, occur in showers, and are heard during inspiration alone. They resemble the sound produced by the crackling of salt in the fire or by rubbing the hair between the fingers close to the ear. "One can compare it to the sound salt produces, when one makes it crackle by heating it gently in a pan, to that given by a dry bladder, when one inflates it, or better still to the sound which one hears on pressing between the fingers the tissue of a normal lung distended with air" (Laennec). Crepitant rales are produced by the passage of air into alveoli which are filled with fluid or are collapsed. The sound suggests that they are produced by the separation of the viscid surfaces of the alveoli.

The crackling sound produced by the bell of the stethoscope rubbing on the hairs of the chest may be mistaken for crepitant rales. In case of confusion, the hair should be moistened and plastered down or shaved off.

Subcrepitant rales suggest a relationship to crepitant rales. They are small, moist rales larger than crepitant rales. Bushnell stresses the importance of distinguishing crepitant and subcrepitant rales from other small rales. "This distinction which is almost universally neglected by systematic writers, enables the diagnosis of pneumonia to be made with accuracy, even though the pneumonic patch be small, and is of special value in the diagnosis of tuberculous pneumonia. The distinction is made by the size of the rale—crepitant and subcrepitant rales are smaller than other similar rales that appear in showers."

Crepitant rales are heard in lobar pneumonia during the stages of engorgement and resolution, in pulmonary edema and in the early stages of pulmonary tuberculosis.

4. **Atelectatic Rales.** When a person whose breathing is habitually shallow is asked to take a deep breath, the examiner often hears at the bases of the lungs a few rales which sound precisely like crepitant rales. After the person has taken a few deep breaths the atelectatic rales disappear.

This type of rale, although having the same tonal quality as crepitant rales, indicates no disease, but simply that the person examined is not using all his pulmonary tissue in breathing. For the reason that these sounds indicate no pathologic lesion, some observers refer to them as "so-called crepitant rales." Other observers, believing that they are produced by the rush of air into collapsed air vesicles which produce this sound when they are suddenly distended and their sticky surfaces forced apart, regard them as a variety of crepitant rales which may be produced in the same manner. Bushnell believed that the sound often called atelectatic rales are produced by a separation of the diaphragmatic from the costal pleura and the "surfaces being moist, their separation is attended by sounds that characterize the peeling off of one moist and slightly tacky surface from another." He prefers to call these sounds "marginal sounds." In proof of the correctness of his theory he refers to the phenomenon known as "reversible crepitation." When a person lies on the right side and breathes deeply, crepitations may be heard over the lower side, while they are absent over the upper side. If he now changes his position and lies on the left side, crepitations are heard over the left side, while none are heard over the upper right side. When the subject lies on one side, the diaphragm on the lower side makes a deeper and more vigorous descent during inspiration, and this, according to Bushnell, produces marginal sounds with especial distinctness.

Whatever the cause of atelectatic rales, the student should remember that they have no pathologic significance. They are commonly missed, since the observer usually examines the upper parts of the chest first, and by the time he has proceeded to examine the bases, the atelectatic rales have disappeared.

Atelectatic rales are often heard when a patient complains of pain at the base of the lungs and the examiner listens first over this area. At first he may suspect pleurisy, but as the patient breathes deeply, the atelectatic rales clear up, while the friction rub of pleurisy does not so readily disappear.

5. **Consonating or Tinkling Rales.** Most of the rales we hear are not loud, but soft, and give the impression that they are produced rather deep within the substance of the lung. There is another type of rales which is distinctly louder, conveys an impression of nearness, and seems to be produced directly under the bell of the stethoscope. This type of rale is called consonating, the term used by Skoda, who believed that its intensity was increased by consonation or the sympathetic vibration of the pulmonary tissue surrounding the place of production. They are pathognomonic of consolidation. Most observers now believe that these rales have a loud, clear quality and seem near to the ear because they are better transmitted through a consolidated area, just as bronchial breathing is. They are heard under the same conditions as bronchial breathing.

Consonating rales are heard better with a monaural wooden stethoscope than with a flexible rubber-tubed binaural stethoscope, and for that reason are more emphasized by Continental physicians than by their American colleagues. They are also designated by many observers as tinkling rales and often have a distinctly metallic quality.

Consonation is rather a quality of rales than a basis of classification. Thus, rales fall into two large classes, dry and moist. Moist rales may be either consonating or nonconsonating. Consonating rales are rales usually heard through an area of consolidation.

The following scheme of classification of rales may prove helpful, although it would not be universally accepted without controversy.

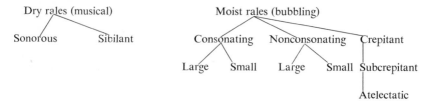

Amphoric and metallic rales have been described, associated with cavities and hydropneumothorax, respectively.

PLEURAL FRICTION RUB

The pleural friction rub was heard by Hippocrates, who observed that in pneumonia "the lung is congealed to the ribs and squeaks like a leather strap." Laennec described it as a "dull sound similar to that produced by rubbing the finger against a bone under the stethoscope" and noted that "on applying the hand one feels a sensation similar to that heard through the stethoscope." Laennec believed that this sound was produced by an interlobular emphysema of the lungs. Raynaud and Stokes later gave the true explanation and proved that it was due to roughening of the pleural surfaces.

Normally the pleural surfaces are smooth and glistening, and no sound is produced as the visceral pleura slips over the parietal pleura in respiration. If the pleural surface is roughened by an inflammatory process, a rubbing sound is produced. The character of the sound varies with the inflammatory lesion present. When the surface of the pleura is markedly roughened, the pleural friction is rough and harsh. When the pleural surface is only slightly roughened, the sound is softer and fainter.

The movement of the visceral pleura over the parietal pleura is greatest in extent at the bases of the lungs and decreases as one passes upward. At the apices of the lungs the movement is practically absent. For this reason the pleural friction is best heard at the bases, is not so marked in the upper parts of the lung, and is rarely heard at the apices.

The pleural friction rub may vary greatly in intensity, varying from a loud creaking noise, sounding close to the ear, to a soft, almost inaudible rub or "click." It is often heard during inspiration and expiration. It is rarely, if ever, heard during expiration alone.

The pleural friction rub is pathognomonic of acute fibrinous pleurisy, whether due to pneumonia, tuberculosis, neoplasm or some acute inflammation of the pleura. The sound is increased by pressure of the bell of the stethoscope upon the chest, may vary from time to time in intensity, and may disappear for a short time only to reappear with increased intensity. It disappears when the patient holds his breath. Occasionally muscle sounds are confused with the pleural friction rub.

Soft pleural friction rubs may be confused with crepitant rales. Crepitant rales, however, are not increased in intensity by pressure upon the bell of the stethoscope and are often modified if the patient coughs, when they may increase in intensity or disappear altogether for a time.

HIPPOCRATIC SUCCUSSION

This classical sign was first described by Hippocrates in empyema. "Set the patient on a stool, which is not wobbly, someone should hold his hands, then shake him by the shoulders and listen to see on which side a noise is heard" (Fig. 245).

Laennec was the first to recognize that Hippocratic succussion is due to the presence of both air and fluid in the chest and to point out that even a large

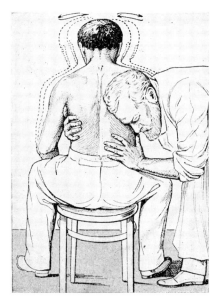

FIG. 245. Hippocratic succussion. (Letulle.)

amount of fluid in the chest produces no splashing sound, when the patient is shaken, unless there is also air present. Air is necessary to produce a splashing sound. A bottle full of water can be shaken violently without the production of a splashing sound; a bottle half-filled with water gives a splashing sound when agitated violently.

This splashing sound is often heard by the patient when he walks or climbs stairs. At other times he feels the displacement of the fluid caused by change in posture. Morgagni described a patient who "said that when she moved her chest she felt a splashing within."

The succussion is best elicited by following the ancient method of Hippocrates, shaking the patient by the shoulders and listening with the ear or stethoscope against the chest. The splashing sound caused by disturbing the level of fluid is easily heard.

Hippocratic succussion is pathognomonic of pneumohydrothorax. One possible exception may be mentioned. We have heard a splashing sound on listening over the chest of a patient with a diaphragmatic hernia when shaken by the shoulders. Here the succussion was caused by the presence of air and fluid in the stomach, which was in the thoracic cavity. In this patient the history and particularly the x-ray examination cleared up the diagnosis.

FALLING-DROP SOUND

When one listens over a chest which contains both fluid and air, one occasionally hears a sound like that produced "by a drop of water which one lets fall into a carafe three-quarters empty" (Laennec). This sound is probably due, as Laennec suggested, to a drop of liquid falling into the accumulation of fluid at the bottom of the pleural cavity. Others have suggested that the sound is due to rales produced in the collapsed lung.

LUNG-FISTULA SOUND

In patients with hydropneumothorax, who have a fistula of the lung opening

below the level of the fluid, respiration may force bubbles of air out into the fluid. This produces a characteristic bubbling or gurgling sound.

This sign is usually heard in hydropneumothorax, but is not pathognomonic of this condition. It was observed by Gerhardt in a patient with an abscess which developed from a carcinoma of the esophagus and broke into the bronchus. He regarded the sign as more the proof of a bronchial fistula than of pneumothorax.

VOCAL RESONANCE

When a normal person speaks or whispers "one, two, three" or "ninety-nine," the voice sounds are heard as a soft confused murmur. The sound is loudest over the upper parts of the lungs, and over the areas where the trachea and larger bronchi are nearest the surface of the chest. Its intensity in various parts of the chest is comparable with that of the vocal fremitus. It is more marked in thin-chested persons than in the fat or muscular, more marked in those with deep voices and more marked in men than in women.

Increased Vocal Resonance. If there is an area of consolidation in the lungs, the voice sounds are increased over this area. This phenomenon is known as bronchophony or pectoriloquy, terms coined by Laennec.

Bronchophony (βρόγχος—brogchos = air passage, + φωνή—phone = voice) means literally the sound of the voice as heard over a large normal bronchus. Laennec also used the term "laryngophony" and noted that the bronchophony over areas in the chest often resembles, and is nearly as intense as, laryngophony.

Pectoriloquy (*pectus*—breast, + *loqui*—speak) is defined usually as the sound of spoken words through the chest wall. Laennec first noted this phenomenon: "holding the stethoscope below the middle of the right clavicle, I had the patient speak, his voice seemed to come out directly from his chest and pass completely through the central canal of the stethoscope. This transmission of the voice took place only in a space about an inch square. In no other part of the chest could I find the same thing."

Laennec's differentiation between bronchophony and pectoriloquy is not clear, and much confusion persists regarding these two terms. A practical and workable differentiation is to call the increased vocal resonance bronchophony, when the sounds are loud and clear, but the words themselves indistinguishable; pectoriloquy when we can make out the individual words distinctly.

The vocal resonance may be tested by either speaking or whispering. Most observers find whispering of greater value. A small area of whispered pectoriloquy in a patient with pneumonia may be present before bronchial breathing can be detected. Both bronchophony and pectoriloquy indicate consolidation of lung tissue. "Bronchophony has clinically the same importance as bronchial breathing, and all that was said concerning the causation of bronchial breathing, holds for bronchophony" (Edens).

D'Espine's Sign. "The first signs of bronchial adenopathy are given exclusively by auscultation of the voice and are observed almost always in the immediate neighborhood of the vertebral column, between the seventh cervical vertebra and the first thoracic vertebra either in the subspinal fossa or lower in the interscapular space. They consist in a timbre added to the voice which one could call whispering in the first stage and bronchophony in the more advanced stage" (d'Espine).

Diminished Vocal Resonance. Diminished vocal resonance is found under the same pathological conditions as diminished vocal fremitus. An occlusion of a bronchus interfering with the transmission of the voice sounds to the lung parenchyma, atelectasis, fluid in the chest, thickening of the pleura are the most common causes.

Egophony. "Egophony resembles pectoriloquy in that it also consists of loud resonance of the voice beneath the stethoscope. It is only rarely, however, that the voice appears to enter the tube of the instrument, and it very seldom passes right along it in the evident manner which characterizes perfect pectoriloquy. The voice is higher pitched and sharper than the patient's natural voice, and has, so to speak, a silvery tone; it produces the illusion that someone is speaking in the patient's chest. It possesses, moreover, one constant characteristic from which it has seemed to me suitable to name the phenomenon; it is quavering and jerky, like the bleating of a goat and, as may be judged from the foregoing description, it is also similar in timbre to the noise made by that animal. This characteristic is subject to only slight variations, which the reader may picture to himself exactly if he calls to mind the effect produced by a chip placed between the teeth and the lips of a person speaking, the sound of the voice when transmitted through a cracked reed, or the stammering nasal tone of a Punch and Judy showman. This last comparison is often strictly accurate, especially in the case of men with a rather deep voice" (Laennec). This phenomenon Laennec named egophony from αἴξ—aix = goat, + φωνή —phone = voice.

Egophony is most commonly heard over moderate-sized pleural effusions, usually near the inferior angle of the scapula. It is often heard over the area where Skodaic resonance is present. It is occasionally heard over an area of consolidation in the lungs.

The student may imitate egophony by counting one, two, three, and while continuing the count, suddenly closing both nostrils tightly with the fingers. This change to a marked nasal quality (popularly and falsely called "talking through one's nose") resembles the change in the vocal resonance when the stethoscope passes to an area where egophony is heard.

THE COIN SIGN

This sign, called in French "signe du sou" (sign of the sou) or "bruit d'airain"

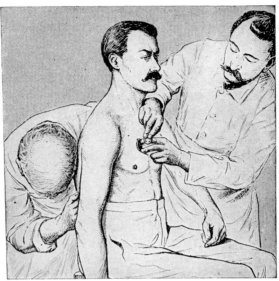

Fig. 246. Method of eliciting coin sound. (Letulle.)

(sound of brass), is elicited by placing a large coin on the chest wall and striking it with another coin, while the observer listens over the back at a point directly opposite that where the coin is struck. When the coin is struck over the normal side of the chest, a rather flat, clicking, poorly transmitted sound is heard; but when the test is carried out over the side of a pneumothorax, the sound has a striking metallic, ringing quality. It reminds one of the sound produced when a pebble is dropped into a deep well. This coin sign when present is pathognomonic of pneumothorax, but may be absent (Fig. 246).

BIBLIOGRAPHY

D'Espine, M. A.: Le diagnostic précoce de la tuberculose des ganglions bronchiques chez les enfants. Bull. Acad. de Méd., Paris *57*:167, 1907.

Fahr, George: The acoustics of the bronchial breath sounds. Arch. Int. Med. *39*:287, 1927.

Heise, Fred H.: The physics of percussion and auscultation of the chest. Med. Rec. *90*:191, 1916.

Pottenger, F. M.: Auscultation. Am. Rev. Tuberc. *56*:1, 1947.

Rappaport, Maurice B., and Sprague, Howard B.: Physiologic and physical laws that govern auscultation and their clinical application. Am. Heart J. *21*:257, 1941.

Sewall, Henry: The origin of the "new leather" and "dry friction" sounds heard on auscultation. Am. J. M. Sc. *137*:364, 1909.

CHAPTER 8

PHYSICAL FINDINGS IN DISEASES OF THE LUNGS

AFTER THE DISCUSSION in the two preceding chapters of the various normal and abnormal findings in the chest, a brief consideration of the physical findings in certain pulmonary diseases will emphasize the association and correlation of the physical signs in these diseases. Again we should remember the classic statement of Skoda that "the findings of percussion and auscultation depend never upon the disease itself, but always upon the changes produced in the organs."

ACUTE BRONCHITIS

Inspection. In general the respiratory rate is not increased, although, when the fever is high, the patient may show tachypnea and, at times, dyspnea.

Palpation. When the bronchitis is severe, a rhonchal fremitus may be felt, especially on deep inspiration.

Percussion. In uncomplicated bronchitis the percussion note over the chest is everywhere resonant.

Auscultation. In the early stages of acute bronchitis the breath sounds may be enfeebled or harsh, and musical rales of the piping, sibilant or sonorous type

are commonly heard. These rales are variable and may disappear on coughing. In the later stages of acute bronchitis, as the amount of bronchial secretion increases, the predominant type of rale is the small and the large, moist rale. They are usually large, loud, widely scattered throughout the lungs, not fine or localized at the apex as in tuberculosis.

BRONCHIECTASIS

Inspection. Many patients with bronchiectasis appear to be in perfect health. They usually give a history of coughing up large amounts of sputum on arising in the morning, but may have had little expectoration during the day. The sputum is abundant, gray or grayish-brown, purulent and semifluid, and has a fetid or sweetish, sickening odor. Patients with marked bronchiectasis of long standing usually show clubbing of the fingers (Fig. 448). The chest on inspection may show no abnormalities, although patients with marked unilateral bronchiectasis may show diminished respiratory movements on the affected side.

139

Palpation. Palpation usually discloses no abnormalities, although at times rhonchi may be felt. When there is a large bronchiectatic cavity near the surface, an increased vocal fremitus is occasionally, but rarely, felt.

Percussion. Most patients with bronchiectasis show no abnormalities on percussion. When marked dilatations or cavities are near the surface of the lungs, they may give a tympanitic percussion note.

Auscultation. The auscultatory findings in bronchiectasis show great variations in different patients. Variations in the same patient may be detected, particularly before and after a paroxysm of coughing.

Many varieties of rales are commonly heard, especially at the bases, the moist bubbling rales predominating. Over a bronchiectatic cavity, bronchophony with cavernous or amphoric breathing may be heard after coughing. When a bronchiectatic cavity is filled with exudate, the breath sounds over it are distant or absent.

It should be emphasized that a deep-seated bronchiectasis may show no physical signs. In many cases the diagnosis is certain only after the instillation of lipiodol into the bronchus, this procedure producing a characteristic picture in the roentgen plate.

EMPHYSEMA

Inspection. The patient with emphysema commonly shows a moderate cyanosis of the lips and of the lobes of the ears, this cyanosis increasing on slight exertion. The chest on inspection shows a marked increase in the antero-posterior diameter, which may be greater than the lateral diameter, so that the chest, when viewed laterally, has a barrel shape (Fig. 247). The sternum and costal cartilages are prominent; the costal angle is widened to 90 degrees or more. "The appearance is somewhat as if the chest was in a permanent inspiratory position" (Osler). Hoover's sign may be present. The shoulders appear elevated, the neck shortened. Small di-

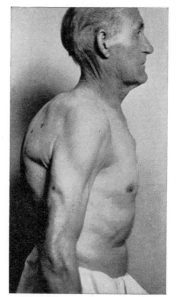

FIG. 247. Barrel chest with kyphosis.

lated venules may be seen on the skin along the line of attachment of the diaphragm. The apex beat of the heart is not visible.

Respiration is shallow, inspiration being short and feeble, while expiration is more prolonged. During inspiration the chest is elevated as one piece. There is little or no general expansion. The respiratory movements seem energetic and forceful, but are really feeble and lacking in force.

Palpation. The vocal fremitus is faint, but is usually present. As a rule, the apex beat cannot be felt.

Percussion. The percussion note is greatly increased; hyperresonance and, at times, a drumlike tympanitic note may be elicited. Absolute cardiac dulness is absent or greatly reduced in area (Fig. 248), and the area of relative cardiac dulness is diminished as well. The area of lung resonance is increased down to the costal margin, while the upper limit of liver dulness is lowered.

After deep inspiration followed by forced expiration, percussion over the bases of the lungs in the back shows little change in the lower limits of lung resonance.

Auscultation. On auscultation the breath sounds are feeble. Expiration is

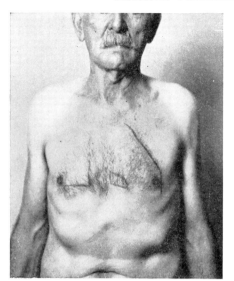

FIG. 248. Small area of absolute cardiac dulness in emphysema.

commonly prolonged and may be four times as long as inspiration. Expiration may be harsh and accompanied occasionally by harsh sibilant rales. Accentuation of the second pulmonic sound is commonly present.

INTERSTITIAL EMPHYSEMA

Interstitial emphysema of the lungs was first described adequately by Laennec. It may be the result of trauma to the chest, after a blow or laceration of the lungs, and often after the induction of therapeutic pneumothorax. It also occurs after severe paroxysms of coughing, in pneumonia and bronchial asthma, after straining at stool, during childbirth, after heavy lifting, and also spontaneously without trauma or any unusual distention of the lungs.

Inspection. Nothing distinctive.

Palpation. Crepitation of the subcutaneous tissues of the neck.

Percussion. Area of cardiac dulness may be diminished or replaced by a tympanitic percussion note.

Auscultation. Crunching, crackling, bubbling sound heard over heart, synchronous with systole.

BRONCHIAL ASTHMA

Patients who are victims of bronchial asthma may be subjectively and objec-tively perfectly well except during attacks. An attack lasts from a few minutes to several hours and presents a characteristic picture.

Inspection. During an attack of asthma the patient is cyanotic, sweats, and has a feeble pulse and cold extremities. The chest is full and fixed and shows little expansion on inspiration. Inspiration is short, expiration markedly prolonged. Coughing is difficult and tight at first; later it is more violent. The sputum is thick and tenacious, and consists of small, round, gelatinous masses of mucus—the "perles of Laennec."

Palpation. On palpation a rhonchal fremitus is usually felt.

Percussion. The percussion note over the chest during an attack of bronchial asthma is usually markedly hyperreso-nant. The area of lung resonance is increased, the area of absolute cardiac dulness obliterated. Here, on percussion, the marked distention of the lungs produces the same signs as in emphysema.

Auscultation. On auscultation the inspiration is feeble and poorly heard, expiration is markedly prolonged and harsh (Fig. 242). During both inspiration and expiration a large number of musical rales—sibilant, sonorous and whistling—are heard throughout the chest. Every variety of musical rale may be heard simultaneously. These rales are commonly so loud and numerous that it is not necessary to apply the stethoscope to the chest in order to hear them; they can be heard at some distance from the patient.

Later during an attack of asthma moist rales usually appear and may become as numerous as the musical rales. As the attack subsides, the rales often disappear with startling rapidity.

PLEURISY

Pleurisy, or pleuritis, is an inflammation of the pleura which leads to a fibrinous effusion, with or without serum, to the formation of pus or to adhesions. It is usually accompanied by fever of a varying degree. Three clinical varieties of this condition are recognized.

Acute Fibrinous Pleurisy; Pleuritis Sicca

Most cases of acute fibrinous pleurisy are of tuberculous origin. Acute fibrinous pleurisy may occur, however, in influenza, lobar pneumonia or rheumatic fever, or may result from a general infection or appear as an extension from disease in some neighboring organ.

Inspection. The patient often shows signs of distress and lies on the affected side. The respiratory rate is increased and the movements of the chest are markedly diminished over the side of the involvement. The patient has a shallow cough which does not bring up any sputum.

Palpation. Palpation often reveals nothing, but may confirm the lessened expansion of the chest on the affected side. At times a pleural friction may be felt. The vocal fremitus shows no change.

Auscultation. On auscultation the breath sounds are not so well heard over the affected side, probably because of the diminished respiratory movements. Over the area of pleuritis a friction rub is heard, which varies greatly in intensity. It is louder on inspiration and may be heard only on inspiration, but at times is audible during expiration as well. It is intensified when the patient takes a deep breath as well as often by pressure on the bell of the stethoscope. At times it is loud, creaking and rough. Fine crackling rales may also be heard with deep inspiration.

Pleurisy with Effusion; Pleuritis Exudativa

The exudate may be serous, *pleuritis serosa;* serofibrinous, *pleuritis serofibrinosa,* or purulent, *pleuritis purulenta,* empyema. The physical findings are essentially the same in these three types.

Inspection. The patient usually lies on the affected side, thus allowing freer expansion of the normal lung. If the amount of the effusion is large, he may be more comfortable in the sitting posture, and may show marked dyspnea.

The movements of the chest during respiration are diminished on the affected side, and in large effusions the affected side appears much fuller than the normal one and the intercostal spaces may actually bulge instead of being depressed. When the effusion is on the right side, the cardiac impulse may be displaced beyond the left mammillary line even into the left axilla; when the effusion is on the left side, the cardiac impulse may disappear under the sternum or even appear to the right of the sternum.

Palpation. Palpation first confirms the observations made on inspection: decreased mobility with bulging of the intercostal spaces on the affected side and displacement of the cardiac impulse. The vocal fremitus is absent or markedly diminished over the effusion.

Percussion. In small effusions and in early stages of any pleural effusion the percussion note may be unchanged. As more fluid accumulates, the percussion note becomes less and less resonant, and finally becomes dull (Fig. 207). This dulness has a peculiar flat, wooden quality, and the resistance to the percussing finger is marked, particularly on direct percussion. The "feel" on percussion and the note obtained are different from the dulness obtained in consolidation of the lung.

Above the fluid the percussion note may have a definitely tympanitic quality —Skodaic resonance (Fig. 225). When the patient is in the erect position, the upper line of dulness is not horizontal, but is higher in the back than in front. At the base of the normal lung on the back there is usually a triangular area of dulness—Grocco's sign (Fig. 226). When the effusion is moderate, shifting dulness may be demonstrated by marking out the upper level of the dulness, first in the sitting and then in the recumbent posture.

When the effusion is on the right side, the dulness extends into and cannot be demarcated from the liver dulness; when the effusion is on the left, Traube's semilunar space may be obliterated (Fig.

217). A right-sided pleural effusion displaces the heart to the left and the cardiac dulness toward the left axilla; a left-sided pleural effusion increases the cardiac dulness to the right of the sternum (Fig. 250). In a left-sided pleural effusion the dulness extends into that of the cardiac dulness, and percussion of the left cardiac border may be impossible.

Auscultation. Early in the disease a friction rub may be heard, which, however, soon disappears. The breath sounds are diminished or absent over the area of the effusion (Fig. 202). Distant tubular breathing is often heard over the effusion. Above the area of dulness the breath sounds are usually harsh, loud, often tubular in character, and may be accompanied by moist, bubbling rales. In a left-sided pleural effusion the inflammatory process may extend to the pericardium, producing a pleuropericardial friction rub heard with each heart beat.

The vocal resonance is diminished or absent over the effusion. The whispered voice may be intensified—bronchophony—and the voice often has a curious nasal twang, the egophony of Laennec, especially just above the level of the effusion. The voice sounds may be better transmitted through a serous than through a purulent fluid. Baccellis' statement, that whispered sounds are not transmitted through a purulent fluid, is disputed by most authorities.

The differentiation between a serous, serofibrinous and purulent effusion is best made with the exploratory needle.

Chronic empyema is frequently accompanied by an irregular temperature of the septic type, marked anemia and a progressive loss of weight. The pus may disappear by absorption, by perforation of a bronchus when the pus is expectorated, and by perforation of the chest wall—*empyema necessitatis* (Fig. 249). Empyema most commonly follows lobar pneumonia. It is seen, however, as a complication of appendicitis, perirenal abscess and of pulmonary tuberculosis.

Pulsating pleurisy is a remarkable

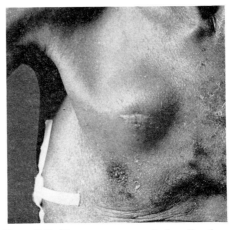

FIG. 249. Empyema necessitatis. Bandage shows site of attempted thoracentesis.

phenomenon, usually a pulsating empyema and commonly a pulsating empyema necessitatis. In this condition the cardiac impulse is transmitted through the effusion.

Interlobar empyema can usually be diagnosed only by the roentgen ray.

Hydrothorax due to cardiac disease, renal disease or other causes presents the same physical findings in the chest as those of pleurisy with effusion, since the physical conditions are identical. In hydrothorax due to cardiac disease other physical findings are often striking. The patient usually shows marked cyanosis, severe dyspnea, edema of the feet and legs, ascites and an enlarged tender liver as well as other evidence of cardiac disease.

Thickened Pleura

Chronic pleurisy, or thickened pleura, is commonly of tuberculous origin, and not infrequently is the result of a serofibrinous or purulent pleural exudate which has not been removed. The physical findings are fairly characteristic.

Inspection. The chest often shows retraction on the affected side. Litten's sign is absent on the side of the thickened pleura.

Palpation. The vocal fremitus is diminished or absent over the affected side.

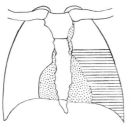

LEFT PLEURAL EFFUSION
HEART PUSHED TO RIGHT

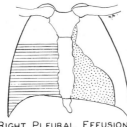

RIGHT PLEURAL EFFUSION
HEART PUSHED TO LEFT

FIG. 250. Effect of pleural effusion on cardiac dulness.

Percussion. The percussion note is dull or flat on the side of the thickened pleura. The heart may be pulled toward the affected side.

Auscultation. The breath sounds are markedly diminished on the side of the chronic pleurisy. Occasionally a creaking, leathery friction rub is heard on auscultation.

The signs of a thickened pleura closely simulate those of pleural effusion. The heart, however, may be pulled toward the involved side in pleural thickening. This cannot, however, always be satisfactorily demonstrated by percussion. Shifting dulness, if present, decides the diagnosis in favor of pleural effusion. Aspiration of the chest may be necessary for diagnosis. The roentgen ray usually permits differentiation between the two conditions.

PNEUMOTHORAX

Pneumothorax may follow a wound in the chest, may appear spontaneously, especially in tuberculosis following the rupture of an air vesicle or bronchiole, or may supervene as a complication of pneumonia and of empyema. In most patients an effusion in the chest occurs

later, so that we have a hydropneumothorax.

Inspection. In acute spontaneous pneumothorax or pneumothorax following perforation of the chest wall, the patient shows marked dyspnea, extreme cyanosis, a feeble, rapid heart action and a fall in blood pressure. In other instances the onset may be so insidious that the patient is not aware of the condition until hydropneumothorax has developed and he hears splashing within his chest.

The appearance of the chest is striking on the side of the pneumothorax, the chest being immobile and the normal intercostal depressions having been obliterated. The cardiac impulse is displaced to the left in a right pneumothorax and to the right in a left pneumothorax.

Palpation. The vocal fremitus is diminished or abolished over the affected side.

Percussion. The percussion note over the affected side is usually hyperresonant or tympanitic. Sometimes, however, it is dull, and mistakes in diagnosis have frequently been made on the erroneous assumption that the percussion note in pneumothorax is always hyperresonant.

At the base of the lung on the side of the pneumothorax, the percussion note is dull when fluid is present.

Auscultation. The breath sounds are markedly diminished or absent on the affected side and exaggerated on the normal side. At the end of inspiration a metallic tinkling sound is often heard. The breath sounds may be amphoric, and, if an open fistula is present, a gurgling sound—the "water-whistle murmur"—may be heard.

In many patients the "coin sound" is obtained over the pneumothorax (Fig. 246), and, when fluid is present, the "Hippocratic succussion" may be heard on shaking the patient (Fig. 245).

PULMONARY ATELECTASIS

Small areas of pulmonary atelectasis may occur in several pulmonary diseases, the areas often being so limited in extent as to give no physical findings. Lobar pneumonia, pleural effusion, pneumothorax and obstruction of a bronchus are the usual causes of collapse of the lung. Massive collapse or acute massive pulmonary atelectasis of the lung is a condition of much interest and in the great majority of cases follows a surgical operation.

MASSIVE COLLAPSE OF THE LUNG

Inspection. The signs of massive collapse usually appear suddenly. The patient looks anxious, the respiratory rate is increased, there is severe dyspnea, cyanosis, prostration, and often pain in the lower part of the thorax. The chest on the affected side looks flat, the intercostal spaces narrowed and depressed, the respiratory movements are markedly diminished, while there is increased expansion over the normal side. The trachea is deviated and the point of maximal impulse displaced toward the affected side.

Palpation. The vocal fremitus is usually decreased or absent over the affected side.

Percussion. Percussion shows that the heart is displaced toward the affected side. This is the most important physical finding. In right-sided collapse of the lung the cardiac dulness on the left may entirely disappear. The percussion note over the affected lung is usually dull, but occasionally is tympanitic.

Auscultation. The breath sounds are usually harsh, tubular in quality and distant. Rales may or may not be present.

The collapse of the lung is most frequently confused with postoperative lobar pneumonia. In doubtful cases the demonstration of displacement of the heart toward the affected side is conclusive evidence of massive pulmonary collapse.

The condition, especially when it follows surgical operation, may appear suddenly and then disappear within a few hours. It commonly disappears in a week or ten days. Occasionally, in massive collapse, there is a persistent

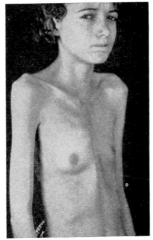

Fig. 251. Atelectasis of left lung.

atelectasis and the chest may become unusually flat and depressed on the affected side (Fig. 251). Massive collapse of the lungs is frequently seen in bronchiogenic carcinoma.

LOBAR PNEUMONIA

The onset of this disease is usually sudden, often accompanied by a chill and a rapid rise in temperature.

Inspection. Dyspnea is almost invariably present and the respiratory rate is increased. The patient's nostrils dilate with inspiration and contract with expiration. The patient often gives a grunt with each expiration. Cyanosis of the tip of the nose, ears and fingertips is commonly present, and in severe cases there may be marked cyanosis of the face. In some patients, however, the face may be flushed. Coughing is usually present. It may be severe and associated with sharp pain in the affected side. The sputum at first is mucoid, but later becomes bright red and then rusty brown—the classic "rusty sputum" of pneumonia. The respiratory movements are decreased on the affected side and increased on the normal side. The affected side often looks larger and fuller than the normal side.

Palpation. The diminished respiratory excursions on the affected side are often better felt than seen. Mensuration of the chest from the midsternal line to the spinal line may show the volume of the affected side to be greater than that of the normal side.

A pleural friction fremitus may be felt because of a coexisting acute pleuritis.

The vocal fremitus is greatly increased over the pneumonic area. If, however, the bronchus to this area is filled with exudate, the vocal fremitus may be diminished, and, for this reason, the patient should be asked to cough before this test is carried out.

Percussion. In a well-developed pneumonia the percussion note is dull or flat over the affected area. This flatness is, however, not the "wooden" flatness produced by fluid, and the sense of resistance to the percussing finger is not so great. Over the normal lung tissue just above the area of consolidation the percussion note often has a tympanitic quality— Skodaic resonance.

Auscultation. In the early stages of lobar pneumonia the breath sounds may be diminished or suppressed. Fine crepitant, consonating rales may be heard which seem unusually close to the ear. The consonating quality of these rales should be emphasized, since such rales are pathognomonic of consolidation.

With the development of frank consolidation, the crepitant rales disappear, the breath sounds become tubular, expiration being harsh and markedly prolonged (Figs. 203, 239). If the larger bronchi are filled with secretion, tubular breathing may disappear until a paroxysm of coughing empties the bronchi.

The expiratory grunt may be transmitted through an area of consolidation with great intensity. The vocal resonance is increased and the voice sounds may have a curious nasal tone—the egophony first described by Laennec in plural effusion.

During resolution the patient looks more comfortable, the cyanosis and tachypnea disappear, the areas of dulness on percussion become smaller, and on auscultation numerous small and large moist rales are heard in increasing numbers, while the harsh tubular breathing gradually disappears and normal vesicular breathing reappears.

BRONCHOPNEUMONIA

The physical findings of bronchopneumonia are at the onset those of an acute bronchitis. Indeed, they may remain so throughout the course of the disease when the areas of bronchopneumonic consolidation are so small that they cannot be demonstrated by physical examination. In such cases it is a safe clinical rule that if a patient has the physical findings of an acute bronchitis, accompanied by a high temperature and symptoms of more serious illness, he probably has bronchopneumonia.

Often, however, the small bronchopneumonic patches coalesce and extend until a larger area of consolidation like that in lobar pneumonia appears. The physical findings then are those of lobar pneumonia. It is often difficult to determine, when an area of consolidation is detected, whether the disease began as bronchopneumonia or as lobar pneumonia. Here the history may be the decisive factor in diagnosis.

In central pneumonia, where the process is deep seated, the patient may show no abnormal physical findings in the chest, although his respiration is rapid, and he has a cough and blood-tinged sputum. Later this process may extend to the surface of the lung and the characteristic findings of consolidation be discovered. At times this process remains central and can be determined only by the roentgen ray.

PULMONARY TUBERCULOSIS

The study of pulmonary tuberculosis more than that of any other disease led to the discovery and development of percussion and auscultation. Gaspard Laurent Bayle, the friend and older colleague of Laennec, used to some extent the direct application of the ear to the chest in the diagnosis of tuberculosis. He published a book which marks the beginning of the modern era in the study of pulmonary tuberculosis and which also profoundly influenced young

Laennec. Laennec continued Bayle's observations, and much of his famous work on mediate auscultation is devoted to the physical signs of pulmonary tuberculosis. At times no disease may be easier to diagnose; at other times no disease more difficult.

Acute Miliary Tuberculosis

Acute miliary tuberculosis was first adequately described by Bayle, who spoke of miliary tubercles, a term first suggested by Manget in 1700, because the lesions were the size of millet seeds. Pathologic changes in the size of millet seeds could scarcely be expected to produce marked physical signs. In some patients the picture is that of a gradually developing infectious disease with malaise, fever and prostration. Commonly, the patients have an annoying cough, often with little or no expectoration. This type is frequently mistaken for typhoid fever, particularly since the spleen is often enlarged. In other patients the disease may develop rapidly with the signs of acute meningitis. This latter type of miliary tuberculosis is the commoner variety in children, in whom tubercular meningitis warrants the diagnosis of miliary tuberculosis.

The miliary tubercles in the lungs produce no physical findings. If the patient has an old tubercular cavity or an old tubercular infiltration of the lungs, these may be detected by physical examination. If the miliary tuberculosis develops into a tuberculous bronchopneumonia, the signs of the latter appear. The diagnosis of acute miliary tuberculosis of the lungs is made by the roentgenogram, not by physical examination.

Acute Pulmonary Tuberculosis

Acute pulmonary tuberculosis is known to the laity as galloping consumption, to the physician as phthisis florida. While chronic pulmonary tuberculosis is a disease the duration of which is measured by years, the duration of acute pulmonary tuberculosis is measured by weeks. Occasionally, however, the acute process subsides and the acute tuberculosis becomes chronic. Acute pulmonary tuberculosis occurs in two forms, the bronchopneumonic form and the lobar form.

The bronchopneumonic type occurs most commonly in infants and young children, less commonly in adults. In adults with chronic ulcerative tuberculosis, acute tuberculous bronchopneumonia may be engrafted on the chronic process, especially after aspiration of the contents of a tubercular cavity. Tuberculous bronchopneumonia may begin suddenly with a chill and a sharp rise in temperature, or gradually and more insidiously with slight fever which, however, soon becomes high and continuous in type. The physical signs are indistinguishable from those of the ordinary acute bronchopneumonia.

The lobar type of tubercular pneumonia is rare in children and usually seen in adults. The onset is often sudden, with a chill, rapidly rising temperature and pain in the side. Physical examination shows involvement of one or more lobes of the lung with signs of consolidation, increased vocal fremitus, dulness on percussion, at first suppressed breath sounds followed by well-marked bronchial breathing. "At this time," as Osler remarked in the first edition of his *Practice,* "as a rule, no suspicion enters the mind of the practitioner that the case is anything but one of frank lobar pneumonia. . . . Between the eighth and tenth day, instead of the expected crisis, the condition becomes more aggravated, the temperature is irregular, and the pulse more rapid. There may be sweating, and the expectoration becomes muco-purulent. Even in the second and third week, with the persistence of these symptoms, the physician tries to console himself with the idea that the case is one of unresolved pneumonia, and that all will yet be well. Gradually, however, the severity of the symptoms, the presence of physical signs indicating softening, the existence of elastic tissue and tubercle bacilli in the sputum present the mournful proofs that the case is one of acute pneumonic phthisis." This mournful experience can usually be avoided by an early and careful examination of the patient's sputum.

Chronic Pulmonary Tuberculosis

The older writers commonly called this disease *consumption* or, when they preferred a foreign or more scientific sounding term, *phthisis,* which is simply a derivation of the Greek word for consumption. Yet they frequently stressed the inadequacy of these terms, since many of their patients showed no wasting, but were on the contrary well nourished as the patient shown in Figure 252. The term *tuberculous phthisis,* introduced by Bayle, and its subsequent alteration to tuberculosis, not only avoided this dilemma, but was more accurate, since it referred to tubercles, the essential pathologic lesion in the disease.

Laennec's epochal work on tuberculosis considered mainly tuberculosis in its more advanced stages. Fournet, his contemporary and successor, wrote the first book on the early diagnosis of tuberculosis. "His attempts to connect the various early changes in the physical

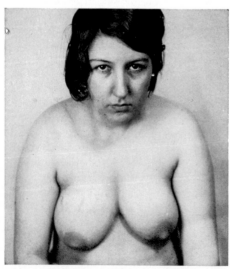

FIG. 252. Healthy-looking, somewhat obese young woman found on examination to have advanced pulmonary tuberculosis with cavitation.

signs with the different stages of the early disease are," as Skoda said, "completely theoretical. But he did yeoman service" (Lawrason Brown). Skoda's book pointed out that pulmonary tuberculosis may be diagnosed in its first stages.

First Stage or Minimal Tuberculosis

The symptoms in the early stages of pulmonary tuberculosis may be of great assistance in the diagnosis. A gradual loss of weight, a slight, annoying, unproductive but continuous cough, an evening rise in temperature, are all suspicious symptoms. The history of a former attack of pleurisy is significant. Hemoptysis may appear in the early stages.

Inspection. The majority of patients in the early stages of tuberculosis show normal-looking chests. A very early physical sign is drooping of the shoulder and deficient expansion of the chest over the apex on the affected side.

The typical tuberculous chest, which is often seen, is long and narrow, the intercostal spaces are wide, the ribs are more vertically placed than normal, and the costal angle is narrow. "Scapulae, having the appearance of wings" were noted by Hippocrates (Fig. 253).

Palpation. The value of palpation in this stage is not great. The tactile fremitus shows little or no difference on the two sides. There may be, however, a rigidity of the muscles over the affected area, as pointed out by Pottenger. One of the greatest values of palpation is to confirm the difference in expansion on the two sides. This is easily determined by watching for the difference in movement during respiration of two hands placed on either side of the chest.

Percussion. Theoretically, there should be and is a difference in the resonance in comparing the affected side of the chest with the normal side. In practice, however, this difference may be difficult to determine, since resonance is a relative term and there is normally a difference in the resonance at the two apices. Unless this difference is marked, percussion of the apices to detect the changes in resonance in early tuberculosis is usually of little value. A retraction of the isthmus of Krönig (p. 113) on one side may, however, point out immediately the presence and location of an early tuberculous lesion.

Auscultation. One of the earliest changes in normal auscultation is the appearance of granular breathing. Granular breathing is a rough "spluttering" type of respiration, characteristic when heard, but difficult to describe. As Landis remarks, "One gets the impression that rales are about to be heard, but as a matter of fact are not."

In early tuberculosis, rales are not heard during ordinary quiet respiration. After deep inspiration, however, dry crackling rales may be heard above and below the clavicle and above the spine of the scapula on the side involved. These rales can often be demonstrated by having the patient cough after a deep expiration. If the dry crackling rales are limited to one apex and do not disappear after deep breathing and coughing, there is strong evidence for the existence of early pulmonary tuberculosis.

Second Stage, or Moderately Advanced, Tuberculosis

In this stage the loss of weight is more obvious, temperature elevations more marked and anemia quite noticeable, in spite of the flushed cheeks which may be present. The cough is more constant and now productive.

Inspection. The clavicle on the affected side is prominent and the supraclavicular and infraclavicular fossae are deep. The diminished expansion on the affected side is obvious. In testing for Litten's sign, there may be a lessened excursion of the diaphragm on the side which contains the more advanced changes.

Palpation. The vocal fremitus may be increased on the affected side.

Percussion. The impaired resonance over the affected apex is now quite obvious. If the other apex is involved, it too may show some impairment in resonance. Krönig's isthmus shows more contraction at the affected apex. Percussion at the bases shows a diminution in expansion on the side more markedly involved.

Auscultation. The breath sounds are now definitely bronchovesicular. In areas which show marked infiltration the breath sounds are clearly bronchial. Cavernous, or amphoric, breathing may appear as the result of cavity formation. A pleural friction rub may be heard. Medium-sized rales are heard, the result

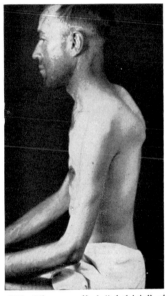

FIG. 253. The so-called "phthisic" chest.

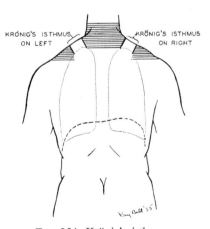

KRÖNIG'S ISTHMUS ON LEFT   KRÖNIG'S ISTHMUS ON RIGHT

FIG. 254. Krönig's isthmus.

of an accompanying bronchitis and caseation. The rales may be numerous or sparse. The more numerous the rales, the more extensive are the areas of softening, and as a rule this means a more serious prognosis.

Third Stage, or Advanced, Tuberculosis

The diagnosis of advanced pulmonary tuberculosis is often possible almost at a glance. It is, however, often very difficult to determine the exact extent of the pulmonary lesion because of the varied pathologic changes which have taken place.

Inspection. A patient in this stage of pulmonary tuberculosis presents the classic picture of emaciation and wasting, from which it received the name of consumption or phthisis. The cheeks are flushed, the flushing being often more marked on the side of the more advanced lesions and occurring particularly with the elevation in temperature. The fingernails may be curved over the tips of the fingers, and clubbed fingers are seen in approximately one-fifth of the cases. Both apices show retraction, and the chest may be flattened. The heart may be pulled over toward the affected side, a dislocation which is obvious on looking for the point of maximal impulse.

Palpation. If there is a cavity at the apex, the vocal fremitus will be increased in this area. The degree and location of the increased vocal fremitus depend upon the degree and location of the infiltration beneath. Rhonchi may be palpated.

Percussion. Over areas of cavitation the percussion note will be tympanitic and high-pitched, and may have an amphoric character. Cracked-pot resonance may be elicited. In areas near the cavity where the lung is heavily infiltrated, the percussion note is dull. As one passes on to the more healthy lung areas, the percussion note may be hyper-resonant as the result of compensatory emphysema.

Flatness may result from a large area of consolidation or from a complicating pleural effusion. With consolidation, the vocal fremitus is increased, while rales and bronchial breathing are heard. In pleural effusion the characteristic absence or diminution of the vocal fremitus and breath sounds is noted. Pleural effusion is sometimes mistaken for advanced pulmonary tuberculosis.

Auscultation. The most distinctive lesion of the third stage of pulmonary tuberculosis is cavitation, which shows the characteristic cavernous or amphoric breathing, exaggeration of the whispered and spoken voice and rales, the latter being coarse and bubbling or having a metallic quality. If the cavities are dry, rales may be absent. The auscultatory findings over the other areas of the lung depend upon the degree of involvement. Rales are usually widely diffused, and over areas of infiltration bronchovesicular or bronchial breathing may be heard.

Pulmonary Fibrosis

Pulmonary fibrosis has also been called chronic pneumonia, interstitial pneumonia, cirrhosis of the lung and fibroid phthisis. Fibroid tuberculosis is a distinct form due to infection with the tubercle bacillus. The physical findings are similar in all cases of pulmonary fibrosis, regardless of the etiology, since the underlying pathologic changes are identical.

Pulmonary fibrosis is essentially a chronic disease. The patients usually give a history of chronic cough with some expectoration, dyspnea on exertion and occasional attacks of hemoptysis.

Inspection. The affected side is usually shrunken, often motionless. There is often a marked scoliosis, the angle being away from the affected side. Litten's sign is absent on the affected side, but present on the normal side. Displacement of the heart towards the affected side may be apparent from the location of the point of maximal impulse. Clubbing of the fingers may be present.

Palpation. The vocal fremitus may be increased or diminished over the affected side.

Percussion. The percussion note shows impairment over the affected side, increased resonance over the normal side.

Auscultation. The breath sounds are diminished in intensity over the fibrotic lung. Fine crackling rales may be heard, or they may be absent.

CARCINOMA OF THE LUNGS

Carcinoma of the lung, formerly considered a rare disease, is now recognized with increasing frequency. Carcinoma almost invariably arises from the bronchi and extends by direct invasion of the surrounding tissues, or by metastases, to more distant parts of the lungs or to other organs. This disease is frequently mistaken for pulmonary tuberculosis, lung abscess or bronchiectasis.

The physical signs are varied and by no means pathognomonic. The patient not infrequently dies from metastases to other organs before any abnormal physical signs in the chest have become evident. Occasionally a patient is operated upon for a brain tumor and the diagnosis established by study of sections from the cerebral metastasis. The frequency of cerebral metastases in carcinoma of the lungs has long been recognized. Bayle, in 1810, described a patient "in a state bordering on idiocy," who showed at autopsy cancer of the lung with metastasis to the brain. When the carcinoma extends to the surface of the lung, we find increased vocal fremitus, impaired resonance, harsh or tubular breathing and rales—the classic signs of consolidation, whether due to tuberculosis, lobar pneumonia or carcinoma. Frequently carcinoma of the lungs causes obstruction of the bronchus, producing atelectasis, which shows characteristic physical findings—impaired resonance, diminished intensity of breath sounds, and displacement of the heart and trachea toward the affected side.

Carcinoma of the lung should be suspected in patients over fifty years of age who have considerable expectoration, which is at times bloody, who show varying but definite pathologic findings in different areas of the lung, and in whom pulmonary tuberculosis can be excluded. The history of a gradual, insidious onset is the rule. The diagnosis can be established only by the roentgen ray, by bronchoscopic examination or by identification of tumor cells in the sputum. The clinical history with characteristic roentgen ray findings may suffice for the diagnosis. If we defer diagnosis until definite abnormal physical findings are present, it is often too late for effective surgical treatment.

ABSCESS OF THE LUNGS

Abscess of the lung may be a complication of bronchopneumonia and of bronchiectasis. It also commonly follows inspiration of microorganisms from the buccal cavity after tonsillectomy or extraction of teeth. The aspiration of foreign bodies, such as pins, beans and peanuts, into the bronchi is also a frequent cause, since they are seldom sterile.

The onset of abscess of the lung is usually acute, with a chill and rapidly rising fever. Copious purulent sputum soon appears and with it a distressing paroxysmal cough. In chronic cases the acute symptoms subside, but the cough and expectoration continue as well as an irregular temperature.

The physical findings in the early stages of lung abscess may be slight, or pathologic changes may be entirely lacking, since the abscess is commonly deep-seated. Impairment of the percussion note and fine rales may be present. In chronic cases the signs of extensive infiltration or of consolidation may be present, with impairment of the percussion note and numerous fine or bubbling moist rales. At this stage the physical signs closely resemble those of advanced pulmonary tuberculosis, a disease with which it is commonly confused. Clubbing of the fingers is frequently seen in chronic lung abscess.

The diagnosis of lung abscess may be suspected from the history and physical findings, but is usually established by roentgen rays. The history, together with the age of the patient, helps differentiate it from carcinoma of the lungs, while an examination of the sputum differentiates it from pulmonary tuberculosis.

INFARCTION OF THE LUNGS

Infarction of the lung is due to an occlusion of the pulmonary artery, or its branches, by an embolus or thrombus. Thrombi may arise in one of the systemic veins, in the right auricle, in the right ventricle or in the pulmonary artery itself, and, becoming dislodged, produce pulmonary embolism. Pulmonary embolism may occur in chronic heart disease, in typhoid fever and occasionally as a tragic sequel to abdominal operations and to childbirth. The thrombosis of any systemic vein may lead to pulmonary embolism.

Small infarctions may give rise to no symptoms; infarctions of moderate size cause pleuritic pain, dyspnea, cyanosis, cough and bloody expectoration; while large infarctions commonly produce sudden death. The physical findings in infarction of the lung are not characteristic. If the infarcted area is near the periphery of the lung, there may be some impairment of percussion note on percussion, and on auscultation a friction rub, crackling rales and enfeeblement of the breath sounds.

EDEMA OF THE LUNGS

Edema of the lungs is common in congestive heart failure with failing compensation, in lobar pneumonia and in the late stages of chronic nephritis. Acute edema of the lungs usually appears quickly in pulmonary infarctions of moderate or large size, and it may also appear rapidly, with little or no warning, in cardiac disease, especially in mitral stenosis, in chronic nephritis, in hypertensive cardiovascular disease and occasionally following thoracentesis, when an excessive amount of fluid is withdrawn.

In acute edema of the lungs the onset is sudden and the patient becomes cyanotic and dyspneic. The skin is cold and sweaty, and a severe cough appears. The expectoration is watery, frothy and foamy, and may later be blood-tinged. The percussion note may be impaired, and, on auscultation, numerous rales are heard all over the chest; fine moist rales early in the attack, course bubbling rales later. The respiration is often so noisy and rattling that the rales can be heard at some distance from the patient. The rales are commonly more numerous on the right side and a right-sided pleural effusion is commoner than a left.

SUMMARY

The following findings are the outstanding physical signs in the diseases of the lungs we have just considered.

Acute Bronchitis. Early in the disease musical rales are heard, later small and large moist rales. There is a purulent expectoration. The patient's temperature is seldom markedly elevated.

Bronchiectasis. Patients usually give a history of expectorating large amounts of purulent, fetid sputum, particularly on arising in the morning. Clubbed fingers are common. As a rule, there is no dulness over the chest on percussion. Numerous moist bubbling rales are present.

Emphysema. The patient commonly shows dyspnea, some cyanosis, deep chest of the so-called "barrel" shape, and shallow respiration. The percussion note over the lungs is hyperresonant, and the area of cardiac dulness is reduced. Auscultation reveals nothing pathognomonic.

Bronchial Asthma. Attacks are paroxysmal, accompanied by great dyspnea and a wheezing cough which at first is very tight. The sputum is thick and tenacious. Rhonchi are felt over the chest on palpation. Percussion usually shows a hyperresonant note. On auscultation, rales of all types are heard over the chest, those of the musical variety being most numerous. These rales are often heard at some distance from the patient.

Pleurisy. Acute fibrinous pleurisy has as its characteristic feature diminution of respiratory movement over the involved side and a friction rub. Pleurisy with effusion shows a diminished vocal fremitus, percussion note from dull to flat, breath sounds diminished or absent, over the involved area. Skodaic resonance is often heard above the fluid level, and on auscultation egophony is heard in the same location. Percussion shows that the heart is pushed away from the side of the effusion, and Grocco's triangular area of dulness may be demonstrated over the back.

A thickened pleura shows contraction of the chest on the involved side with diminution of the respiratory movements. The percussion note is dull or flat over the thickened pleura. Percussion of the heart shows it to be drawn toward the affected side. The breath sounds are usually diminished over the thickened pleura. Occasionally a friction rub is heard.

Pneumothorax. The chest on the affected side is immobile, the intercostal depressions are obliterated, and percussion usually shows a hyperresonant or tympanitic note. Occasionally, however, the percussion note is dull. Percussion of cardiac dulness shows the heart to be pushed away from the side of the pneumothorax. On auscultation the breath sounds are markedly diminished over the affected side and exaggerated on the normal side. The "coin sound" is commonly present, and in hydropneumothorax the "Hippocratic succussion" may be elicited.

Pulmonary Atelectasis. Pulmonary atelectasis is clinically most important as a massive collapse of the lung. In this condition the patient shows severe dyspnea, cyanosis, prostration, and diminution of respiratory movements on the affected side. The vocal fremitus is usually decreased. The percussion note on the affected side is usually dull. Percussion of the heart shows it to be displaced toward the affected side, the reverse of pneumothorax.

Lobar Pneumonia. Lobar pneumonia generally has a characteristically sudden onset. Dyspnea, cyanosis and cough appear early. Inspection shows the respiratory movements to be decreased over the affected side. The vocal fremitus is greatly increased over the involved area, where percussion shows a dull or flat note. Auscultation in the early stage shows diminution or suppression of the breath sounds. After consolidation the breath sounds are harsh and have a characteristic tubular character.

Bronchopneumonia. The signs of bronchopneumonia in the early stages are essentially those of acute bronchitis. As the disease progresses and consolidation appears, the signs are those of lobar pneumonia. It is often impossible to differentiate by physical examination alone between bronchopneumonia and lobar pneumonia.

Chronic Pulmonary Tuberculosis. The findings in chronic pulmonary tuberculosis vary with the degree of lung involvement. In the early stages the signs may be slight indeed. Persistent fine, moist rales at the apex are significant. In advanced tuberculosis with extensive consolidations, the physical findings are those of consolidation due to any cause—increased vocal fremitus, dulness on percussion, and harsh or tubular breathing.

When cavitation is present, we may obtain cracked-pot resonance or amphoric resonance on percussion and on auscultation hear amphoric breathing over the cavity.

Carcinoma of the Lungs. Carcinoma of the lungs shows no pathognomonic findings. When consolidation is present, we see the classic findings of increased vocal fremitus, impaired resonance, and tubular breathing. When the tumor obstructs the bronchus, we have the physical findings of atelectasis with impaired resonance, diminished intensity of the breath sounds and the mediastinal shift toward the side of the lesion.

Abscess of the Lung. Abscess of the lung may be suspected from the history. Copious, purulent sputum and a persistent cough are suggestive. The most common physical findings are impairment of the percussion note and fine or bubbling moist rales. In many patients the abscess is so deep that it produces few or no changes in the physical findings.

Infarction of the Lung. Pulmonary embolism and infarction of the lung are dramatic causes of sudden death. Smaller infarctions produce dyspnea, cyanosis and bloody expectoration. Such patients may show impairment of the percussion note over the infarcted area, friction rub and crackling rales.

Edema of the Lungs. The most marked findings in edema of the lungs are cyanosis, dyspnea and frothy expectoration. On auscultation bubbling rales are heard throughout the chest, these rales often being heard at some distance from the patient.

ROENTGEN RAY IN DIAGNOSIS OF PULMONARY DISEASE

The use of the roentgen ray in the diagnosis of pulmonary disease has not only aided enormously in the accuracy of our diagnosis, but has influenced profoundly our concepts of the origin and development of many pathologic lesions in the lungs. While this subject is a specialty in itself, a few references to its contributions will be made.

Bronchiectasis. In bronchiectasis the lungs may show evidence of generalized fibrosis at the bases. After injection of lipiodol or iodized oil into the bronchi, the walls of the latter are clearly shown with their irregular surfaces, bulblike dilatations and general coarseness in outline as compared with the smooth surface of normal bronchi with their feathery outlines. Such a roentgen picture in bronchiectasis usually permits the diagnosis without equivocation.

Pleurisy. Acute fibrinous pleurisy may show some cloudiness over the affected area. In pleurisy with effusion the effusion is shown as a dense shadow which changes in intensity with change of the patient's position. The upper level of the fluid is usually sharply delineated. In large effusions displacement of the heart toward the normal side is obvious.

Pneumothorax. The chest on the affected side shows an absence of the normal lung markings. The outlines of the collapsed lung are clearly seen. The displacement of the heart toward the normal side is clearly seen. When there is an accompanying hydrothorax, the fluid is seen to splash on shaking the patient.

Pulmonary Atelectasis. In this condition the collapsed lung is seen as a dense shadow. The drawing over the heart toward the collapsed lung is usually apparent.

Lobar Pneumonia. The areas of consolidation are clearly seen as dense shadows. Such areas of consolidation are often visible in the roentgen plate when they are too deeply situated to give clear physical signs. Many unsuspected areas of consolidation are revealed only by the roentgen ray. Similarly small areas of consolidation in bronchopneumonia are diagnosed only by the roentgen ray.

Chronic Pulmonary Tuberculosis. The physician of today would enjoy the reactions of Bayle, Fournet and Laennec if they could but see the great advances and refinements in the diagnosis of pulmonary tuberculosis which the roentgen ray has achieved. Miliary tuberculosis is diagnosed by the presence of numerous minute shadows in the lung parenchyma, whereas Bayle diagnosed the condition at autopsy. Incipient tuberculosis is seen in the small but clearly defined infiltration at the apex, while Fournet faced a skeptical profession who doubted his ability to diagnose early tuberculosis. The areas of infiltration, consolidation and cavitation are shown in roentgen plates with the clarity almost of diagrammatic drawings, a precision which Laennec, even with his great skill in examining the chest, could not attain.

Carcinoma of the Lung. A neoplasm in the pulmonary tissue often casts a clear shadow in the roentgenogram, often allowing a positive diagnosis when the history and physical findings at most permit a tentative one. Areas of atelectasis supervening on carcinoma are easily recognized.

Abscess of the lung and infarction of the lung produce areas of consolidation or infiltration which cast clearly recognizable shadows.

BIBLIOGRAPHY

Bayle, G. L.: Recherches sur la Phthisie Pulmonaire. Paris, Gabon, 1810.

Brown, Lawrason: The Story of Clinical Pulmonary Tuberculosis. Baltimore, Williams & Wilkins, 1941.

Cecil, Russell L., and Loeb, R. F.: A Textbook of Medicine. 9th ed. Philadelphia, W. B. Saunders Co., 1955.

Fishberg, Maurice: Pulmonary Tuberculosis. 2d ed. Philadelphia, Lea & Febiger, 1919.

Graham, E. A., Singer, J. J., and Ballon, H. C.: Surgical Diseases of the Chest. Philadelphia, Lea & Febiger, 1935.

Hamman, Louis: The diagnosis of pulmonary tuberculosis. Am. Rev. Tuberc. *1*:207, 1917.

Musser, John H. (M. E. Wehl, Ed.): Internal Medicine, Its Theory and Practice. 5th ed. Philadelphia, Lea & Febiger, 1951.

Norris, George William, and Landis, Henry R. M.: Diseases of the Chest and the Principles of Physical Diagnosis. 6th ed. Philadelphia, W. B. Saunders Co., 1938.

Osler, Sir William: Modern Medicine. 3rd ed. Re-edited by Thomas McCrae. Philadelphia, Lea & Febiger, 1927, Vol. 4.

Osler, Sir William: The Principles and Practice of Medicine. New York, D. Appleton & Co., 1892.

Pottenger, Francis Marion: Clinical Tuberculosis. 2d ed. St. Louis, C. V. Mosby Co., 1922, Vols. 1 and 2.

Pottenger, Francis Marion: Tuberculosis in the Child and the Adult. St. Louis, C. V. Mosby Co., 1934.

Pullen, Roscoe L.: Medical Diagnosis, Applied Physical Diagnosis. 2d ed. Philadelphia, W. B. Saunders Co., 1950.

CHAPTER 9

INSPECTION, PALPATION AND PERCUSSION OF THE HEART

In BEGINNING OUR EXAMINATION of the heart, it is helpful to keep in mind the gross anatomy of the normal heart and the manner in which it is projected against the chest wall (Fig. 255). The right ventricle occupies the largest area,

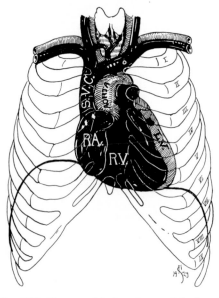

FIG. 255. Topographical anatomy of the heart.

156

the right auricle a smaller area, and the left ventricle a relatively thin strip. In cardiac disease these relationships may be profoundly altered.

INSPECTION

On inspection of the heart we look first for the *point of maximal impulse* (P.M.I.), which is often incorrectly called the apex beat. This thrust of the heart was first carefully studied by William Harvey, who wrote in his *De Motu Cordis:* "The heart is lifted, and rises up to the apex, so that it strikes the chest at that moment and the beat may be felt on the outside." The impulse that we see and feel on the normal chest wall is the impulse, not of the apex, but that of the left ventricle proximal to the apex. The apex itself is covered by the lung, and is usually 0.5 cm. to the left of the point of maximum impulse. The correctness of this statement has been repeatedly proved by percussion and by the roentgen ray. The importance of this observation is obvious. The point of maximum impulse does not represent the extreme left border of the heart as the apex does.

The apex of the heart does not move appreciably up or down during systole. The transverse diameter shortens more than the longitudinal diameter. As Hirschfelder has shown, the movements of the heart during systole push the apex of the heart against the chest wall, while the anterior and right wall of the heart move inward toward the septum (Fig. 256). Thus, during systole, we have a protrusion of the left ventricle, but a retraction of the right. This observation is important, since, if the right ventricle is hypertrophied, or not covered by the lung, systolic retraction may be more obvious than systolic protrusion.

The point of maximum impulse is best seen in patients with a thin chest wall. In patients who are markedly emaciated the impulse may be so widespread and seem so forceful that cardiac disease may be suspected when none is present. In patients with marked development of the chest musculature, or in obese persons, it is seen with less distinctness. In a person with an emphysematous chest the cardiac impulse may not be seen at all. In dextrocardia the cardiac impulse is on the right instead of on the left side.

Point of Maximum Impulse. The first question which confronts the examiner is the position of the point of maximum impulse. When present, it is normally located in or about the fifth costal interspace inside the left midclavicular line. However, as Niehaus and Wright

have pointed out the "overall demonstrability of the apex for all ages and weights, and both sexes, is only 24.6 per cent instead of the implied 100 per cent."

The point of maximum impulse normally changes during deep inspiration and on change in position. When a patient takes a deep inspiration and holds his breath, the point of maximum impulse moves downward from the fifth to the sixth interspace. When the patient lies on his right side, it moves slightly toward the right, and when he lies on his left side it moves about 2 cm. toward the left. The absence of mobility leads one to suspect an adherent pericardium. However, as Broadbent pointed out, we should remember that a deep inspiration may bring the lungs over the heart so that the impulse disappears altogether. Disappearance of the impulse on inspiration does not necessarily mean that the heart is freely movable. Similarly, when the patient lies on the right side, change in the point of maximum impulse may only mean that another part of the heart has been brought in contact with the chest wall and not that the apex has shifted.

Marked enlargement of the heart produces a displacement of the point of maximum impulse to the left. Under such conditions it is outside the mammillary line, often in the anterior axillary line or even in the mid-axillary line. In mitral disease the impulse is displaced laterally, while in aortic disease it is displaced both laterally and downward (Fig. 257).

Any pathologic process affecting the position of the heart may produce a displacement of the point of the maximum impulse. A right-sided pleural effusion displaces it toward the left axilla, while a left-sided pleural effusion displaces it toward the right (Fig. 250). Pleural adhesions, mediastinal tumors and pneumothorax may produce similar displacements.

The *character of the impulse* may give information of great value. In aortic insufficiency the cardiac impulse has a

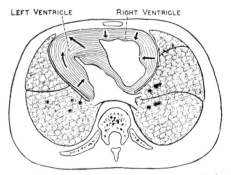

LEFT VENTRICLE   RIGHT VENTRICLE

FIG. 256. Movements of the heart producing protrusions and retractions during systole. (After Hirschfelder.)

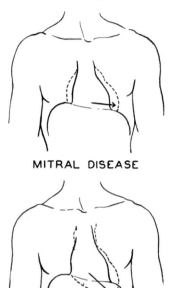

MITRAL DISEASE

AORTIC DISEASE

FIG. 257. Displacement of apex in mitral and aortic disease.

characteristic appearance almost sufficient for diagnosis. There is a slow, vigorous lifting of the interspace, the so-called "dome-shaped" or rounded heaving thrust.

The *force of the impulse* should be studied. The force as well as the heart rate is often increased in persons who have normal hearts, but are very nervous because of the examination. In such persons, as the examination proceeds and the patient becomes more composed, the heart rate slows, the intensity of the cardiac contractions diminishes and the force of the impulse lessens. The force of the impulse by no means coincides with the force of the cardiac contraction. A soft, flabby, dilated heart may make greater excursions in systole than a smaller, more powerfully contracting heart, and thus show not only a larger area of pulsation, but appear to contract more powerfully.

The *amplitude* of the point of maximal impulse depends in part upon the thickness of the chest wall, whether it lies under the rib or the interspace, and upon the character and thickness of the lung which covers it. The extent of the cardiac impulse depends largely upon the force and volume of the systole. In aortic insufficiency when the heart beats forcefully, the area is extensive, but, as previously mentioned, a dilated, flabby, weakly contracting heart may also show a large area of cardiac pulsation.

"Herzstoss." In some patients there is no definite point of maximum impulse seen or felt. The whole precordium, or a considerable part of it, rises *en masse* during systole. This phenomenon is called "Herzstoss" by the Germans in contradistinction to "Spitzenstoss" (apex beat). The term "Herzstoss" has found its way into English medical terminology, for lack of an accurate and suitable English word. It is seen especially in flat-chested patients with hypertrophied hearts.

Systolic Retraction. This phenomenon, also described as a "negative cardiac impulse," was first studied by Skoda, who considered it a sign of adhesive pericarditis. It should be remembered, however, that during systole there is normally some retraction of the intercostal spaces near the point of maximum impulse. If the point of maximum impulse lies under a rib, the observer sees only the retraction of the intercostal spaces. According to some observers, this reaction of the precordium is due to negative intrathoracic pressure produced by a hypertrophied right ventricle or by an unusually forcible action of the heart.

Systolic retraction is a normal occurrence. Eden's advice is sound: that before we make a diagnosis of adhesive pericarditis, we should be sure "that not only the interspaces, but also the ribs themselves are retracted during systole."

Diastolic Heart Beat. "The diastolic heart beat is an outward thrust that can be seen and felt during diastole, occurring in the absence of a normal apical systolic impulse, and accompanied by a proto-diastolic sound" (Wood). This sign, first described by Skoda in 1852 and by Friedreich in 1864, has been recently studied by Wood and his associates. It is usually associated with a systolic retraction of the precordium and a sudden diastolic emptying of the cervical veins. The diastolic heart beat, when accompanied by an absent systolic apex impulse, a systolic retraction of the precordium, and a sudden diastolic emptying of the cervical veins, is a pathognomonic sign of pericardial scar.

Broadbent's Sign. The sign, first observed by Sir William Broadbent and first published by his son Walter Broadbent in 1895, is of value in the diagnosis of adherent pericardium. Walter Broadbent described four cases "in each of which there is visible retraction, synchronous with the cardiac systole, of the left back in the region of the eleventh and twelfth ribs, and in three of which there is also systolic retraction of less degree in the same region of the right back." Sir William Broadbent later noted that "this indication is not infallible, as the tugging has been observed when the heart was hypertrophied without adhesions."

Rate and Rhythm. Inspection of the cardiac impulse with careful observation of the rate and rhythm of the cardiac contractions is of extreme importance.

The rate is increased in a variety of conditions producing *tachycardia* such as hyperthyroidism, acute febrile diseases and severe anemias. The most striking type of tachycardia is that known as paroxysmal tachycardia, in which the heart has paroxysms of rapid beating with a rate of 200 or over, usually appearing suddenly and ceasing just as suddenly as it began. This extremely rapid heart action, obvious at the point of maximum impulse, is also extremely forceful and accompanied by forceful pulsations of the entire precordium. The heart rate is slowed in heart block, the slow rate of 40 or 50 being readily recognized by the cardiac impulse.

In cardiac irregularities, information of extreme importance can be obtained by inspection of the cardiac impulse alone. Indeed, one may say without exaggeration that the important clinical varieties of cardiac irregularities can be diagnosed by inspection of the cardiac impulse.

Sinus arrhythmia, called formerly by Mackenzie "the youthful type of irregularity," is readily recognized. The heart beats more rapidly during inspiration than during expiration.

Extrasystoles or, more accurately, premature contractions, also called, inaccurately, "dropped beats," are easily seen at the point of maximum impulse. The heart beats regularly for a time, then there is a pause, and after a moment the beats resume their normal rhythm. The premature contraction may or may not be seen, but the longer pause following it is obvious.

Auricular fibrillation is readily recognized by inspection of the point of maximum impulse. This condition was formerly called "delirium cordis"—cardiac delirium. This term describes the behavior of the heart very well. Inspection shows that the cardiac action is utterly irregular both in force and rhythm, strong impulses alternating with weak impulses at times, then followed by a series of strong beats; pauses of varying lengths, alternating with runs of rapid beats in which the heart seems to be racing.

King has called attention to a "visible apical reduplication" as an important diagnostic sign in bundle-branch block. He found this sign in 84 per cent of his cases. This double or "bifid" thrust may be recorded by a cardiogram (Fig. 258). It may also be made very evident by fastening a light straw upon the chest

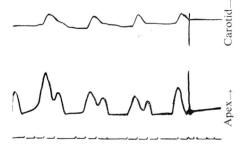

FIG. 258. "Bifid" apex thrust. (King.)

over the point of maximum impulse. We have used this method, following King's suggestion, to demonstrate this finding before groups of students.

A presystolic gallop rhythm may also produce a reduplication of the cardiac impulse. Here, however, according to King, there is a presystolic lift preceding the ventricular impulse; in block the split is in the main ventricular lift. King's differentiation seems to be demonstrated by his tracings.

The significance and explanation of these variations in the rate and rhythm of the cardiac contractions will be further discussed when we consider the pulse.

The Precordium. The precordium and the anterior surface of the chest should be carefully examined for the presence of abnormal pulsations. Marked pulsation in the first and second right interspaces outside the sternal border should make one suspicious of aneurysm of the ascending arch of the aorta. In

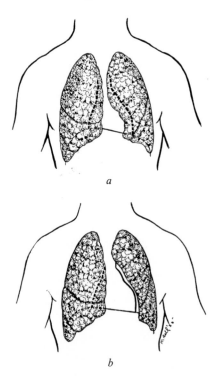

a

b

Fig. 259. Increase in area of cardiac pulsation by retraction of the left lung: *a*, lung of normal size; *b*, markedly retracted lung.

aneurysms such a pulsation is expansile. Marked pulsation at the base of the heart is seen in aortic insufficiency, in a dilated aorta or a saccular aneurysm. It may be due at times to the extremely forceful action of a violently beating heart. In aneurysm of the ascending aorta and of the sinus of Valsalva there may be diffuse heaving of the sternum. Pulsation in the third, fourth and fifth left interspaces suggests dilation of the left ventricle. Marked pulsation in the sternal notch occurs in aortic insufficiency and aneurysms. More commonly it is due to arteriosclerosis of the aorta, an "uncoiled aorta."

A marked retraction of the left lung due to fibrous tuberculosis may uncover a large area of the heart and produce a wide and forceful area of cardiac pulsation (Fig. 259).

PALPATION

The first aim of palpation should be to confirm inspection. In those patients in which we have not been sure of the location of the point of maximum impulse, palpation makes us certain. Often one is unable to see the impulse, but can feel it, and in that way gain information regarding the location and size of the heart. The various disturbances in rate and rhythm which have been observed can be confirmed by palpation.

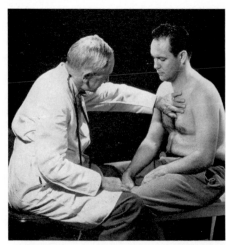

Fig. 260. Palpation of base of heart.

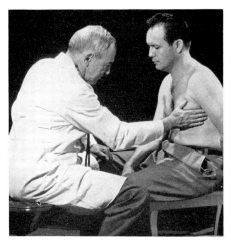

FIG. 261. Palpation of the point of maximum impulse.

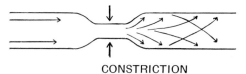

CONSTRICTION

FIG. 262. Production of thrill in a tube by constriction.

Palpation gives us a better impression of the force of the heart beat than does inspection. Often the impulse appears both forceful and extensive, but on palpation proves to be weak, though present over a large area.

Pericardial Friction Rub. On palpation over the precordium a friction fremitus may be felt in fibrinous pericarditis. This fremitus is synchronous with the heart beat and is not affected by respiration. It is produced by the roughened visceral and parietal pericardium rubbing upon each other. This sign was described by Hope as a "vibratory tremour generally perceptible to the hand." When a pericardial effusion follows fibrinous pericarditis, the friction rub disappears.

Thrills. Corrigan showed that thrills could be produced by attaching a piece of rubber tubing to a water faucet, turning on the water and constricting the tubing at a certain point. This constriction produces numerous eddies, twists and turns in the current of the stream below the constriction, thus causing vibrations in the wall of the tubing. These vibrations are felt as thrills and heard as murmurs. Above the constriction there are no eddies, and as a result no thrills or murmurs (Fig. 262).

Presystolic Thrill. The presystolic thrill felt near the apex of the heart is pathognomonic of mitral stenosis. Corvisart, who first noted this sign, described it as "a thrill particularly difficult to describe, felt by the hand when applied to the pericardial region." Laennec with more imagination described it as "frémissement cataire" (cat's purring tremor) and added that it "may be compared quite accurately to the vibration which accompanies the sound of satisfaction which a cat makes when one strokes it with the hand." Laennec remarked that a similar sensation may be produced by stroking the palm of a gloved hand with a rough brush.

The presystolic thrill of mitral stenosis is usually felt only over a small area at or near the point of maximum impulse. It is as a rule better felt in a heart which is beating forcefully. It may not be felt when the patient is lying quietly in bed, but may be brought out by moving the patient up and down rather rapidly a few times and thus producing more active cardiac contractions, and also by turning the patient on his left side.

The novice and, for that matter, the more experienced observer may have difficulty in timing the thrill. Careful examination, however, will reveal that the thrill precedes the systolic shock or thrust by just a fraction of a second, and is therefore presystolic in time. Simultaneous auscultation of the heart will convince the examiner that he feels the thrill just before he hears the first heart sound.

Systolic Thrills. A systolic thrill may be felt over the precordium with its maximum intensity at the aortic area in aortic stenosis. This thrill is usually rough and purring, and commonly of greater intensity than any other thrill felt over the heart. Some observers have maintained that the diagnosis of aortic stenosis cannot be safely made in the absence of this sign, but this is an extreme view. This systolic thrill of aortic stenosis is felt in the carotid and brachial arteries and is transmitted in the direction of the blood flow.

In pulmonary stenosis a rough systolic thrill is felt over the pulmonary area and from here is transmitted upward and diagonally toward the left clavicle and downward over the precordium.

In aneurysm of the ascending aorta, which produces a definite area of pulsation, a systolic thrill may be felt over this area. More characteristic, however, is the diastolic shock due to forcible closure of the semilunar valves, which, when present, is often of great intensity and is a valuable sign of aneurysm.

PERCUSSION OF THE HEART

Percussion of the heart was first performed by Auenbrugger, who observed on percussing the chest that "where the heart is located the sound obtained has a certain fullness showing clearly that the more solid portion of the heart, located there, dulls somewhat the ringing resonance." Corvisart used this method and discusses its value in his translation of Auenbrugger and in his treatise on heart disease. Laennec learned the procedure from his master, Corvisart. It was used and further developed by Piorry and Skoda.

Percussion of the cardiac outlines has been the cause of more controversy than almost any other subject in the field of physical diagnosis. Some distinguished students of physical diagnosis have in recent years stated that percussion of the cardiac outlines is so notoriously unreliable that they no longer attempt it, but rely solely upon the position of the point of maximum impulse as the only reliable index of the point to which the heart extends on the left. They also find that the only reliable guide to the size of the heart is the x-ray picture. Unfortunately, in many instances no cardiac impulse is visible, and in many instances the use of the x-ray is impossible. The physician always has his fingers and ears with him at the bedside of the patient, even when he is miles away from an x-ray laboratory.

A study of Figure 263 may explain in part this "defeatist" attitude on the part of certain physicians. This diagram of Moritz illustrates graphically the different results obtained by competent

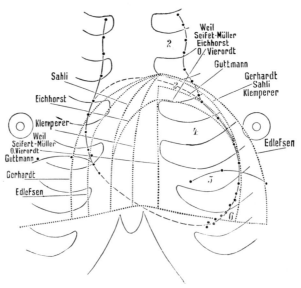

FIG. 263. Cardiac outline in percussion, according to various authors. (Moritz.)

observers who have recorded their views as to the outlines of the normal heart, obtained on percussion.

This difference of opinion is explained in part by the remark of Friedrich Müller that "we must not explore the chest by percussing our ideas into it." Many of these ideas we obtain by a study of the cardiac outlines in textbooks of anatomy rather than in roentgenograms. In one instance we see the inert heart hardened by formalin and distended to its maximum by embalming fluid injected under pressure, while the roentgenogram shows the heart as it is during life. A similar example is seen in comparing the pictures of the stomach, as portrayed commonly in textbooks of anatomy, with those obtained by studying the stomach under the fluoroscope or in the roentgen plate.

Much of the distrust of percussion arises from demanding of the method more than it will give. Percussion of the cardiac outlines is accurate only to a limited extent, but when we recognize these limitations, it is a valuable method of examination. Differences in opinion between two examiners as to the extent of cardiac dulness are to be expected. One observer, on percussing the heart, may consider it enlarged, while a second observer disagrees. Similar differences of opinion may exist between two roentgenologists who examine the same plate of a patient's chest or between two pathologists who see the same heart at autopsy. Careful percussion will usually reveal whether the heart is approximately normal in size or whether it is definitely or markedly enlarged. More than this we cannot expect of the most refined percussion.

Method of Percussion. Many beginners, in attempting to outline the cardiac dulness, strike too forcibly and thus fail to hear the slight change in the percussion note caused by the thin layer of overlying lung. One should use the lightest percussion possible and, with experience, rely more and more upon the vibratory sense. In percussing one should begin at the side and percuss

toward the sternum, since it is easier for the ear to appreciate a change from resonance to dulness than vice versa (Fig. 264). Similarly, the plessimeter finger recognizes more readily a change from the vibration over a resonant area to a diminished vibration over a dull area.

Personally, we prefer to hold the plessimeter finger parallel to the outlines of the heart rather than at right angles to it (Fig. 265), although good results may be obtained with the latter position. When the plessimeter finger is held parallel to the cardiac outlines, a larger number of vibrations cross the outlines than when the plessimeter finger

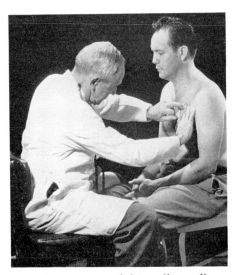

Fig. 264. Percussion of the cardiac outline.

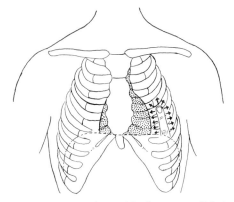

Fig. 265. Percussion with finger parallel to cardiac outlines.

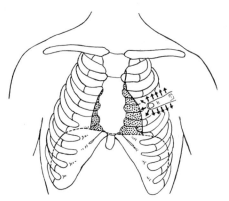

FIG. 266. Percussion with finger at right angle to cardiac outline.

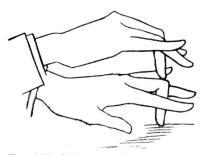

FIG. 267. Orthopercussion. (Külbs.)

is held at right angles to the cardiac outlines (Fig. 266).

Certain refinements and modifications of the ordinary methods of percussion have been devised by several observers. The *orthopercussion* method of Plesch is carried out by flexing the left middle finger to a right angle, placing the pulp of the finger on the area to be percussed, and then striking the flexed finger at the distal end of the first phalanx (Fig. 267). The *threshold method* of Ewald and Goldscheider consists in diminishing the strength of the percussion stroke over a flat area until no sound is heard, and then percussing with the same force until a sound becomes audible, when an area of resonance is encountered. It is based on the principle that a transition from no sound to sound is more readily perceived than a transition from a weak sound to a stronger one. Both these methods are recommended in the percussion of absolute cardiac dulness. These refinements of the ordinary methods may give excellent results in

the hands of experienced observers. The beginner should first master thoroughly the ordinary method; later he may experiment with its variants. He should follow the advice of Skoda and strike "with the middle finger bent in the form of a semicircle, avoid striking or grazing with the fingernails. In carrying out this percussion the movement should be only in the wrist and not in the shoulder, elbow, or joints of the hand."

Auscultatory percussion of the cardiac outlines often gives satisfactory results. In carrying out this method of percussion the stethoscope is placed over the lower part of the sternum, above the xiphoid, and the observer rubs or scratches lightly over the surface of the skin, beginning in the left anterior axillary line and gradually moving toward the sternum. At first a soft rubbing or scratchy sound is heard, but just as the border of relative cardiac dulness is reached the sound abruptly becomes intense. The right border of the heart may also be outlined by this method.

Cardiac Outlines. We have already noted in percussion of the chest that the left border of the normal heart and a part of both left and right ventricles are covered by lung tissue. Percussion over this part of the heart gives a note which is impaired or dull or diminished in resonance, but retains a certain degree of resonance. This area is called *relative cardiac dulness*

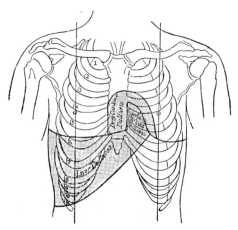

FIG. 268. Diagram of cardiac dulness.

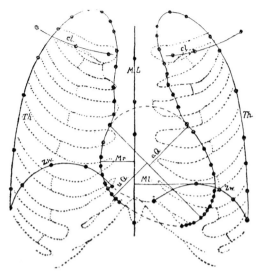

FIG. 269. Teleoroentgenogram of heart. (Seifert and Müller.)

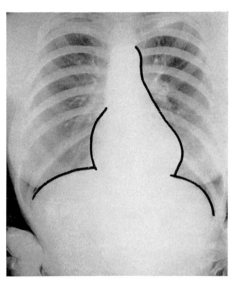

FIG. 270. Roentgenogram of normal heart.

(R.C.D.). As we percuss toward the sternum we presently encounter an area where the heart is no longer covered by the lung, there is no trace of resonance, and the percussion note is flat. The area is spoken of as the area of *absolute cardiac dulness* (A.C.D.). Most observers agree on these details. In an average normal man the relative cardiac dulness extends from 8 to 10 cm. to the left of the midsternal line in the fifth intercostal space inside the mammillary line.

Agreement is not so general in regard to the right border of the heart. Figure 268 is an illustration widely copied and used as an illustration in textbooks of physical diagnosis. Though we agree with the outlines of absolute (deep) cardiac dulness and the outlines of relative (superficial) cardiac dulness to the left, the line of cardiac dulness on the right is shown as identical with the right margin of the sternum. We believe that percussion over the sternum throws the entire sternum into vibration and makes it difficult, if not impossible, to mark out a line of relative cardiac dulness under the sternum. An examination of the teleoroentgenogram (Fig. 269), however, shows that in the fourth and fifth right interspaces the heart emerges from the sternum and lies to the right of it. This is easily confirmed by a study of chest roentgenograms (Figs. 270 and 271).

We believe that, on percussion of the normal heart, there is an area of relative dulness in the fourth right interspace to the right of the sternum, usually 4 to 5 cm. from the midsternal line, which represents the right border of the heart. In the interspaces above this, any change in percussion note encountered, as we percuss toward the midline, is due to the sternum (Fig. 272). The size

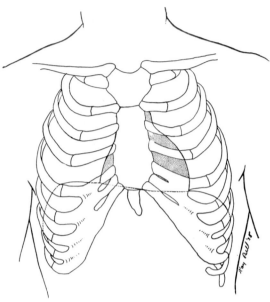

FIG. 271. Cardiac shadow drawn after study of series of normal chest roentgenograms.

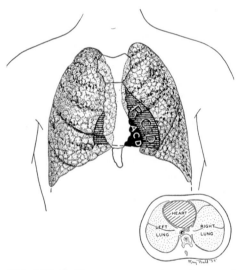

FIG. 272. Outlines on percussion of normal heart.

of the heart should be expressed in terms of centimeters from the midsternal line (M.S.L.), not in reference to the parasternal line on the right or the mammillary line on the left.

In women with large pendulous breasts it is often impossible to outline by percussion the left border of the heart. In most instances, however, if the breast is elevated, the examiner can determine the point to which relative cardiac dulness extends to the left. In some patients with the combination of obesity and large breasts, it may be impossible to obtain any accurate knowledge regarding the size of the heart by percussion.

Physiologic Changes in the Area of Cardiac Dulness. The position of the heart, and with it the area of cardiac dulness, is influenced by the level of the diaphragm. In deep inspiration the diaphragm descends, and the heart with it, producing a decrease in cardiac dulness, while in forced expiration the diaphragm rises and produces an increase in the cardiac dulness (Fig. 273).

In the later months of pregnancy the diaphragm is pushed upward, causing the heart to lie more horizontally and closer to the chest wall, thus increasing the area of cardiac dulness (Fig. 274). In pregnancy the diagnosis of an enlarged heart on the basis of percussion should be made with caution.

In some persons the heart has a vertical position which decreases the area of cardiac dulness, while other normal persons may have a heart which lies more horizontally, thus increasing the area of cardiac dulness.

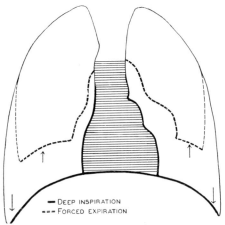

FIG. 273. Change in cardiac outlines produced by respiration.

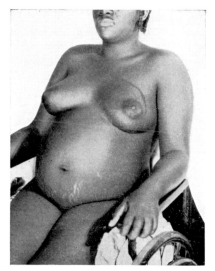

FIG. 274. Cardiac outlines in ninth month of pregnancy. Apparent increase in cardiac dulness due to distention of the abdomen.

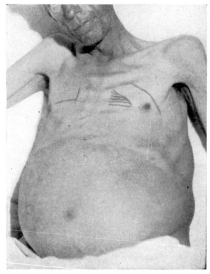

FIG. 275. Increased width of the cardiac dulness due to ascites.

Cardiac Dulness in Abdominal Distention. Just as the enlargement of the uterus in pregnancy causes a certain displacement of the abdominal organs with an elevation of the diaphragm, similarly a variety of pathologic conditions such as ascites, an ovarian cyst, or peritonitis may cause an elevation of the diaphragm with an increase in the area of cardiac dulness which is, of course, due to the position of the heart and not to disease of the heart. The patient shown in Figure 275 had a marked upward displacement of the heart due to ascites and to a large abdominal cyst. The cardiac outlines shown here were verified at autopsy.

Changes in Position of Cardiac Dulness. Any condition, either pushing or pulling the heart to the right or the left, will obviously alter the location of the cardiac dulness. A left-sided pleural effusion will push the heart to the right, and increase the cardiac dulness to the right of the sternum. The left border of the heart in such cases can usually not be made out, since the cardiac dulness fuses with the dulness of the effusion. A right-sided pleural effusion pushes the heart to the left, increasing the cardiac dulness on that side (Fig. 250).

In pneumothorax as well as in pleural effusion the heart is displaced toward the normal side, but in massive collapse of the lung the heart is displaced toward the affected side. This is a valuable diagnostic point.

Pleural adhesions may pull the heart to either side with resulting changes in cardiac dulness similar to those produced by pleural effusions.

Decrease in the Area of Cardiac Dulness. A decrease in the relative cardiac dulness may occur in pulmonary emphysema. In most cases of pulmonary emphysema an increase in relative

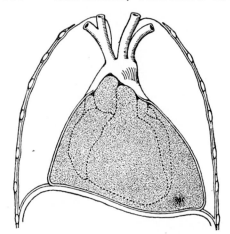

FIG. 276. Diagram of pericardial effusion. (Külbs.)

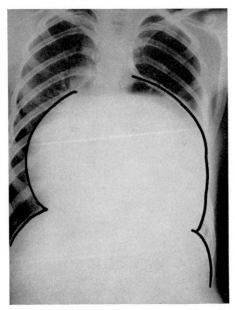

FIG. 277. Roentgenogram of pericarditis with effusion. Note large shadow and small area of air above fluid, the result of a small paracentesis.

cardiac dulness cannot be demonstrated. The absolute cardiac dulness is, however, usually decreased in emphysema (Fig. 248), since the lung is increased in size and covers a greater area of the heart than normal. Indeed, in many cases of pulmonary emphysema no absolute cardiac dulness can be made out on percussion.

Atrophy of the heart rarely, if ever, produces a decrease in the area of cardiac dulness.

Increase in the Area of Cardiac Dulness. An increase in the area of cardiac dulness is most strikingly seen in patients with cardiac disease. This increase is usually more marked than the increase due to changes in the position of the heart. It should be emphasized, however, that we cannot detect by percussion an appreciable increase of the cardiac dulness in hypertrophy of the heart unless there is an accompanying dilatation. The hypertrophied heart in many cases of chronic glomerulonephritis cannot be determined on percussion; the hypertrophied and dilated heart in aortic insufficiency is easily outlined.

Cardiac Enlargement. Enlargement of the left ventricle produces an increase in the relative cardiac dulness to the left and often downward on this side. Enlargement of the left ventricle appears in aortic insufficiency, in aortic stenosis, in mitral insufficiency, in long-standing hypertension and in chronic nephritis.

Enlargement of the right ventricle causes an increase in the relative cardiac dulness to the left and upward, often as high as the second rib, and to the right of the sternal margin. Enlargement of the right ventricle with congestion or obstruction in the pulmonary circulation is seen in mitral stenosis, in pulmonary insufficiency and in tricuspid insufficiency.

Pericardial Effusion. When there is a considerable effusion into the pericardial sac in exudative pericarditis, the cardiac dulness is increased in all directions and assumes the form of a triangle with the apex at the level of the first or second intercostal space (Fig. 276) or a general globular enlargement (Fig. 277).

Rotch's Sign. As Rotch pointed out in 1878, a large pericardial effusion produces dulness in the fifth right interspace and changes the cardiohepatic angle, which is normally a right angle, to an obtuse angle. Figure 278 is taken

A Large Amount of Liquid has been Introduced into the Sack

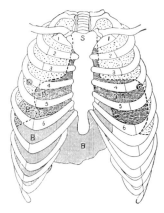

B—Liver.

B¹—The portion of the liver which is covered by the right lung.

C—Lung.

D—The area of percussion flatness caused by a large effusion.

S—Sternum.

—Nipple.

1, 2, 3, 4, 5, 6—Ribs.

- - - Broken line—Border of lung.

Fig. 278. Rotch's sign. (Rotch's original illustration).

from Rotch's original communication, and Figure 350 shows a boy with a large pericardial effusion who shows an obtuse cardiohepatic angle. The outlines shown in Figure 350, obtained on percussion, were verified shortly afterward at autopsy.

Adhesive Pericarditis. Adhesive pericarditis leads to cardiac enlargement, the degree of enlargement depending somewhat upon the extent of the adhesive process. Some of the largest hearts seen clinically or at the autopsy table are in patients suffering from adhesive pericarditis. The relative, and especially the absolute, cardiac dulness are both markedly increased to the left and to the right (Fig. 351).

Increase in the Absolute Cardiac Dulness. Increase in the absolute cardiac dulness without demonstrable cardiac enlargement occurs when the left lung is retracted and a larger area of the ventricle is exposed. It also occurs in mediastinal tumors when the heart is pushed up against the chest wall and a larger area of the ventricle comes into direct contact with the anterior surface of the chest.

Increased Retrosternal Dulness. An increase in the area of retrosternal dulness is seen in tumors lying in the anterior mediastinum and in dilatation of the aorta in aortic aneurysms. Figure 279 shows marked increase in retrosternal dulness due to a mediastinal

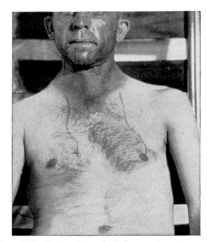

Fig. 279. Retrosternal dulness due to mediastinal tumor.

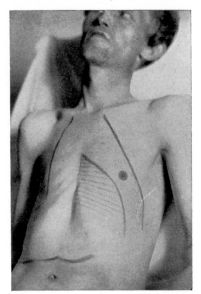

Fig. 280. Increased retrosternal dulness in dilatation of aorta.

ond and third costal interspace due to an aneurysm of the ascending arch of the aorta. Over such an area of dulness an expansile pulsation is usually seen.

tumor. This tumor lay mainly on the right side and produced obstruction to the venous outflow in the right arm with consequent enlargement of the arm. Figure 280 shows an increase in the retrosternal dulness in a patient suffering from mitral and aortic disease with marked widening of the aorta. Figure 364 shows an area of dulness to the right of the sternum in the sec-

BIBLIOGRAPHY

Broadbent, Sir William: Heart Disease. London, Baillière, Tindall & Cox, 1900.

Corvisart, J. N.: Essai sur les Maladies et les Lesions Organiques du Coeur. Paris, Migneret, 1806.

Corvisart, J. N.: Nouvelle Méthode pour Reconnaître les Maladies Internes de la Poitrine. Paris, Migneret, 1808.

Hope, J.: A Treatise on the Diseases of the Heart. London, John Churchill, 1839.

King, John T.: The clinical recognition and physical signs of bundle-branch block. Am. Heart J. *3:*505, 1928.

Lewis, Thomas: Clinical Disorders of the Heart Beat. London, 1914.

Mackenzie, Sir James: Diseases of the Heart. London, H. Frowde, 1921.

Rotch, T. M.: Absence of resonance in the fifth right intercostal space, diagnostic of pericardial effusion. Boston M. and S. J. *99:*423, 1878.

Seifert, Otto, and Müller, Friedrich: Taschenbuch der medizinisch-klinischen Diagnostik. 15th ed. Wiesbaden, J. F. Bergmann, 1912.

Senac, J. B.: Traité de la Structure du Coeur. Paris, Jacques Vincent, 1749.

Vaquez, Henri: Diseases of the Heart. Philadelphia, W. B. Saunders Co., 1924.

Wood, F. C., Johnson, J., Schnabel, T. G., Jr., Kuo, Peter T., and Zinsser, H. F.: The diastolic heart beat. Tr. A. Am. Physicians *64:*95, 1951.

CHAPTER 10

AUSCULTATION OF THE HEART

ONE OF THE FIRST OBSERVATIONS of the heart sounds is that of William Harvey. "It is easy," he wrote, "to see, when a horse drinks, that water is drawn in and passed to the stomach with each gulp, the movement making a sound, and the pulsation may be heard and felt. So it is with each movement of the heart, when a portion of the blood is transferred from the veins to the arteries, that a pulse is made which may be heard in the chest."

The scientific study of the heart sounds began with Laennec's investigations on auscultation and its application to the diagnosis of cardiac disease. "Normally, this sound is double, and each beat of the pulse corresponds to two successive sounds: one clear, abrupt, like the clapping of the valve of a bellows, corresponds to the systole of the auricles; the other duller, more prolonged, coincides with the pulse beat as well as with the sensation of shock . . . and indicates the contraction of the ventricles."

ORIGIN OF THE HEART SOUNDS

Laennec, as we see, believed that the first sound ("clear, abrupt") was due to auricular systole, while the second sound ("duller, more prolonged") was caused by ventricular contraction. Magendie, the great French physiologist, advanced the interesting but quite erroneous theory that the first sound was produced by the impact of the apex of the heart against the ribs during systole, and that the second sound was caused by the shock of the anterior surface of the heart against the sternum. This theory was soon proved to be incorrect, since both sounds remain when the sternum and ribs are removed.

James Hope, in 1835, after enumerating nine "erroneous or defective" theories, gave the explanation of the causes of the heart sounds which is still most widely accepted in the textbooks of today. According to Hope, the first sound is caused by two components: the closure of the auriculoventricular valves and the muscular contraction of the heart. The second sound is produced by the closure of the semilunar valves. There has been unanimity of opinion that the second sound is valvular in origin, and many authorities still adhere to the view of Hope that the first sound has a muscular and a valvular component. Orías and Braun-Menéndez support this view.

William Dock, however, produced evidence that the first heart sound is

171

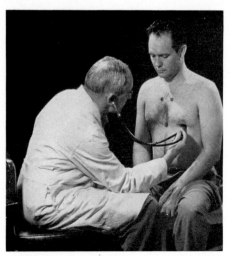

FIG. 281. Auscultation of the heart at the mitral area. Three solid circles indicate tricuspid, aortic and pulmonary areas.

due to the sudden tension of the previously slack fibers of the auriculoventricular valves. His experiments on dogs indicate that there is no muscular element in the first heart sound and that ventricular systole produces no sounds, if tension of the auriculoventricular valves is prevented.

The weight of evidence now favors the view that both the first and second normal heart sounds are mainly valvular in origin. The first sound is produced normally mainly by tension of the auriculoventricular valves (mitral and tricuspid), the second sound by tension of the semilunar valves (pulmonary and aortic). It should be noted, however, that in complete heart block,

during contraction of the auricle, sounds can be heard and also recorded.

CHARACTER OF THE NORMAL HEART SOUNDS

The first sound occurs with the apex impulse and corresponds to the beginning of ventricular systole. The second sound occurs at the end of systole and marks the beginning of ventricular diastole.

The first tone is definitely deeper and longer. The difference in tone, their duration and the relative time intervals, is illustrated in Figure 282. They can be recorded with the proper instruments (Fig. 283).

Over the ventricles of the heart the first sound is louder than the second sound and lower in pitch with a vibration frequency of 57 to 70 per second. Over the base of the heart the second sound is louder than the first sound, but higher in pitch with a vibration frequency of 90 to 100 per second.

It is usually possible, because of the rhythm of the heart, to distinguish between the first and second sounds. The pause between the first and second sounds is much shorter than the pause between the second sound and the next following first sound. If one is in doubt, he can place his finger at the point of maximum impulse and recognize the first sound, which is synchronous with the cardiac impulse, or he can place his hand flat over the point of maximal impulse and listen through his hand

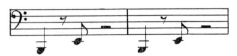

FIG. 282. The rhythm of the normal heart sounds. (After Edens.)

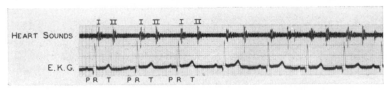

FIG. 283. Phonogram of normal heart sounds at mitral area.

with the stethoscope, as suggested by Dr. David Riesman. The carotid pulse is likewise a reliable sign, since it appears immediately following the first sound.

The heart sounds are sometimes heard at a certain distance from the chest. Corvisart noted this occurrence and Laennec studied it with care. "In more than twenty patients in whom I have heard the heart beats at a distance from two inches to two feet from the chest, three or four at the most were suffering from organic diseases of the heart. All the others showed nothing but purely nervous palpitations; many indeed only showed it after they had walked rather quickly or climbed the stairs rapidly" (Laennec).

Third Heart Sound. Thayer, in 1908, called attention to a third heart sound which is heard at the apex, particularly when the subject lies upon the left side. It is best heard when the heart beats slowly after having been accelerated, and it follows the second sound by approximately 0.18 second. It has no pathologic significance and was found by Thayer in 65 per cent of normal persons under forty-five years of age. It is often loud in mitral stenosis and in dilatation of the ventricle. This sound was first noted by Barie in 1893, but Thayer's studies first called general attention to it. Its cause is not definitely known. Thayer believed that it was caused by a sudden tension of the mi-

tral valve during diastole, while Vaquez explains it as due to distention of the ventricle produced by the rush of blood into this cavity in diastole.

REDUPLICATION OF THE HEART SOUNDS

Both the first and second heart sounds are composite sounds, the first sound being produced by the mitral and tricuspid valves, the second sound by the pulmonic and aortic valves. Since each sound is produced by two sets of valves, any condition interfering with their simultaneous action produces a splitting or doubling of the first or second sound.

Reduplication of the first sound, heard usually at the apex, is present in arteriosclerosis of the heart valves and is believed by Vaquez to be frequently a precursor of the gallop rhythm. It is often heard in children and in thin-chested persons.

Reduplication of the second sound is often heard in children and in normal adults, being heard at the end of inspiration and disappearing during expiration. Pathologically, it is heard in mitral stenosis and in adhesive pericarditis. Bouillaud called it the drum sound (*bruit de rappel*).

RHYTHM OF THE HEART

When the heart action is weakened and the diastolic pause shortened, the

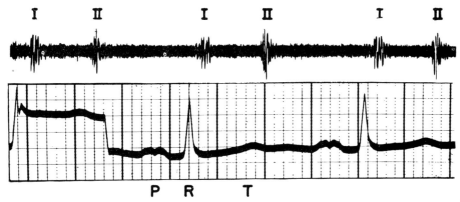

Fig. 284. Phonogram of normal heart sounds at pulmonary area. Note that second sound is louder than first sound but of shorter duration. Electrocardiogram standard lead No. 2.

heart sounds become evenly spaced and, on auscultation, resemble the ticking of a clock. For this reason such a rhythm is referred to as a "tic-tac rhythm" or "pendular rhythm." Because of its resemblance to the sounds of the fetal heart, it is also called "fetal rhythm" or *embryocardia*. Fetal rhythm is heard particularly in cardiac dilatation and is frequently a bad prognostic sign.

The diagram shown in Figure 285 indicates the character of the sounds in reduplication, in fetal rhythm and in gallop rhythm. Figure 286 is a phonogram of the fetal heart sounds.

Gallop   Rhythm. Gallop   rhythm (*bruit de galop*) was so named by Bouillaud. The first published description of it was, however, by his pupil Potain. "It is characterized," as Potain pointed out, "by the presence of a double sound during the first period." The

name is a "very expressive term" and is "marvelously adapted to the sound it describes." Potain called attention to its characteristics, that "it precedes the first sound by a very short time but longer than that which separates the two parts of a reduplicated sound, much shorter than the short silence (between the first and second sounds). The sound is dull, much more so than the normal sound. It is a shock, a perceptible elevation, scarcely a sound. If one applies the ear to the chest, it affects the tactile sensation more perhaps than the auditory sense. If one attempts to hear it with a flexible stethoscope, it lacks only a little, almost always, of disappearing completely. The place where one perceives it best, is a little below the apex of the heart, somewhat toward the right, but sometimes one can distinguish it throughout the entire precordial regions. The sound results

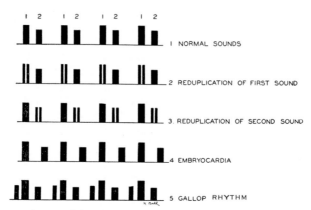

FIG. 285. Diagram of normal heart sounds and certain variations, and of certain abnormal heart sounds.

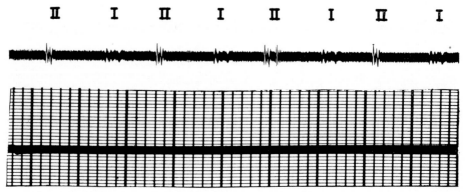

FIG. 286. Fetal heart sounds.

from the abruptness with which the dilatation of the ventricle takes place during the presystolic period, a period which corresponds to the contraction of the auricle. It appears to be an indirect consequence of the excessive arterial tension which interstitial nephritis produces."

Subsequent studies over a period of sixty years have confirmed Potain's findings. Gallop rhythm is heard most commonly in arterial hypertension and in chronic nephritis.

The gallop rhythm has been well termed "the cry of the heart for help." It is of grave, though not necessarily of fatal, import.

Potain divided the gallop rhythm into three varieties, presytolic (late diastolic), mesodiastolic, and protodiastolic (early diastolic). The view advanced by Wolferth and Margolies is that the mesodiastolic is due to a merging of the presytolic and protodiastolic gallops which occurs as the diastole shortens during tachycardia.

The *presystolic gallop rhythm* is the commoner of the two, and electrocardiographic studies show that in this type the extra sound is related to auricular contraction. This has led some observers to believe that in certain cases of arterial hypertension the contraction of the strain becomes audible. The sound is probably valvular in origin.

The *protodiastolic gallop rhythm* is produced by an extra sound which appears early in diastole, and is obviously not related to auricular contraction.

The time of occurrence of the extra sound of the gallop rhythm is altered by the rate of the heart. When the heart rate is increased, the diastole becomes shorter and the extra sound is heard sooner after the second heart sound.

In many cases a protodiastolic gallop rhythm is confused with an exaggerated normal third heart sound. The third heart sound is nearly always protodiastolic in time and occurs soon after the second heart sound. Normal presystolic third heart sounds have been recorded in phonograms, but are usually inaudible.

From the clinical standpoint the view of Oppenheimer and Mond and of Bramwell would seem sound. According to these observers the extra sound in the gallop rhythm is almost invariably presystolic and synchronous with auricular contraction (Fig. 287), while the third heart sound follows the second sound and occurs early in diastole (Fig. 288).

In the last analysis, as Wolferth and Margolies have emphasized, "the only available criterion for distinguishing between physiological third heart sounds and gallop rhythm is the status of cardiac function." When the physiological third heart sound is heard, there is no "cry of the heart for help."

Systolic gallop is less common than diastolic, but cannot be called rare. Its origin is unknown, and it is heard as frequently in apparently normal as in diseased hearts. When the sound has a clicking quality, it is spoken of as a midsystolic click (Fig. 289).

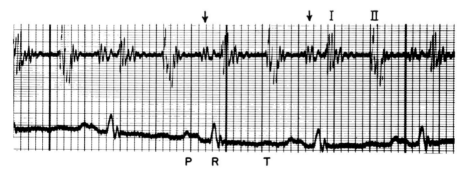

FIG. 287. Presystolic gallop following auricular contraction. Extra sound marked by arrow.

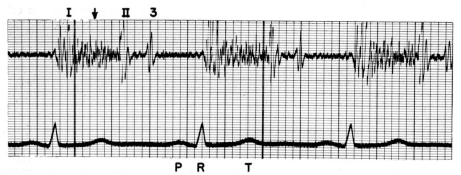

FIG. 288. Third heart sound (3) in mitral disease. Systolic murmur, marked by arrow, also present.

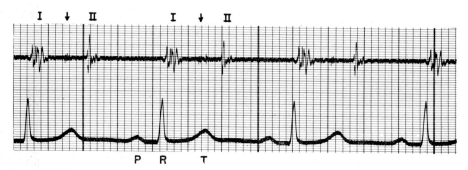

FIG. 289. Midsystolic click marked by arrow in patient with mitral disease.

VALVE AREAS

The areas over the heart where the sounds of the valves are heard with the greatest intensity do not correspond to the anatomical location of the valves, as is seen in Figure 290. The mitral valve area is located in the fifth left intercostal space, the pulmonary valve area is in the second left intercostal space, the aortic valve area at the right second rib and in the right second intercostal space, the tricuspid area over the sternum at the junction of the gladiolus or corpus sterni to the xiphoid process.

Abnormal sounds or murmurs produced at the various valves are usually heard at these valve areas, although their maximum intensity may be elsewhere and their distribution may be quite different from that of the normal sounds. These important features of abnormal valvular sounds will be discussed later.

CHANGES IN THE INTENSITY OF THE HEART SOUNDS

When the patient stands, the sounds are usually louder than when he is sitting. On deep inspiration the intensity of the heart sounds is diminished, since the layer of lung tissue covering the heart is thicker. On expiration the lung contracts and the heart sounds are louder. The heart sounds are louder than normal when there is an increased activity of the heart as the result of exercise, nervousness, cardiac neuroses, paroxysmal tachycardia, or hyperthyroidism.

There are normal differences in intensity between the heart sounds at the various valvular areas. Vierordt found marked variations in the sounds of the heart in the different valvular areas in different patients, but found the first mitral sound almost invariably the loudest. He also observed that in patients from forty to fifty years of age the second aortic tone was usually louder than the second pulmonic. Bock gives the following scale of intensity of the heart sounds: loudest, the first mitral sound, followed by second aortic sound, and then the second pulmonic tone. Of greater interest is a comparison of the relative intensity of the second sound at the pulmonary and aortic areas. Creighton found in a study of 100 cases that up to the age of twenty the second pulmonic tone was louder, from twenty to thirty the two tones were of equal intensity, while from fifty years on the second aortic tone was louder.

Increased Intensity of the Heart Sounds. The mitral first sound is greatly accentuated in mitral stenosis, as well as the second pulmonary sound. The second aortic tone is accentuated, especially in arterial hypertension whether "essential" or due to chronic nephritis, in arteriosclerosis of the aortic valves and in many cases of polycythemia vera. In lobar pneumonia the second pulmonic tone is often accentuated. This is regarded as a favorable prognostic sign.

Decreased Intensity of the Heart Sounds. This may be due to a decrease in the contractile power of the heart or to a poor conduction of the heart sounds to the surface. In typhoid fever, in any condition of exhaustion or weakness, the sounds may be faint because of the relatively weak cardiac contractions. In cardiac failure and myocardial infarction the first mitral tone may be markedly diminished in intensity. Among the conditions causing a poor conduction of the heart sounds to the surface of the chest are emphysema, pleural thickening, tumors in the anterior mediastinum, and pericardial effusion. A gradually decreasing intensity of the heart sounds in patients who have shown a pericardial friction rub is presumptive evidence that fluid is accumulating in the pericardial sac.

FRICTION SOUNDS

Friction sounds heard over the heart and synchronous with the heart beat are pathognomonic of fibrinous pericarditis. Collin, who first called attention to this sign, described it as a "sound analogous to the creaking of new leather. This sound continued for the first six days of the disease, but disappeared as soon as the local symptoms indicated a slight liquid effusion into the pericardium."

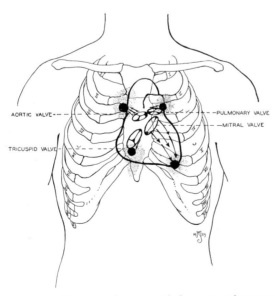

AORTIC VALVE

PULMONARY VALVE

MITRAL VALVE

TRICUSPID VALVE

FIG. 290. Anatomical location of heart valves and of the areas where sounds are best heard.

The *pericardial friction rub* is synchronous with the heart beat and unaffected by respiration, which should distinguish it from a pleural friction rub. The sound is almost always double, but as a rule it does not coincide strictly with any period of the cardiac cycle. Ordinarily friction sounds are heard partly during systole and partly during diastole, and for this reason are described as "riding astride" the two heart sounds. When they follow each other at a definite interval they form a to-and-fro rhythm. Pericardial friction sounds are not transmitted, and as Stokes, one of the pioneers in their study, noted nearly a century ago, "in many instances we find that on removing the stethoscope but a single inch from the spot where the sound is heard, it totally ceases, although we still hear the ordinary sounds of cardiac pulsation."

The pericardial friction rub changes in intensity with the position of the patient, increasing in intensity when the patient sits up. Pressure on the bell of the stethoscope produces an increase in the loudness and distinctness of the friction sounds. This modification produced by pressure varies with the elasticity of the chest and is marked in children and in poorly nourished adults.

The character of the friction rub varies in different patients or at different times in the same patient. The sound has been compared in different instances to the rasping of wood, the grating of nutmeg, the rustling of silk, the crackling of parchment, the creaking of new leather.

"It may strike the reader," Hope remarked, "as rather incredible that so many varieties of rubbing murmur should be produced by a single affection; but his doubts will cease on finding that he may closely imitate nearly the whole, even the creaking sound, by rubbing a damp finger, with various degrees of force, and in various positions, against the back of his hand, while he listens with a stethoscope applied to the palm."

CARDIAC MURMURS

Cardiac murmurs were first described in 1819 by Laennec, who believed they were always produced by valvular lesions and added that "their situation, and the time at which they are heard, indicates obviously which orifice is affected." Later he denied any value to blowing murmurs in diagnosing valvular lesions, since he saw patients who had cardiac murmurs, but showed no valvular lesions at autopsy. In this, Laennec, as Potain remarked, fell into a second error greater than the first.

Bouillaud, Gendrin, Skoda, Hope, Forbes and Stokes continued the studies begun by Laennec. James Hope's "Diseases of the Heart," which first appeared in 1831, contained an account of all the pathognomonic heart murmurs which we recognize today, each correctly described and its pathological significance correctly recognized. All these observers heard extracardiac as well as cardiac murmurs and speculated as to their causes. Potain first studied systematically extracardiac murmurs, classified them and advanced explanations as to their causes. The mistake made by earlier observers was largely due to their attempt to determine from the character of the murmur alone whether or not it arose from organic disease of the heart. Potain showed that, with a few exceptions, there was no such single characteristic, but that only a careful study of the individual murmur and of its associated physical findings leads to a correct differential diagnosis.

Murmurs are either systolic or diastolic in time, occurring with either systole or diastole. They are also commonly designated according to the valve area in which they are best heard, as, for example, mitral systolic. Murmurs occurring late in diastole and just before systole are usually designated as presystolic.

Mechanism of Production of Organic Heart Murmurs. Murmurs may be produced in a tube through which a fluid is flowing by four methods: first, by increasing the rate of flow through the tube; second, by producing a constriction in the tube; third, by causing a dilatation in the tube; and fourth, by inserting a taut string or membrane which vibrates as the fluid flows past (Fig. 291). All four of these mechanisms are found in the production of heart murmurs in patients. In anemia, in hyperthyroidism, in early hypertension and after violent exercise the heart rate is increased and a systolic murmur may be heard over the heart. The mitral orifice in mitral stenosis is narrowed and corresponds to the experimental constriction. In mitral insufficiency with dilatation of the ventricle, the mitral orifice is dilated as in the experimental dilatation of the tube. In a rather uncommon lesion, rupture of the mitral leaflet or of the papillary muscle, the condition corresponds to the vibrating membrane in the flowing current.

The normal valves of the heart must fulfill two functions: they must prevent the back flow of the blood, and they must offer no impediment to the forward flow of the blood. Healthy heart valves fulfill these requirements perfectly. During ventricular systole the mitral and tricuspid valves are closed and allow no blood to regurgitate, the aortic and pulmonary valves lie flat against the vessel walls and allow the blood free passage. During diastole the two sets of valves change their role. The aortic and pulmonary are hermetically sealed and prevent a regurgitation from the aorta and pulmonary artery, while the mitral and tricuspid valves are open and allow free passage of the blood from the auricles to the ventricles (Fig. 292). In a normal heart we hear only the sounds produced during the closure of the valves.

In a heart with an insufficiency of a valve, the valve does not close completely during the period of closure, and an opening is left through which a part of the blood regurgitates. This back current of the blood sets the valves and the ventricular wall adjacent into vibration and a murmur results—the murmur of insufficiency. If a valve is stenotic or narrowed, the valve fails to open completely during the period when

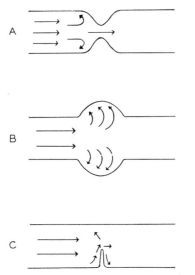

FIG. 291. Method of production of heart murmurs: *A,* constriction of rubber tube; *B,* dilatation of tube; *C,* vibrating flap in lumen.

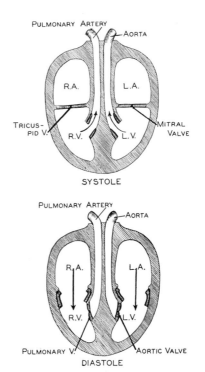

FIG. 292. Diagram of position of heart valves during systole and diastole.

it should be normally wide open, and the blood passing through this narrowed orifice encounters resistance, vibrations are set up in the valve, and the murmur of stenosis appears.

Transmission of Heart Murmurs. Murmurs are usually transmitted best in the direction of the blood stream by which they are produced. Thus the murmur of aortic stenosis is well heard in the carotid arteries, while the murmur of aortic insufficiency is well heard along the left sternal border and at the apex.

In the transmission of murmurs from the mitral orifice, the papillary muscles of the heart play an important role. DeSautelle and Grey have shown that the murmur of mitral insufficiency is loudest over that part of the ventricles where the papillary muscles are inserted. They also found that if the papillary muscles are cut off and sewed to another part of the wall, the murmur is then loudest over this area. This role of the papillary muscles may explain why the murmur of mitral insufficiency is loudest at the apex, although the flow of the blood producing the murmur is in the opposite direction.

Character of Murmurs. The character of a murmur depends upon the velocity and tension of the blood as it passes through an orifice, upon the character of the orifice itself, upon the width of the orifice and from the resonating character of the surrounding structures. Hirschfelder has ingeniously compared a valvular orifice to the larynx with its vocal cords. When the cords are closely approximated, a high note is produced; when they are wider apart, the note is low; when they are lax and wide apart, the air moving over them produces no sound (Fig. 293). This diagram explains those cases, at first puzzling to the student, in which a marked valvular insufficiency is found at the autopsy of a patient who during life showed no cardiac murmur.

Murmurs are occasionally so loud that they are heard by the patient himself and may be heard several feet away from the patient. This phenomenon was well known to Corvisart and Laennec and has been frequently observed. In a patient under our care recently a rasping, systolic, aortic murmur could be clearly heard by a group of students standing at the foot of his bed.

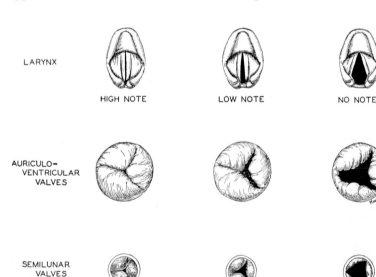

FIG. 293. Similarity between sounds produced at heart valves and in the larynx. (Modified after Hirschfelder.)

Cardiac murmurs may change in intensity with respiration. Just as the normal heart sounds are feebler during deep inspiration, when the heart is more nearly covered by the lungs, and stronger during expiration, when the lungs are contracted, so cardiac murmurs may be more intense during expiration than inspiration. Any condition interfering with the transmission of the heart sounds to the chest wall will weaken the intensity of murmurs.

Usually it is not difficult to determine whether a murmur is due to insufficiency or stenosis of a valve. A murmur proves the inability of a valve to close completely at the time it should close or its inability to open completely at the time when it should be open. A systolic murmur is produced by insufficiency of the auriculoventricular valves (mitral and tricuspid) or by stenosis of the semilunar valves (aortic and pulmonary). A diastolic murmur is due to stenosis of the auriculoventricular valves or insufficiency of the semilunar valves. Fortunately, the observer does not have to make his diagnosis solely from the murmurs present, but has other accessory signs such as the presence or absence of thrills, the character of the radial, brachial and carotid pulse, the size and shape of the heart and the character of the heart sounds in the different valvular areas, or sounds heard over vessels to aid him in arriving at a correct diagnosis. These accessory signs may be more important at times than the presence of a cardiac murmur. The correct diagnosis of a heart lesion takes all these factors into consideration.

The most common valvular lesions are located in the mitral and aortic valves. Mitral insufficiency, mitral stenosis and aortic insufficiency are by far the most common valvular lesions encountered. It is upon these three lesions that the student should concentrate particularly. Familiarity with other lesions should also be attained, but the student should first be sure that he is not meeting the more common lesions

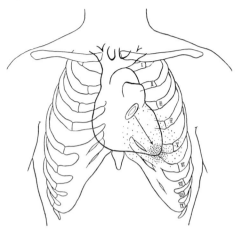

FIG. 294. Location of murmur in mitral insufficiency.

before he diagnoses the uncommon ones.

Mitral Insufficiency. The murmur of mitral insufficiency is systolic in time and best heard near the apex of the heart, but is also commonly heard over the greater part of the precordium (Fig. 294). It is transmitted by papillary muscles upward and outward toward the axilla and may be heard in the back on the left side. Laennec, who first heard and described it, compared it to the sound of a bellows—"bruit de soufflet." Stokes and other physicians of his time described the murmur as the "bellows murmur." Later writers refer to it as the blowing murmur of regurgitation (Fig. 295).

This lesion is usually a complication of rheumatic endocarditis, and pathologic investigations indicate that changes in the mitral leaflet play only an accessory role, the lesion being produced mainly by retraction of the papillary muscles, which prevents the leaflets from rising during systole, and lasts throughout systole. It is usually soft and blowing, decreases rapidly and has been compared to a jet of steam. Occasionally it is musical, more rarely harsh (Fig. 296).

Since a mitral insufficiency is rarely found at autopsy except in association with mitral stenosis, some observers

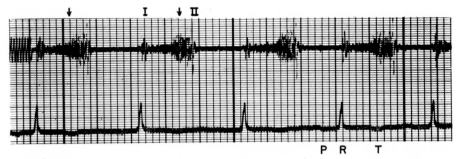

FIG. 295. Systolic murmur heard at apex in mitral insufficiency. The murmur, marked by arrow, begins immediately after the first sound and builds up in intensity until the second sound appears.

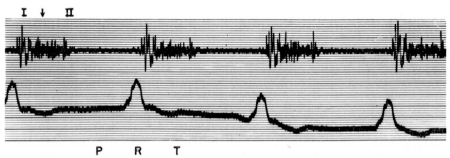

FIG. 296. Systolic murmur at apex in mitral insufficiency. Murmur, marked by arrow, heard throughout systole.

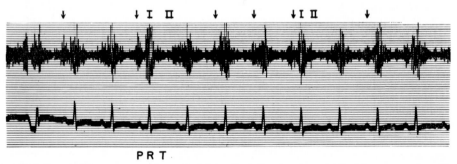

FIG. 297. Presystolic murmur, also called late diastolic murmur, marked by arrow, in mitral stenosis.

have doubted the existence of a pure mitral insufficiency or have regarded it as a rare lesion. Most cardiologists disagree with such an opinion. Reid's advice is sound: "A systolic murmur completely masking the first sound is generally reliable evidence of organic mitral regurgitation, but it is a good rule to hold that an apical systolic murmur, whatever its transmission or quality, is insufficient evidence of organic mitral insufficiency unless in addition

there is evidence of cardiac enlargement of persistent type."

Mitral Stenosis. The murmur of mitral stenosis was heard by Laennec, who described it as "bruit de scie ou de râpe" (noise of a saw or a grater) and compared it also to the noise produced by a wood file. Bertin pointed out its association with mitral stenosis, and Hope extended these observations.

Laennec's comparison of the sound with that produced by a saw or a

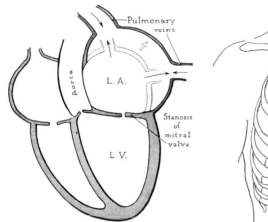

FIG. 298. Diagram of mitral stenosis. Stenosis of mitral valve produces increased pressure within left auricle which dilates this auricle.

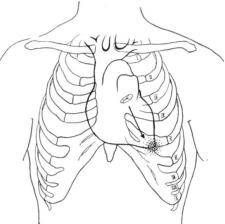

FIG. 299. Location of murmur in mitral stenosis.

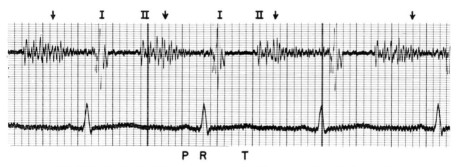

FIG. 300. Early diastolic murmur, marked by arrow, in mitral stenosis.

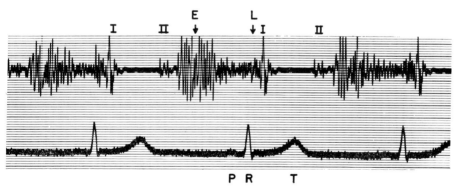

FIG. 301. Early diastolic murmur (E) and late diastolic murmur (L) in mitral stenosis. Early diastolic murmur much louder.

grater or a wood file is excellent. It is a harsh, rumbling sound preceding the first sound, occurring usually in late diastole, just preceding the systole of the heart and therefore presystolic (Fig. 297). The sound is produced by the obstruction to the flow of blood through the narrowed mitral valve during diastole. It is best heard on light pressure of the bell of the stethoscope and with the patient lying on his left side.

The rumble is purring, crescendo, rapidly increasing in intensity and ending with a loud snapping first sound.

This first sound was so greatly accentuated in a patient described by Graves that it was audible 6 feet from the chest wall.

The murmur is loudest near the apex and is not so widely transmitted as the murmur of mitral insufficiency (Fig. 294). Like the presystolic thrill it may at times be present only after the patient exercises.

The murmur of mitral stenosis may begin in mid-diastole, or even in early diastole, and continue until the appearance of the first sound, or it may be short in duration and appear only just before the beginning of systole. At times two distinct murmurs may be present, one in early diastole (protodiastolic) and another in late diastole (presystolic or telediastolic). The first type of murmur, which is of relatively long duration, commonly persists in auricular fibrillation (Fig. 300), while the second type of brief duration invariably disappears. This is not surprising. The murmur in early diastole is caused by the flow of blood during diastole from the left auricle into the left ventricle through the narrowed mitral lumen. This flow continues in auricular fibrillation. The presystolic rumble is produced by the powerfully contracting left auricle forcing the blood through the constricted mitral orifice, just before ventricular systole. This auricular contraction is absent in auricular fibrillation. The first type of murmur is by some referred to as diastolic, while the second type is called presystolic. The difference in the mode of production of these two murmurs is shown in Figure 302.

At the base of the heart, auscultation at the pulmonic area shows a marked accentuation of the second pulmonic sound.

Mitral stenosis is in most instances produced by endocarditis complicating rheumatic fever or chorea. The typical lesions with the characteristic physical findings appear usually about ten years after the endocarditis. At first the lesion is a mitral insufficiency with

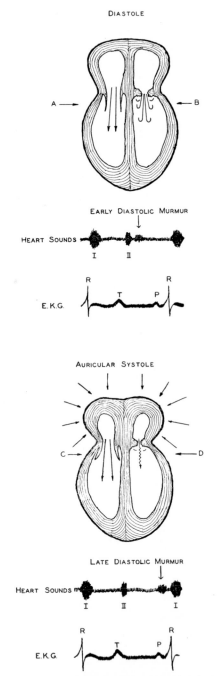

FIG. 302. *A*, Blood flowing through normal valves in diastole *produces no murmur; B,* blood flowing through stenosed valves in diastole *produces early diastolic murmur; C,* blood flowing through normal valves during auricular systole *produces no murmur; D,* blood flowing through stenosed valves in auricular systole *produces late diastolic (presystolic) murmur.*

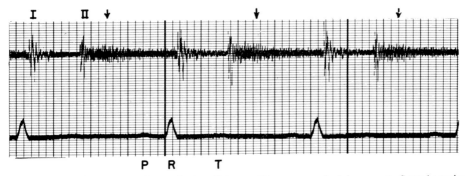

FIG. 303. Diastolic murmur in aortic insufficiency. Murmur marked by arrow. Sound tracing at aortic area. Electrocardiogram standard lead No. 3.

typical findings; later the scarring about the valve increases, producing stenosis, the valve being often described as a "fish mouth" valve.

Mitral stenosis is usually associated with mitral insufficiency with the result that one hears on auscultation a presystolic rumble leading up to a snapping first sound which is followed by a blowing systolic murmur (Fig. 296).

In atrial fibrillation complicating mitral stenosis the presystolic rumble disappears. This absence of a rumble led Mackenzie in the early studies of this condition to surmise that the auricle "enormously distended . . . like an over-distended bladder, had become paralyzed." Mackenzie's observation that the presystolic rumbling disappears in auricular fibrillation was correct, since this murmur is late in diastole. The diastolic murmur which may persist is early in diastole.

Aortic Insufficiency. The murmur of aortic insufficiency was first clearly described by James Hope in 1831. Hope observed that "when there is regurgitation through the permanently open aortic valves, a murmur accompanies the second sound" and noted further that "it was louder and more superficial opposite to and above the aortic valves than about the apex," that it was "prolonged through the whole interval of repose," that it had "the softness of the bellows murmur, an inferior degree of loudness, and a lower key, like whispering the word *awe* during inspiration. It often becomes musical."

The murmur of aortic insufficiency accompanying the second sound and lasting through the whole interval of repose is diastolic in time, as the phonogram in Figure 303 demonstrates. The distribution of the murmur is especially in the direction of the regurgitant stream, as shown in Figure 304. In many patients the murmur is often loudest along the left sternal border at the second, third and fourth ribs and their interspaces. In some patients it may be heard at the left sternal border, but not clearly over the aortic valve area.

The murmur of aortic insufficiency is usually soft and blowing, but quite distinct, so that there is ordinarily little question whether the student hears it. Either he hears it or he does not. Often

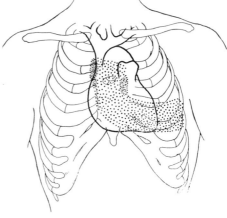

FIG. 304. Distribution of murmur in aortic insufficiency. Points at which dots are closer together indicate greater intensity.

the murmur is inaudible when listening with the stethoscope, but is clearly heard when the examiner places his ear directly on the chest wall at the aortic area or over the sternum. Occasionally it is so faint that it can be heard only when the patient holds his breath after a deep expiration. In that unusual complication, rupture of an aortic cusp, the soft diastolic murmur may suddenly become musical or harsh and rasping.

Aortic insufficiency is usually due to a rheumatic endocarditis, to syphilis or to arteriosclerosis. The statistics in reference to the relative frequency of rheumatic and syphilitic aortic insufficiency show some variations. Osler states that syphilis "is the most important cause, certainly in young adults and middle-aged persons."

Flint Murmur. This murmur was first described by Austin Flint, Sr., in 1862 in two patients, who showed a diastolic aortic murmur, but also had a marked presystolic murmur at the apex. At autopsy both patients showed aortic lesions, but normal mitral valves. Flint's observations have since been repeatedly confirmed and the importance of his observations has been generally appreciated. The Flint murmur is often heard in aortic insufficiency.

Flint's explanation of the murmur is as follows: "In cases of considerable aortic insufficiency, the left ventricle is rapidly filled with blood flowing back from the aorta as well as from the auricle, before the auricular contraction takes place. The distention of the ventricle is such that the mitral curtains are brought into coaptation, and when the auricular contraction takes place the mitral direct current passing between the curtains throws them into vibration and gives rise to the characteristic blubbering murmur. The physical condition is in effect analogous to contraction of the mitral orifice from an adhesion of the curtains at their sides." No better explanation has been suggested since (Fig. 305).

It is often extremely difficult to decide whether a patient suffering from aortic disease and showing a presytolic apical rumble has aortic insufficiency with a Flint murmur or aortic insufficiency with mitral stenosis. On the *basis* of pathologic findings the diagnosis of aortic insufficiency with a Flint murmur is more often correct. Clinical experience checked by necropsy observations teaches the physician that a single diagnosis is more often correct than a multiple diagnosis. A presystolic thrill is usually absent in a Flint murmur and usually present in mitral stenosis. The character of the pulse may aid. If it is small, instead of bounding, there is probably a mitral stenosis present.

Aortic Stenosis. Aortic stenosis is a comparatively uncommon lesion. It was first recognized clearly by Hope, who observed that it was systolic in time, well heard over the sternum at the level of the third rib, well heard upward for 2 inches or more and louder in these areas than below the level of the valves. "Its pitch or key is usually that of a whispered *r,* from being superficial, and it accordingly conveys the idea of being pretty near to the ear."

The murmur of aortic stenosis is a

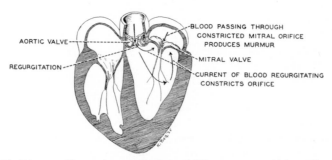

FIG. 305. Diagram illustrating production of Flint murmur. (After Hirschfelder.)

loud systolic murmur most intense over the aortic areas, transmitted from there to the first right interspace and along the course of the arteries. It is usually loud and distinct over the carotid and brachial arteries. It is also well heard, but is not loud over the pulmonary area and over the body of the heart (Fig. 306). The murmur of aortic stenosis is the loudest usually heard in valvular heart disease and may be audible several feet away from the patient.

The murmur of aortic stenosis cannot arise until the blood begins to flow into the aorta, and as a result the murmur does not appear until a brief interval after the beginning of systole. This is well shown in the phonogram (Fig. 307).

Aortic stenosis may be the result of an old rheumatic endocarditis or of arteriosclerosis. Exceptionally, it is ap-

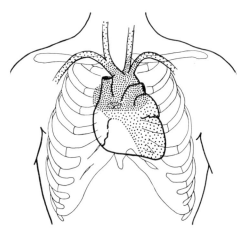

FIG. 306. Distribution of murmur in aortic stenosis.

parently congenital. In syphilitic diseases of the aortic valves there may be a loud systolic rumble, as well as the signs of aortic insufficiency.

A rough systolic murmur is often heard over the aortic area in aortitis and in marked atheroma of the aorta. In aortitis this systolic murmur may appear before the diastolic murmur of aortic insufficiency appears. Frequently in aortitis with aortic insufficiency both systolic and diastolic aortic murmurs are heard. Syncope frequently occurs in aortic stenosis, and sudden death is not uncommon.

Pulmonary Stenosis. Pulmonary stenosis is a valvular lesion infrequently seen, but one of the most common of all congenital heart lesions. It may be congenital or may be acquired as the result of endocarditis. According to Hirschfelder, 82 per cent of all cases showed evidence of other congenital cardiac lesions.

The murmur of pulmonary stenosis (Fig. 308) is systolic in time, rasping, best heard at the left border of the sternum in the second interspace and is propagated toward the left clavicle, usually disappearing at the level of the clavicle. It is sometimes heard in the left interscapular area. The systolic murmur of pulmonary stenosis is usually accompanied by a systolic thrill at the second left interspace.

Congenital pulmonary stenosis with a defect of the interventricular septum is associated commonly with a marked cyanosis; acquired pulmonary stenosis, rarely.

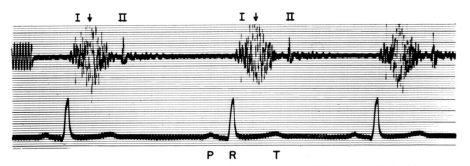

FIG. 307. Systolic murmur over aortic area in aortic stenosis. Murmur marked with arrow.

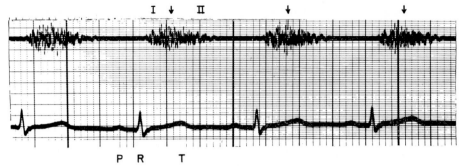

FIG. 308. Murmur of pulmonary stenosis heard at pulmonic area. Systolic in time, harsh in tone. Murmur marked with arrow.

Pulmonary Insufficiency. Pulmonary insufficiency is a rare disease occurring either as a congenital lesion or as a result of endocarditis. The murmur is soft, diastolic and best heard along the left sternal border at the third interspace and heard as far down as the xiphoid process.

The Graham Steell Murmur. Graham Steell in 1889 showed that in some patients with mitral stenosis an excessive pressure is produced in the pulmonary artery which causes dilatation of that artery with insufficiency of the pulmonary valve. This produces a soft diastolic murmur along the left border of the sternum. This murmur is, however, exceptional and occurs in only 4 per cent of the cases of mitral stenosis.

Tricuspid Stenosis. This lesion is also excessively rare and not often diagnosed. In 26,000 admissions at the Johns Hopkins Hospital this condition was found in only 7 cases, in all of whom other cardiac lesions were present. A rumbling presystolic murmur is present over the lower part of the sternum and along the left sternal border.

Tricuspid Insufficiency. Organic tricuspid insufficiency is rare, most of the cases seen being examples of relative tricuspid insufficiency. The murmur of tricuspid insufficiency is a soft, low-pitch systolic murmur of greatest intensity over the lower part of the sternum. Pulsation of the liver occurs often and is a valuable diagnostic sign.

Tricuspid insufficiency, while rare in the organic form, is one of the commonest of lesions in the functional form due to dilatation of the ventricle from other heart lesions. Autopsy records also show that it is one of the most commonly missed of all lesions, because it is commonly mistaken for, or not differentiated from, a coexisting mitral insufficiency, and also because a widely dilated tricuspid orifice produces no murmur.

THE MURMURS OF CONGENITAL HEART DISEASE

Pulmonary Stenosis. This is the most common primary congenital lesion, comprising more than one half of all cases of congenital heart disease. The murmur of pulmonary stenosis has already been discussed.

Interventricular Defect. Perforation of the interventricular septum was first described by Henri Roger in 1879 and has since been known as Roger's disease. Roger described the murmur as: "A loud murmur, audible over a large area, and commencing with systole, is prolonged so as to cover the normal tic-tac. It has its maximum at the upper third of the precordial region. It is central like the septum, and from this central point gradually diminishes in intensity in every direction. The murmur does not vary at any time, and it is not conducted into the vessels." A phonogram of this murmur shows that it begins the instant systole appears and lasts throughout systole (Fig. 357). Most systolic murmurs begin a brief

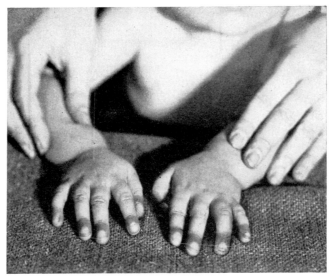

FIG. 309. Clubbing of fingers with pigmentation.

instant after the onset of systole and do not occupy the entire period of systole. In addition to this murmur there is a systolic thrill in the third left interspace.

The murmur of an interventricular defect may be confused with that of pulmonary stenosis, but the former is louder in the third than in the second interspace and is propagated transversely and never upward to the clavicle.

The term "tetralogy of Fallot" is applied to the combination of four pathologic states: pulmonary stenosis, interventricular septum defect, dextroposition of the aorta, and hypertrophy of the right ventricle. "This is the most common cause of marked congenital cyanosis met in adults" (Levine). Most of these patients survive for only a few years, but occasionally patients fifty or more years of age are seen. The blood shows a marked polycythemia, counts of 10,000,000 or more being frequently seen. In children there is usually marked clubbing of the fingers, often with brownish pigmentation above the fingernails (Fig. 309). Many adults suffering from congenital heart disease with marked cyanosis show this combination of conditions at autopsy (Fig. 310).

Patent Ductus Arteriosus (Botallo). The murmur of a patent ductus arte-

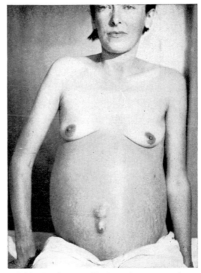

FIG. 310. Patient suffering from tetralogy of Fallot. Marked cyanosis of the lips, and ascites.

riosus is best heard at the second or third left intercostal space near the sternum, and is transmitted to the left clavicle, to the vessels of the neck and often backward to the left interscapular area. It is continuous, with systolic accentuation, and is described as a "machinery murmur" or, according to Vaquez, "resembles the sound of a train in a tunnel." This machinery murmur, when present, is diagnostic of the condition, but it is often absent.

The diagnosis of congenital heart disease is often aided by the presence of marked cyanosis and clubbing of the fingers in the patient. Congenital lesions are often multiple in the same patient.

FUNCTIONAL MURMURS

In contrast to organic murmurs, which are produced by pathologic changes in the heart valves, there is a group of murmurs which are not due to such changes and the significance or importance of which it is often difficult to determine. These murmurs are most commonly spoken of as functional, accidental or hemic, and form a group the explanation of which has resulted in an almost endless controversy. These murmurs confused Laennec so much that he finally came to the erroneous conclusion that no murmurs are of any value in the diagnosis of cardiac disease. Potain made the most exhaustive study of functional murmurs. His studies covered a period of nearly thirty years —from 1865 to 1894. He found such murmurs present in one-eighth of all the patients seen on his hospital service. They were present in practically all cases of Graves' disease, in 50 per cent of the cases of chlorosis, 5 per cent in measles and scarlet fever, 10 per cent in pulmonary disease. He found the murmurs commoner in young persons, the greatest frequency being between the ages of twenty and thirty, while there was a rapid decrease in frequency after the age of thirty.

The student should not gain the impression that functional murmurs are truly "accidental" and to be altogether disregarded. Often they may, quite often they may not, be disregarded. A relative insufficiency of the mitral valve due to an enlarged left ventricle produces a systolic murmur which is functional in so far as there is no organic pathological process on the mitral leaflets. Such a murmur, however, may be of as great as or greater importance than the systolic organic murmur of an almost perfectly functioning mitral valve.

The most satisfactory classification of these murmurs is into intracardiac and extracardiac.

Intracardiac Functional Murmurs. Intracardiac functional murmurs are commonly due to the same mechanism that produces organic valvular murmurs, but differ in the important respect that the changes in the valves are functional and may be transient, while organic murmurs due to anatomical lesions are permanent.

The best-known example of these functional murmurs is the murmur of relative tricuspid insufficiency. The tricuspid valve in several diseases in which the pressure in the pulmonary circulation is markedly increased may become insufficient with dilatation of the tricuspid ring and of the right ventricle. This increased pressure is observed in pulmonary sclerosis, in mitral stenosis and insufficiency, in adherent pericardium and in myocarditis. If the patient's condition improves, the tricuspid insufficiency disappears; if he dies, the autopsy reveals a dilatation of the tricuspid rings, but normal valve cusps. This type of functional insufficiency producing a systolic murmur has long been recognized. In recent years it has been shown that at the aortic area a functional insufficiency may occur, especially in arterial hypertension, which produces a diastolic murmur, and that a functional insufficiency of the mitral valve is not uncommon with the production of a systolic murmur. Both these murmurs occur most commonly during cardiac failure and disappear with improvement in cardiac tone.

A presystolic murmur is sometimes heard at the apex in patients who have an obstruction to the pulmonary circulation, but no lesions of the mitral valve. We have seen three such patients who were suspected of having mitral stenosis, but showed at autopsy extensive pulmonary fibrosis and perfectly normal mitral valves. This murmur has been studied recently by Wyckoff and Bunim.

The functional systolic murmurs at

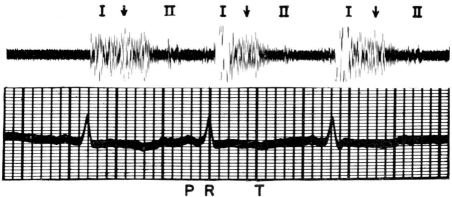

FIG. 311. Systolic murmur in severe anemia following gastric hemorrhage. Systolic murmur marked by arrow. Sound record at apex.

the apex of the heart have aroused particular discussion. Extremely loud systolic murmurs may be heard at the apex which, because of their intensity, the inexperienced observer feels sure are due to mitral disease, and yet at autopsy the mitral valves may show only a slight enlargement of the mitral ring or, indeed, none at all. Such experiences are extremely common.

These systolic murmurs are heard frequently in Graves' disease and in severe anemias (Fig. 311). In both conditions the heart action is rapid, even "delirious," and this tachycardia, according to some, produces the murmurs, possibly by defective valve closure. The systolic murmurs heard in severe anemias, which are often loudest at the base of the heart, were thought by Bouillaud to be due to the decreased viscosity of the blood in anemia, and this observation forms the basis for the theory of "hemic murmurs"— murmurs produced by changes in the blood itself.

"Hemic murmurs," however, at times are due to dilatation of the heart with a relative mitral insufficiency. Such an example is seen in Figure 312, which shows a roentgenogram of a patient's heart who was suffering from a severe secondary anemia with a marked cardiac dilatation and a loud systolic murmur. When the patient's anemia improved, the cardiac dilatation disappeared and with it the systolic murmur (Fig. 313).

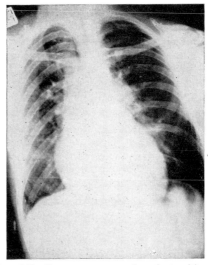

FIG. 312. Roentgenogram of patient with severe anemia, showing marked cardiac dilatation.

White believes that such terms as "hemic" and "accidental" should be omitted. He adds, "conditions like anemia act by causing cardiac dilatation."

Systolic murmurs at the pulmonary valve area are frequent. White remarks, "It is the commonest of all heart murmurs, and if absent with the subject in the upright position, it can usually be brought out in the normal individual as well as in the cardiac patient by the assumption of the recumbent position, especially in full expiration. Therefore the pulmonary systolic murmur may be

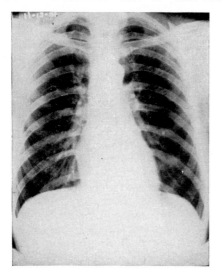

Fig. 313. Same patient after anemia was markedly improved.

considered to be a normal physiological event unless of considerable intensity in the upright position; even then it should be carefully analyzed before being called abnormal." Such murmurs are probably associated with slight displacement or distortion of the pulmonary artery.

Extracardiac Functional Murmurs. These murmurs, better known as cardiorespiratory or cardiopulmonary murmurs, were first described by Laennec and later exhaustively studied by Potain.

Laennec in 1826 noted that "in certain persons the pleura and the anterior borders of the lungs extend in front of the heart and cover it almost entirely. If one examines such a person at the moment when he notes the heart beats are rather forceful, the diastole of the heart compressing these portions of the lung and forcing the air out of them, alters the breath sounds in such a manner that they imitate more or less closely the sound of a saw or that of a soft wood file. But with a little practice it is easy to distinguish this sound from the bellows sound produced by the heart itself. It is more superficial. One hears below the normal sounds of the heart; and on asking the patient to hold his breath, it diminishes markedly or ceases almost entirely."

Potain confirmed these findings and demonstrated that these murmurs are loudest and most commonly heard in those areas where the movements of the beating heart are the most extensive. He also showed that they are heard over the areas where there is retraction of the heart, which produces a small area of increased negative pressure with a sudden expansion of the lung causing air to rush in with the production of a murmur. This retraction is usually systolic, and such murmurs are usually systolic; but occasionally the retraction is diastolic, and in such cases the murmur is diastolic (Fig. 314).

Hamman in 1937 called attention to the presence of a "peculiar crunching, crackling, bubbling sound heard over the heart with each contraction" in interstitial emphysema of the lungs. This sound may appear or disappear with change of position.

Potain also devoted much time to a study of the location on the precordium of organic and functional murmurs. The areas in which these murmurs are most frequently heard are shown in Figure 315.

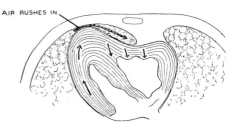

Fig. 314. Relation of heart and lung flap during production of cardiorespiratory murmur.

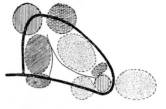

MURMURS ALMOST ALWAYS ORGANIC
MURMURS MOST FREQUENTLY ORGANIC
MURMURS MOST FREQUENTLY FUNCTIONAL
MURMURS ALWAYS FUNCTIONAL

Fig. 315. Heart murmurs. (After Potain.)

SUMMARY

The murmurs of stenosis of the valves are usually due to organic disease of the valves and are accompanied by a thrill.

The murmurs of insufficiency of the valves may be due to organic disease of the valves or to a functional dilatation of the valve rings with normal valve leaflets.

A functional dilatation of a valve may be more serious than organic disease of the valve leaflets.

Cardiorespiratory murmurs are profoundly altered by respiration and by change in the position of the patient.

Organic murmurs may also be somewhat altered by respiration, being weaker during inspiration.

Congenital cardiac defects are often multiple, and the patient may show cyanosis and clubbing of the fingers.

Diastolic murmurs are more often organic than functional.

The diagnosis of a heart lesion may be made in many instances from the auscultatory signs alone, but it is safer to seek the additional aid of inspection, palpation, percussion, examination of the pulse and, when possible, of the roentgen rays.

AUSCULTATION OF THE BLOOD VESSELS

Arteries. In addition to the murmurs produced within the heart and transmitted to the arteries, murmurs may arise in the arteries themselves. A systolic murmur may be produced in a normal artery by deep pressure.

The eddies in an aneurysmal sac may produce over the aneurysm loud systolic murmurs which are transmitted for some distance along the arteries. A rough continuous murmur with a systolic accentuation is heard over an arteriovenous aneurysm.

In both types of aneurysm a systolic thrill often accompanies the systolic murmur.

In stenosis of the aorta, also called coarctation of the aorta (*co* = together, + *arctare* = to press), there is a soft systolic murmur over the innominate, carotid and subclavian arteries and their branches. This murmur is often heard at the angle of the left scapula.

In aortic insufficiency a loud first sound, or pistol-shot sound, and Traube's double sound, may be heard over the femoral arteries without exerting pressure.

Duroziez's sign is the "double intermittent crural murmur" in aortic insufficiency which, as Duroziez noted, "most commonly is not present and it is necessary to produce it by means of compression." On pressing the stethoscope firmly over the femoral artery in aortic insufficiency one often hears this double murmur—"swish-swish."

Veins. A continuous humming or roaring murmur is heard over the jugular vein in some cases of marked anemia and hyperthyroidism. It never ceases, occurs during systole and diastole, and has been called the "humming-top murmur" and the "bruit du diable."

Loud murmurs are occasionally heard in the region of the ensiform cartilage in cirrhosis of the liver over dilated veins produced by a well-developed collateral circulation. Gwyn has described two cases in which a diagnosis of congenital heart disease has been made, in both of which the murmur disappeared on making pressure over the sternum in a certain spot.

BIBLIOGRAPHY

Bock, H.: Ueber die Verwendbarkeit des Differential-Stethoskopes nach Dr. Bock. Berlin. klin. Wchnschr. *46*:544, 1909.

Bramwell, Crighton: Gallop rhythm. Quart. J. Med. *4*:149, 1935.

Bramwell, Crighton: Sounds and murmurs produced by auricular systole. Quart. J. Med. *4*:139, 1935.

Coleman, Warren: The vibration sense in percussion. Tr. A. Am. Physicians *50*:278, 1935.

DeSautelle, W. T., and Grey, E. G.: The relation of the papillary muscles to mitral regurgitant murmurs. Arch. Int. Med. *8*: 734, 1911.

Dock, William: Mode of production of the first heart sounds. Arch. Int. Med. *51*:737, 1933.

Eggleston, Cary: The persistence of a mitral stenotic murmur in the presence of auricular fibrillation. Tr. A. Am. Physicians 43: 36, 1928.

Gwyn, Norman B.: On some venous murmurs found in hepatic cirrhosis and their confusion with murmurs of congenital heart disease. Tr. A. Am. Physicians 45:240, 1930.

Hamman, Louis: Spontaneous interstitial emphysema of the lungs. Tr. A. Am. Physicians 52:311, 1937.

Harvey, William: The Works of William Harvey, M.D., transl. by Robert Willis. London, Sydenham Society, 1847.

Harvey, William: De motu cordis, transl. by Chauncey D. Leake. Springfield, Ill., Charles C Thomas, 1931.

Hirschfelder, A. D.: Diseases of the Heart and Aorta. Philadelphia, J. B. Lippincott Company, 1933.

Joseph, G.: Geschichte der Physiologie der Herztöne. Janus 2:345, 1852.

Laubry, Ch., and Pezzi, C.: Les Rhythmes de Galop. Paris, Gaston Doin, 1926.

Levine, Samuel A., and Harvey, W. Proctor: Clinical Auscultation of the Heart. Philadelphia, W. B. Saunders Co., 1949.

Lewis, J. K., and Dock, W.: The origin of heart sounds and their variations in myocardial disease. J.A.M.A. 110:271, 1938.

Lewis, Thomas: Notes upon the cardiorespiratory murmur and its relationship to other physical signs. Quart. J. Med. 2:178, 1908–09.

Mackenzie, Sir James: Principles of Diagnosis and Treatment in Heart Affections. London, Oxford University Press, 1918.

McKusick, Victor A., Murray, Genevieve, E., Peeler, Robert G., and Webb, George N.: Musical murmurs. Bull. Johns Hopkins Hosp. 97:136, 1955.

Mond, Herman, and Oppenheimer, Enid Tribe: Gallop rhythm in hypertension. Arch. Int. Med. 43:166, 1929.

Orias, Oscar, and Braun-Menéndez, Edvardo: The Heart-Sounds in Normal and Pathological Conditions. New York, Oxford, 1939.

Potain, C.: Clinique Médicale de la Charité. Paris, G. Masson, 1894.

Pullen, Roscoe L.: Medical Diagnosis, Applied Physical Diagnosis. 2nd ed. Philadelphia, W. B. Saunders Co., 1950.

Reid, W. D.: The Heart in Modern Practice. Philadelphia, J. B. Lippincott Co., 1928.

Routier, Daniel, and Van Heerswynghels, J.: A propos du bruit de galop, étude phonocardiographique. Arch. d. Mal. du Coeur 28:629, 1935.

Stokes, William: The Diseases of the Heart and the Aorta. Dublin, Hodges and Smith, 1854.

Thayer, W. S.: On the early diastolic heart sound (the so-called third heart sound). Boston Med. and Surg. J. 48:173, 1908.

Thayer, W. S.: Further observations on the third heart sound. Arch. Int. Med. 4:297, 1909.

Vaquez, H.: Maladies du Coeur. Paris, J. B. Baillière et Fils, 1928.

Vierordt, Herman: Die Messung der Intensität der Herztöne. Tübingen, H. Laupp'sche Buchhandlung, 1885.

Weiss, Otto, und Joachim, Gerhard: Registrierung und Reproduktion menschlicher Herztöne und Herzgeräusche. Arch. f. ges. Physiol. 123:341, 1908.

White, Paul D.: Heart Disease. 4th ed. New York, The Macmillan Company, 1951.

Wolferth, Charles C., and Margolies, Alexander: Gallop rhythm and the physiological third heart sound. Am. Heart J. 8:441, 1933.

Wyckoff, John, and Bunim, Joseph: Observations on an apical diastolic murmur unassociated with valvular disease, heard in cases of right ventricular hypertrophy. Tr. A. Am. Physicians 50:280, 1935.

CHAPTER 11

THE PULSE

PALPATION OF THE PULSE is one of the most ancient and time-honored practices of the medical profession. The physicians of ancient Egypt were familiar with the procedure of palpating the pulse, which is described in the Edwin Smith Papyrus (1600 B. C.) and in the Papyrus Ebers (1550 B. C.). The ancient Chinese distinguished at least twenty-three kinds of pulses and claimed that all diseases could be diagnosed by the pulse, since every disease alters the blood and consequently the pulse. A thousand years later Hippocrates taught his disciples to feel the pulse as a part of their examination of the patient. A century after Hippocrates, Praxagoras of Cos wrote a treatise on the pulse which led later physicians to believe that Praxagoras had discovered the pulse. Herophilus of Alexandria, the pupil of Praxagoras, also devoted much time to the study of the pulse, timed its beats by a water clock, and distinguished several varieties of irregularities in the pulse. He also noted that the beats of the heart and the pulsations of the pulse were synchronous. Rufus of Ephesus, who practiced during the reign of Trajan in the second century, wrote a treatise on the pulse which was lost for centuries, but was discovered and translated by Daremberg in 1845. Of this treatise Broadbent in 1890 wrote: "His description of the different characters of the pulse leaves little to be added at the present day"—a tribute to the genius of Rufus and at the same time a confession of a lack of progress in this field for eighteen hundred years. Rufus described the pulse as frequent or infrequent as regards the rate; quick or slow, referring to individual pulsations; strong or weak, referring to the intensity of the beats; hard or soft, referring to its compressibility. He also noted the intermittent pulse, the vibrating pulse and the dicrotic pulse, was familiar with the bigeminal pulse and studied the effects of the respiratory movements upon the pulse. Paul of Aegina, who practiced during the seventh century of the Christian era, distinguished no less than sixty-two varieties. Among the various types listed we note the pulsus dicrotus, pulsus parvus and pulsus rarus, terms still in general use.

Little progress was made during the succeeding centuries in knowledge of the pulse. Cardinal Cusanus (1401–1464) mentions a *clepsydra*, or water clock, with which one could study the frequency of the pulse in disease. The celebrated Galileo timed the swinging of a pendulum with his own pulse, and

195

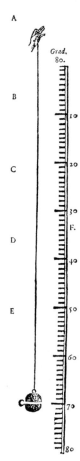

FIG. 316. Santorio's original pulsilogium. The instrument timed the pulse by the swing of the pendulum. The length of the cord which determined the rate of the swing was measured on the scale.

conversely used a pendulum to count the rate of the pulse. Santorio Santorio (1561–1636), better known as Sanctorius, used this invention of Galileo, calling it a *pulsilogium* or *pulse clock* (Fig. 316, 317), and Athanasius Kircher in 1664 described and illustrated a similar instrument. In 1707 Sir John Floyer published his classic "Pulse-Watch," which is a landmark in the history of the pulse. Floyer at first used the common Sea-Minute-Glass, "but because that was not portable, I caused a Pulse-Watch to be made which run 60 Seconds, and I placed it in a Box to be more easily carried, and by this I now feel Pulses." This pulse watch he

Tertium.

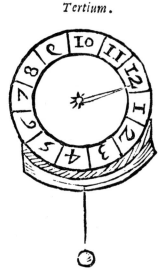

FIG. 317. Santorio's improved pulsilogium. In this instrument the length of the cord is measured on the dial.

always compared with the minute glass which he kept at home as a standard.

Though the ancients were quite familiar with various types of pulses and irregularities of the pulse, they were totally unaware of the mechanism by which these changes were produced. Our knowledge of this mechanism is the result of investigations carried out during the past century. This advance is the result of the labors of Karl Vierordt, the physiologist of Tübingen, who devised the first practical sphygmograph, of Carl Ludwig, the physiologist of Leipzig, who invented the kymograph, of Etienne Jules Marey, the physiologist of Paris, who introduced graphic methods of studying the pulse into clinical medicine, and James Mackenzie, the country doctor of Burnley, who devised an instrument for recording simultaneously the venous and radial pulses. Mackenzie's discovery cleared up many unexplained points, since it enabled him to obtain a record through the jugular vein of what the auricles were doing at the same time the radial pulse recorded the action of the ventricles. Thus the great advance in our knowledge of the pulse during the past century has been due to the use of graphic methods. However, the following quotation from Mackenzie (1926), who did perhaps more than any other in this domain, is significant: "In the examination of the arterial pulse several methods may be employed, as exploration by the fingers, by graphic records and by instrumental measurement of the arterial pressure. By far the most important of these methods is the first. There is a tendency to exalt the others at the expense of the digital, but no apparatus can ever replace the trained finger. No doubt the other methods can give very definite information of a limited kind, but in diagnosing the patient's condition they should only supplement the digital examination."

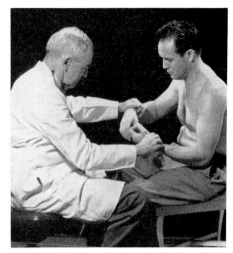

Fig. 318. Palpation of the pulses.

INEQUALITY OF THE PULSES

The Chinese physician of old always felt both pulses of a patient simultaneously as the first procedure in the examination of his patient and laid great stress on a comparison of the two pulses, since he diagnosed diseases of the heart, liver, kidney and intestines from the left wrist and diseases of the lungs, stomach, spleen and kidney from the right wrist. It would be wise for the physician of today to follow his example, but for a different reason. Inequality in the two pulses is readily made out and may be of great diagnostic value. Retardation of the pulse is commonly present in the arteries beyond the aneurysmal sac. An aneurysm of the transverse or descending arch of the aorta causes a retardation of the pulse wave at the left wrist with an artery that feels smaller and is more easily compressed. An aneurysm of the ascending aorta or innominate artery may produce the same changes in the pulse at the right wrist.

A tumor pressing upon any of the large trunks may produce changes in the pulse similar to those of aneurysm. It should, however, be remembered that in some persons there is normally a difference in the size of the two pulses. In some people one radial artery is smaller and the ulnar artery larger by

way of compensation. Some persons have a radial artery that is more superficial at one wrist than at the other. These anatomical differences produce a larger pulse on one side than on the other, but no retardation of the pulse.

In coarctation of the aorta the radial and carotid pulses are large and throbbing, while the femoral, popliteal and dorsalis pedis pulses are scarcely palpable. The pulsations of the abdominal aorta may be difficult to feel, and delayed. This difference is due to stenosis of the aorta, which produces also a collateral circulation between the upper and lower parts of the body mainly through the internal mammary, intercostal, scapular and deep epigastric arteries. These latter vessels are usually markedly dilated and show visible pulsations. The enlargement of the intercostal arteries may produce notching or erosions on the lower border of the ribs which are clearly seen in the x-ray plate. Indeed, the diagnosis is now definitely made by the roentgenologist.

PALPATION OF THE PULSE

In examining the pulse the orthodox procedure is to take the hand of the patient with the palm upward and place three fingers on the radial artery with the index finger nearest the heart. With his fingers in this position the observer is able to feel distinctly the patient's pulse and note its characteristics.

Many misconceptions have arisen as to what the pulse really is. When one observes the carotid pulse, one gets the impression that the carotid artery is alternately expanding and contracting. Mackenzie, however, has shown that if we take two sphygmographic tracings simultaneously, one with the receiver directly over the carotid and the other with the receiver alongside the artery, the tracings are not similar as they should be if the artery alternately dilated and contracted, but one tracing is the reverse image of the other. The carotid really resembles a cord which is alternately tightened and relaxed, tightened or straightened during systole, relaxed during diastole. This movement can often be well observed in a tortuous sclerotic brachial artery, when the brachial pulse is clearly seen as an alternate straightening and relaxation of the vessel. What we see as a carotid pulse is not an alternate dilatation and contraction, but an actual displacement of the whole vessel.

What we feel as the pulse differs somewhat from what we see. We do not feel an expansion of the artery since this, if it really does occur, is so slight that it cannot be registered on the sphygmograph. Also, as Broadbent remarked, "A moment's reflection as to the volume of blood discharged by the left ventricle into the aorta, and a comparison of this with the capacity of the entire arterial system, will convince us that it is altogether inadequate to produce any such expansion of the smaller arteries as will be appreciable to the touch." The pulse we feel is also not due to sinuous movement of the radial artery produced by the alternate cord-like stretching and relaxation.

To feel the radial pulse it is necessary to press it, even if very lightly, against the bone. In palpating the pulse the pressure of the examining fingers flattens the vessel somewhat during diastole, then a wave of blood discharged by the ventricular systole passes along, and the vessel resumes its circular shape. This change from the oval to the circular shape we feel as the pulse. Broadbent gives the following apt comparison: "Such a pulsation can be felt on a large scale by placing the foot on the inelastic leather of a fire engine in action, in which there can be no expansion."

The pulse is largely an index of the heart's action, although, in addition to the action of the heart, the elasticity of the larger vessels and the resistance in the arterioles and capillaries play an important role in determining certain characteristics of the pulse.

CHARACTERISTICS OF THE PULSE

It is a common practice to speak of the force of the pulse. The strength or force of the pulse depends in great measure upon the force of the systole, since the pulse obviously cannot be strong if the ventricular systole is weak or the ventricular filling incomplete. The pulse, however, may be feeble, although the cardiac contractions are very forcible, as in mitral stenosis or in certain cardiac irregularities. The force of the pulse is not, therefore, an accurate index of the force of the cardiac contractions.

The use of the term "force" in relation to the pulse and the description of the pulse as strong and weak are open to serious objections. By the term "strong" one person means the volume of the pulse, while another may mean the pressure within the artery.

The terms "quick" or "slow" are also often ambiguous, since they may refer to the pulse rate or to the character of each individual beat. The ancients were more accurate in their terminology. When referring to the pulse rate they spoke of a *pulsus frequens* or *pulsus rarus* (frequent or infrequent), and when describing the character of the individual beat they used the terms "pulsus celer" or "pulsus tardus" (quick or prolonged).

The pulse is best described according to the following characteristics:

1. Rate—pulsus frequens or rarus (rapid or slow).

2. Size—pulsus magnus or parvus (large or small).

3. Type of wave—pulsus celer or tardus (abrupt or prolonged).

4. Rhythm—pulsus regularis or irregularis (regular or irregular).

5. Tension—pulsus durus or mollis (hard or soft).

Rate

The average rate of the pulse in normal adults is 60 to 80 per minute; in children, 90 to 140; in the aged, 70 to 80.

Tachycardia ($\tau\alpha\chi\acute{v}s$—tachus = swift, $+ \kappa\alpha\rho\delta\acute{\iota}\alpha$—cardia = heart). An acceleration of the pulse, tachycardia or pulsus frequens, is a normal occurrence during and after exercise. One hundred per minute may be considered the upper limit of normal. The pulse rate is decreased during sleep, increased after eating, and during coitus may rise to 140 per minute or more. It changes slightly during respiration, being faster during inspiration than during expiration. Excitement, as everyone knows, produces a temporary increase in the pulse rate, and the physician, in feeling the patient's pulse, should wait two or three minutes before beginning to count the rate. In patients with irritable heart the pulse may be rapid during the physical examination, but fall to normal after the patient is completely relaxed.

In most diseases associated with fever the pulse rate is increased. The pulse rate usually bears a definite ratio to the height of the temperature, the rate being increased on an average of five beats for every degree F. (eight beats per degree C.). An increased pulse rate is usually present in severe anemias, and after a severe hemorrhage the pulse is markedly increased in rate. Atropine increases the pulse rate.

One of the most common causes of a persistent tachycardia is Graves' disease. This disease is also known as Basedow's disease, and more correctly as Parry's disease, since this syndrome was first observed by Caleb Hilliard Parry, forty-nine years before Graves' and fifty-four years before Basedow's publications. In Graves' disease the temperature is commonly elevated, but the increase in the pulse rate is out of all proportion to the elevation in temperature (Fig. 57). Basedow called attention to three outstanding findings in this disease: exophthalmos, tachycardia, and goiter. This combination of signs is often referred to as the "Merseburger triad," named after Merseburg, the home of Basedow.

In vagus paralysis due to increased intracranial pressure (late basilar meningitis) the pulse rate is increased. Persistent tachycardia is an important sign in myocardial disease and almost invariably present in cardiac failure. Tachycardia may be the only pathologic finding in acute and chronic myocardial disease. A fast pulse associated with indistinct and blurred heart sounds suggests myocardial disease.

Paroxysmal Tachycardia. This condition was first described by William Stokes in 1854, but studied more extensively by Richard Cotton in 1867. Cotton's first case showed a pulse rate of 230 per minute, and three weeks after the onset of the attack "the patient entirely recovered; the action of the heart becoming *suddenly* in every respect natural, and the pulse eighty in the minute."

L. Bouveret, in 1889, gave the disease the name of "essential paroxysmal tachycardia," and it is often referred to by the French as Bouveret's disease. According to Bouveret, "each paroxysm begins and ends suddenly, in a few seconds. These sudden transitions from normal rhythm to a tachycardial rhythm, and vice versa, are accompanied sometimes by peculiar sensations in the head or in the precordial region." The tachycardia may, however, attain its maximum several hours or days after its sudden onset and may decrease for several hours before its sudden termination.

A patient may have attacks of paroxysmal tachycardia for many years with no apparent impairment of health. The paroxysmal attacks vary in their duration from a few minutes or hours to days or weeks. Paroxysmal tachycardia may follow coronary occlusion or acute myocarditis. Thyroid disease is a common cause of paroxysmal tachycardia.

Pathognomonic of this disease is the abrupt onset and sudden termination with a pulse rate exceeding 200 per minute. The stimuli producing these attacks may originate in the auricle, in the ventricle or in the auriculoventricular node. This differentiation can be made only with the electrocardiogram. Though the rate is rapid, the beats are regular (Fig. 319).

Bradycardia ($\beta\rho\alpha\delta\acute{v}s$—bradus = slow, $+\kappa\alpha\rho\delta\iota\alpha$—cardia = heart). Slowing of the pulse, bradycardia or pulsus rarus, is noted during convalescence from certain infectious diseases, especially in influenza and often in pneumonia. Icterus usually produces bradycardia. Typhoid fever causes a relative bradycardia, the temperature being markedly elevated while the pulse rate is only slightly increased. The appearance of the bedside chart in typhoid fever is characteristic (Fig. 51). In increased intracranial pressure with vagal stimulation (early basilar meningitis) the pulse rate is decreased.

The classic example of bradycardia is seen in heart block, first described by Morgagni as "epilepsy with a slow pulse," but better known as *Stokes-Adams disease*. Some patients with heart block may have epileptiform attacks when the pulse rate falls below forty per minute. All patients with heart block will have epileptiform attacks when the pulse is slower than sixteen per minute. Other patients have attacks of unconsciousness closely resembling apoplectic attacks. Osler relates that one

patient, the subject of many such attacks, had been bled so often that he had a label inside his coat—"Do not bleed me in an attack." A patient with a pulse rate of fifty or forty per minute should be suspected of having a heart block until proved to the contrary. This disease at times may exist for years with no apparent impairment of health. We observed such a patient once who had a pulse of forty for fifty years and died at the age of eighty-four from pneumonia.

Bradycardia is also common in aortic stenosis and in patients who have been digitalized. Heart block, aortic stenosis and digitalis are the three most common causes of bradycardia.

Some persons can increase the pulse rate at will, while others can decrease the rate. This voluntary control of the pulse rate is rare, and its cause is not well understood. The alteration in rate is probably due to sympathetic or vagus depression or stimulation. Voluntary acceleration of the heart rate has been ascribed by some observers to stimulation of the sympathetic accelerator nerves and by others to depression of the vagus nerve. In a patient whom we studied, voluntary bradycardia was apparently due to pressure of the tensely held neck muscles on the vagus nerves, producing mechanical stimulation of the nerves.

Size

The size of the pulse is dependent upon the degree of filling of the artery during systole and of emptying during diastole. It is a measurement of the pulse pressure—the difference between systolic and diastolic pressures. A *pulsus magnus* has a high pulse pressure, a *pulsus parvus* a low pulse pressure. The collapsing pulse in aortic insufficiency is a good example of the *pulsus magnus*,

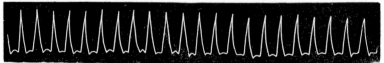

Fig. 319. Radial tracing in paroxysmal tachycardia. Pulse 200 per minute. (Mackenzie.)

while the pulse in aortic stenosis is the classical example of the *pulsus parvus*.

Type of Wave

The type of pulse wave which the palpating finger feels and which is more clearly shown in the sphygmogram depends upon the rapidity with which pulse pressure changes. The term *pulsus celer* does not refer to the pulse rate, inasmuch as it does not mean a rapid pulse, but a quick pulse, one which rises quickly and falls quickly.

Since the size of the pulse and the type of pulse wave are closely related, they will be considered together and some of the classic examples of disturbances in size and type considered.

The Pulse in Aortic Insufficiency. The pulse in aortic insufficiency is a *pulsus magnus et celer*. It is a *pulsus magnus* because it shows a high pulse pressure and a *pulsus celer* because it rises quickly and falls quickly (Fig. 320).

The pulse of aortic insufficiency is one of the most striking of pulses. It was first described by Raymond Vieussens in 1715, who wrote that the "pulse, which appeared to be very full, very fast, very hard, unequal and so strong that the artery of first one then the other arm, struck the ends of my fingers just as a cord would have done which was very tightly drawn and violently shaken." James Hope, more than a century later, described it as a jerking pulse, "the pulse of unfilled arteries." Corrigan wrote a classic paper on aortic insufficiency in which he called attention particularly to the throbbing carotids in this disease and noted that the pulse was "invariably full." Corrigan's description of the pulse was clear and vivid, his description of the clinical picture of aortic insufficiency so complete that it has been customary since his day to speak of the *Corrigan pulse*.

Other terms commonly used in designating this pulse are *collapsing pulse* and *water-hammer pulse*. The term "collapsing" was applied, since the extreme and marked change in pulse pressure imparts to the palpating finger the impression that the pulse has collapsed. The term "water-hammer" is more frequently used than understood. The water hammer was a toy or piece of physical apparatus much used in the nineteenth century. A water hammer consists of a thick glass tube about 1 foot in length half filled with water, the air having been expelled by boiling the water just before sealing the end of the tube with a blow pipe. When such a tube is inverted the water falls down through the vacuum like a solid body, and the hand feels a short hard knock. A similar sensation is often transmitted to the finger by the water-hammer pulse. The term "water-hammer pulse," according to Dock, was not used first by Corrigan, but by Sir Thomas Watson.

Dock thinks that the term "Corrigan pulse should be applied, if at all, to visible phenomena; water hammer to palpatory sensations. As the handling of water hammers has been abandoned, the term should also be given up." It is, however, probably too widely used and too widely referred to, to be abandoned; besides, if we understand what is meant by water hammer, the term is very descriptive.

The water-hammer pulse is produced by a high pulse pressure, the difference

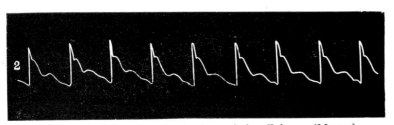

Fig. 320. Radial tracing of pulse in aortic insufficiency. (Marey.)

between the systolic and diastolic blood pressure being often 80 to 100 mm. of mercury as compared with 50 to 60 mm. in the normal person. This pulse is almost always associated with aortic insufficiency, but may be seen occasionally in severe anemias, in arteriovenous aneurysm, in coarctation of the aorta and rarely in Graves' disease.

Though this pulse is well felt with the palpating fingers over the radial, it can often be felt better by grasping the wrist with the entire hand, holding the palm of the examining hand over the flexor surface of the wrist. The water-hammer pulse is usually more striking and more easily felt by holding the patient's hand over his head.

The cause of this pulse has been the subject of much discussion. Vieussens believed that it was due to the quantity of blood which rushed back into the ventricle through the damaged valves during systole. MacCallum brought out evidence to support this mechanical conception. In experiments, the production of a traumatic aortic insufficiency is followed immediately by the appearance of the typical pulse.

The Pulse in Aortic Stenosis. The pulse in aortic stenosis is the antithesis of that found in aortic insufficiency. The pulse of aortic stenosis is a small hard pulse, and it rises and falls slowly—a *pulsus parvus et tardus.* The pulse rate in aortic stenosis is usually slow, often

even when congestive heart failure is present. The sphygmographic tracings show clearly this characteristic pulse (Fig. 321). Aortic stenosis is "said to be the only heart disease in which the absolute diagnosis is determined by the pulse-tracing" (Hirschfelder).

Sphygmographic tracings in aortic stenosis frequently show two other types of pulse, the anacrotic pulse and the *pulsus bisferiens.* These two types of pulse, which are not, however, pathognomonic of aortic stenosis, will be considered later.

The Pulse in Mitral Stenosis. The pulse in uncomplicated mitral stenosis is regular and small, but not feeble. It is the typical *pulsus parvus.* This small size of the pulse is often of great value in diagnosis.

Pulsus Alternans. The classical *pulsus alternans* is a pulse which shows a regular alternation in the size of the beats. This pulse was first described by Ludwig Traube in 1872 as "a succession of high and low pulses, in such a manner that a low pulse follows regularly a high pulse, and this low pulse is separated from the following high pulse by a shorter pause than that between it and the preceding high pulse." Traube illustrated his article with a tracing which is shown in Figure 322. This alternation of the pulse is readily perceived by the palpating finger, and occasionally is so striking that it can be seen on inspec-

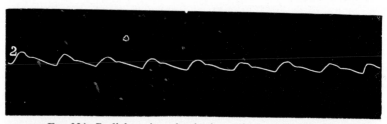

FIG. 321. Radial tracing of pulse in aortic stenosis. (Marey.)

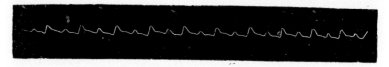

FIG. 322. Traube's tracing of *pulsus alternans.*

tion, particularly of the brachial arteries in elderly arteriosclerotic patients.

Mackenzie regarded *pulsus alternans* as a grave prognostic sign. He states that he had noted this form of irregularity and had published some tracings in his book on the pulse which appeared in 1902. In 1905 Wenckebach called attention to these tracings and, Mackenzie writes, "When I saw his account, I started to re-examine all my patients who had shown this condition (about a dozen), and I found they were all dead."

Pulsus alternans occurs chiefly in elderly patients suffering from myocardial disease, usually the result of arterial hypertension, coronary disease or aortic lesions. When it occurs in the course of an attack of paroxysmal tachycardia or for only a few beats following an extrasystole, it has no sinister meaning. *Pulsus alternans* may follow overdosage with digitalis and, in such cases, disappears when the drug is discontinued.

Dicrotic Pulse. A normal sphygmogram shows a second small wave on the declining wave produced by the radial pulse. In certain fevers, notably typhoid fever, there is a marked relaxation of the arteries, and the dicrotic wave becomes exaggerated (Fig. 323) and can be felt as a small wave immediately following the pulse wave. It is most marked when the diastolic pressure is low. The dicrotic pulse is easily obliterated by slightly increasing the pressure of the examining finger. A dicrotic pulse should always suggest the possibility of typhoid fever, if fever is present.

Anacrotic Pulse. The anacrotic pulse is a pulse which shows in the sphygmogram a small wave on the ascending limb of the pulse wave, analogous to the dicrotic wave on the descending limb (Fig. 324). It was once thought to be characteristic of aortic stenosis, but this view is incorrect. It has no pathological significance. Some observers consider it an artefact. It cannot be felt by the examining finger, and in diagnosis is of no importance.

Pulsus Bisferiens. The *pulsus bisferiens* (*bis* = twice + *feriere* = to beat) is a pulse having two beats and shows at the apex two waves (Fig. 325). According to Broadbent, it differs from the dicrotic pulse in that the dicrotic wave of the dicrotic pulse is easily obliterated, while the *pulsus bisferiens* is brought out by firm pressure. It is common in aortic stenosis, but is found also in arteriosclerosis and in chronic nephritis. Some observers consider it a form of the dicrotic pulse, but Hirschfelder states that the *pulsus bisferiens* is associated with vasoconstriction of the vessels, while the dicrotic

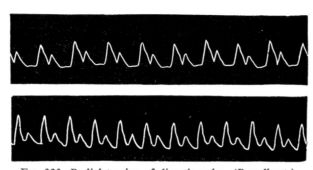

FIG. 323. Radial tracing of dicrotic pulse. (Broadbent.)

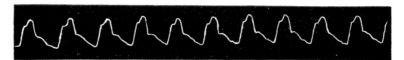

FIG. 324. Radial tracing of anacrotic pulse in aortic stenosis. (Mackenzie.)

pulse is associated with vasodilatation. This is in agreement with Broadbent's procedure for the differentiation of the two. It is commonly associated with reduplication of the first heart sound.

Pulsus Paradoxus. The *pulsus paradoxus* is characterized by a decrease in the size of the pulse or even its momentary disappearance during inspiration. This phenomenon is normally present during forced inspiration, but when it occurs, not as the result of effort, but during quiet respiration, it is pathological. It is found commonly in patients with an adherent pericardium, but has been described also in tumors of the mediastinum, in pleural adhesions and in stenosis of the larynx. Its mechanism has not been satisfactorily explained.

Rhythm

The normal pulse is a series of rhythmic beats following each other at regular intervals—*pulsus regularis*. When the beats follow each other at irregular intervals, pulse is irregular—*pulsus irregularis*.

The presence of an irregularity in the pulse, and therefore in the heart beat, is often the most significant feature of the entire physical examination. We should not forget, however, that a patient with a seriously damaged heart may have a regular pulse and that a patient with an excellent heart may have a definite irregularity.

This simple division of the pulse into *pulsus regularis* and *irregularis* was familiar to Rufus of Ephesus in the second century. Some of his descriptions of irregularities of the pulse almost allow us to make a diagnosis. "The *pulsus caprisans* is when a strong beat is followed by a weak one in such a manner that the artery appears ready for a new diastole without having entirely completed the systole" (extrasystole?). Until the early part of the twentieth century, however, the cause of cardiac irregularity was an unsolved mystery. The man who did most in the solution of this mystery was James Mackenzie, a practitioner in the town of Burnley, England.

Mackenzie at the beginning of his practice saw many patients with irregular pulses. They were much disturbed and asked him what these irregularities meant. Unable to find out in any medical book or by consultation with colleagues, he determined to find out for himself and began taking radial tracings on all his cardiac patients, using a Dudgeon sphygmograph for this purpose. After several years' patient effort he had collected a large number of such tracings, but could make nothing out of them. He then devised an instrument of his own which took simultaneous tracings of the radial artery and of the jugular vein. His subsequent studies of cardiac irregularities were epochal and gave us a clear and entirely new insight into the origin of cardiac irregularities.

Mackenzie's studies of the venous pulse showed that although "the movements in the neck seemed dancing, an analysis of a tracing refers each movement to a definite cause." The venous pulse he found to consist of three waves, one of which he labeled *a* because it was due to the contraction of the auri-

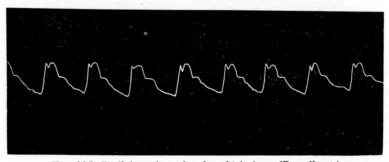

Fig. 325. Radial tracing of *pulsus bisferiens*. (Broadbent.)

cle; the second v, due to contraction of the ventricle; and the third c, produced by the carotid pulse (Fig. 326). The carotid origin of wave c is doubtful, and the v wave is probably produced by ventricular filling.

Mackenzie recognized three common varieties of irregularity. His classification has been since widely adopted.

1. **Sinus Irregularities.** In this type of irregularity the pulse rate is constantly changing, usually with respiration, and the palpating finger notes that the beats are equal in strength. It is seen especially in youthful persons and, for this reason, was called by Mackenzie "the youthful type of irregularity." It is common in infants and can be induced in many persons by forced respiration, the pulse rate being usually increased during inspiration.

This type of irregularity is of vagal origin, stimulation of the vagus producing a momentary slowing. It is common in dogs, in which it can be abolished by section of the vagus. It is called sinus irregularity because the sino-auricular node, at the mouth of the superior vena cava, originates the normal rhythmical stimuli which produce regular cardiac contractions. In this condition the stimuli are produced in an irregular manner.

Sinus irregularity is not pathologic. Mackenzie stated that "Its presence indicates that the heart is healthy."

2. **Premature Contractions.** These have been widely described as extrasystoles, which they usually are not, and also as "dropped beats," an incorrect term, since they are only "dropped" when there is no pulse wave. Mackenzie noted: "In many cases the finger fails to recognise the small pulse beat due to an early occurring systole." The finger receives the impression of a long pause, and then the normal rhythm is resumed. On listening at the apex of

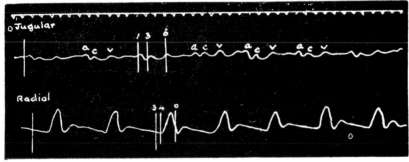

FIG. 326. Radial tracing of normal venous pulse. (Mackenzie.)

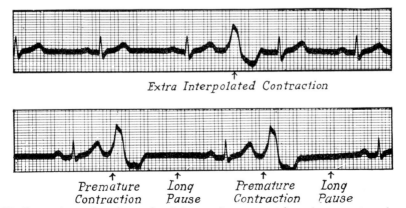

Extra Interpolated Contraction

Premature Contraction   *Long Pause*   *Premature Contraction*   *Long Pause*

FIG. 327. Comparison of an interpolated (or true) extra systole and a premature (so-called) extra systole.

the heart, the premature contraction can usually be heard.

Tracings of such a pulse (Fig. 328) show there is a small beat (the dropped beat) which follows closely after the normal beat and is succeeded by a pause before the next normal beat occurs. It will also be noted that the interval between the normal beat preceding the small beat and the next normal is twice as long as the interval between the normal beats. Mackenzie at first called this beat a "premature systole," but later spoke of it as an "extrasystole." Lewis and other observers have called it a "premature contraction." The term "premature contraction" is more accurate, since in most instances this systole is not an extra, interpolated contraction, but a contraction which has occurred prematurely (Fig. 327).

This premature contraction, as tracings of the pulse and electrocardiograms have shown, may have three points of origin: it may be auricular, ventricular, or nodal (originating at the auriculoventricular node). A ventricular premature contraction is followed by a completely compensatory pause; the pause following an auricular premature contraction is not completely compensatory. This difference may be apparent on palpation.

In diagnosing premature contractions by palpation of the pulse, the important feature is the pause followed by a resumption of the normal rhythm. Premature contractions may appear in severe cardiac disease, but may also be present for years without any apparent impairment of the heart. Mackenzie, after a lifetime spent in studying extra systoles, concluded that "when the extra systole is the only abnormal sign, the prognosis is a favorable one, and where it is associated with other signs, the prognosis is to be based on the other signs."

3. **Pulsus Irregularis Perpetuus.** Irregularities in the pulse have been described for thousands of years, but in 1903 Hering drew attention to a particular type of irregularity which he called *pulsus irregularis perpetuus*—perpetually irregular pulse. Mackenzie encountered this irregularity early in his work on the pulse and gave it the name of the "dangerous form of irregularity."

In this type of irregularity there is a complete arrhythmia, beats follow each other at irregular intervals, and the strength of the individual beats shows great variations. This irregularity in both force and rhythm is readily appreciated by the finger and is graphically shown in a pulse tracing (Fig. 329). This type of irregularity differs from a sinus arrhythmia and extrasystoles in that the former two have a certain regular rhythm which is changed at times by the disturbing irregularity, while the *pulsus irregularis perpetuus* has no regularity at all.

The explanation of this type of irregularity began with the discovery by Mackenzie that tracings of the jugular

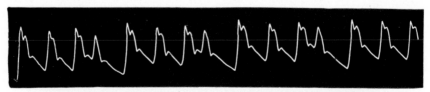

FIG. 328. Radial tracing of premature contractions. (Mackenzie.)

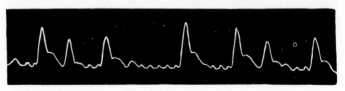

FIG. 329. Radial tracing of *pulsus irregularis perpetuus*. (Norris and Landis.)

veins in these patients showed an absence of the normal *a* wave. In one of his old patients who had a mitral stenosis with a loud presystolic murmur, he saw the appearance of this irregularity coincide with a disappearance of the presystolic murmur. Mackenzie came to the conclusion that this dangerous type of irregularity was due to a paralysis of the auricle which caused a disappearance of the *a* wave because it did not beat and for the same reason was unable to pump the stream of blood through the narrowed mitral orifice with sufficient force to produce a presystolic rumble. He called the disease "paralysis of the auricle" (Fig. 330).

Later investigations showed the irregularity to be due to *fibrillation of the auricles*. This condition of fibrillation was well known to the physiologists and can be produced in a dog's heart by stimulating the auricles with an electrode. As the electric current passes into the auricles, they cease to beat regularly, and, instead, a series of twitchings or fibrillations appear at various points over the auricle. Electrocardiographic studies carried out by one of Mackenzie's colleagues, Thomas Lewis, showed that the electrocardiogram in the *pulsus ir-regularis perpetuus* was identical with that produced by electricity stimulating the dog's auricles. Since this discovery that the cessation of auricular activity was due to fibrillation of the auricles, the condition has been universally called auricular fibrillation.

The extreme irregularity of the pulse in this condition is matched by the extreme irregularity of the heart. This led older writers to speak of "delirium cordis," a very descriptive term for the heart action. Others have referred to an "asystole" of the heart, which is accurate as far as the auricle is concerned, since "it stands still and systole never takes place, and meanwhile the walls quiver with fibrillating contractions" (Mackenzie).

Auricular fibrillation is usually serious. It is seen especially as a complication of mitral stenosis, of hyperthyroidism, and in the hypertensive heart. Mackenzie states that 60 or 70 per cent of all cases of serious heart failure with dropsy owe the failure directly to this condition or have failure aggravated by its presence. Embolism is a frequent occurrence in auricular fibrillation. Auricular fibrillation is not, however, incompatible with many years of relatively good health,

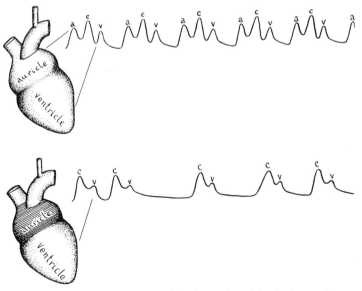

Fig. 330. "Paralysis of the auricle." The auricle is paralyzed in the lower figure, the *a* wave disappears. (The Doctor Explains, Alfred A. Knopf.)

particularly in the absence of a valvular lesion. One of our own patients with auricular fibrillation lived for twenty years after discovery of this lesion, carried on his normal activities, took digitalis regularly and died at eighty of malignant disease.

Pulse Deficit. In auricular fibrillation many of the ventricular beats are so weak that, although they may be heard at the apex, they fail to come through at the wrist. If one counts simultaneously the beats at the apex and at the wrist, the apex rate is faster than the radial pulse. This difference, illustrated in Figure 331, is called the pulse deficit. With cessation of fibrillation, the pulse deficit disappears. Pulse deficit is also frequent with premature contractions.

Heart Block. Mackenzie's jugular pulse tracings showed conclusively that in heart block the *a* wave registers often several auricular contractions before the *v* wave of ventricular contraction occurs (Fig. 332). The "epilepsy with a slow pulse" of Morgagni was due to the fact that all the auricular contractions did

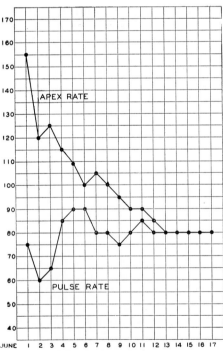

FIG. 331. Pulse deficit. Under digitalis therapy the deficit disappears.

not pass through the bundle of His and produce ventricular contractions, with the result that the radial pulse was markedly slowed.

Pulsus Bigeminus. In *pulsus bigeminus,* the bigeminal pulse (*bi* = two + *geminus* = twin), the beats come in couples or twins, the second beat usually being somewhat weaker. It has also been described as "coupled beats" (Fig. 333).

Pulsus bigeminus may be produced by two quite different mechanisms.

1. *Premature Contractions.* When each normal systole is followed closely by a premature contraction, the premature contraction in turn is followed by a longer pause, and a coupling of the beats occurs. This coupling is readily perceived by the finger and its mechanism clearly seen in an electrocardiogram (Fig. 334).

2. *Partial Heart Block.* When every third auricular contraction fails to pass through and cause ventricular contraction, a similar coupling of the beats occurs (Fig. 335).

Premature contractions are a more common cause of the bigeminal pulse than heart block. A bigeminal pulse is frequently produced by digitalis and disappears when the drug is discontinued. The bigeminal pulse seen in Figure 336 was produced by digitalis intoxication, which caused a heart block.

Pulsus bigeminus is often confused with *pulsus alternans.* In the latter condition, however, the rhythm is regular, while in *pulsus bigeminus* the weaker beat is followed by a pause. At times, however, differentiation may be so difficult that we must have recourse to a blood-pressure apparatus or pulse tracings or the electrocardiogram.

Pulsus Trigeminus. In *pulsus trigeminus* (*tres* = three + *geminus* = twin) every three beats are followed by a pause. This condition may be produced by premature contractions replacing each normal third beat, to a heart block in which each fourth ventricular contraction is missing and, according to Lewis, also to an extrasystole replacing

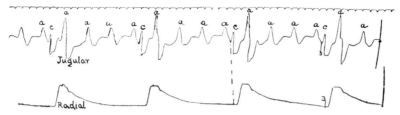

Fig. 332. Jugular wave in heart block. Four auricular beats to one ventricular—4:1 rhythm. (Mackenzie.)

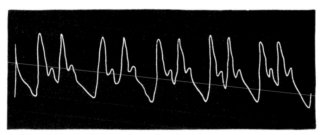

Fig. 333. Radial tracing of *pulsus bigeminus.* (Riegel.)

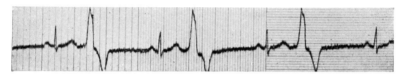

Fig. 334. Electrocardiogram in *pulsus bigeminus*—alternating premature contractions.

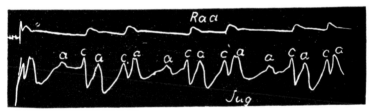

Fig. 335. Coupling of beats due to heart block. Tracing shows a failure of every third auricular contraction to pass through auriculoventricular bundle. (Mackenzie.)

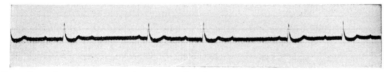

Fig. 336. *Pulsus bigeminus* in digitalis poisoning. Electrocardiogram shows "cradling" or down curve between S and T, characteristic of digitalis effect.

the fourth normal beat, this extrasystole failing to reach the wrist.

Tension

To estimate the tension of the pulse it is necessary to use the fingers of both hands. The index finger of one hand is placed over the distal end of the pulse, and firm pressure is exerted here to prevent the pulse from returning to the radial artery from the ulnar artery through the palmar arch. The index finger and second finger of the other hand are then placed over the radial artery, pressure is exerted with the index finger, and the pulse is felt with the second finger. If the pressure necessary to obliterate the pulse is slight, we have a soft compressible pulse, a *pulsus mollis,* a pulse of low tension. If the pulse is obliterated with difficulty, we have a hard pulse, a *pulsus durus,* a pulse of high tension. The pulse tension corresponds to the diastolic blood pressure.

The normal radial pulse is palpable only during systole and not during diastole. If the diastolic pressure is above 100 mm. of mercury, the artery is palpable throughout the pulse cycle.

It should be remembered that the physician diagnosed high blood pressure and low blood pressure long before satisfactory instrumental measurement of the blood pressure was possible. Sir William Broadbent noted the characteristics of normal low and high tension as follows:

In a pulse of average tension, the vessel only stands out, so as to be felt distinctly, during the actual beat, and subsides gradually or rapidly in the interval; it cannot, therefore, be rolled by the fingers at all periods.

In a pulse of low tension the vessel can scarcely be said to be felt as such at all; it starts up with the beat, and is at once lost again when the brief wave has passed.

In a pulse of high tension, on the other hand, the artery stands out among the structures of the wrist like another tendon, and can be rolled like a cord under the fingers, and followed for some distance up the forearm. While the vessel is thus being rolled about, the pulsation in it may scarcely make itself felt. . . . Pressure, however, brings out the pulsation and develops its force.

The older generation of physicians who estimated the tension of the pulse only with the palpating finger noted a low tension in fevers, in patients with failing hearts and in many anemic and nervous persons; high tension in renal disease, gout, lead poisoning and pregnancy.

A hard pulse or a soft pulse can be determined by palpation, but most attempts to estimate the blood pressure in terms of millimeters of mercury with the fingers fail. For accurate determinations of the blood pressure the sphygmomanometer has replaced the finger. As the late Professor Gibson, a lifelong student of cardiovascular disease, once wrote: "A long training of my fingers beside the sphygmomanometer has taught me how fallacious the finger must always be."

VESSEL WALL

The last procedure in palpating the pulse is to feel the vessel wall. In marked arteriosclerosis of the radial artery the wall of the artery feels hard and irregular on light palpation, the so-called "pipe stem" or "goose neck" artery. The blood should be expressed from the artery, in doubtful cases, by pressing the two second fingers firmly together over the radial and then, keeping them on the artery, draw them 2 or 3 inches apart. If the artery after the blood has thus been forced out can be distinctly felt by the two index fingers, it is definitely thickened.

The most common error made in palpation is to confuse the tension of the pulse with thickening of the vessel wall. In our experience, based on later pathologic examination of the radial arteries palpated by competent clinicians, the diagnoses of "moderate" and "slight" arteriosclerosis are usually wrong.

CAPILLARY PULSE

Capillary pulse is also known as Quincke's pulse, since the observations of Heinrich Quincke focused attention upon this phenomenon.

It is best seen, as Quincke pointed out, "in the area between the whitish, blood-poor area and the red injected part of the capillary system of the nail-bed; in the majority of persons examined, there is, with each heart beat, a forward and backward movement of the margin between the red and white part, and he can convince himself that the increase of the redness follows a moment later than the apex beat and is still clearly systolic and rather rapid, while the backward movement of the edge of the redness seems to take place more slowly. That is, a lingering in the wave which can be seen by the eye, just as palpation and the sphygmograph show it in the pulse waves of the radial artery." "A large and rapidly falling pulse is seen especially in aortic insufficiency, and for this reason, the capillary pulse is especially clear in this condition. Even in a horizontal position of the hand, we see a very clear and rapid appearance and disappearance of the margin between the red and white zone and also a uniform coloration of the nail and lightning-like and evanescent reddening, so that the manner of the appearance and disappearance of the capillary pulse is, for the eye, a characteristic sign of active visibility of the capillary pulse in health, and in addition the transparency of the nails and the proper degree of elasticity of the arteries must be considered."

The pulse is often brought out especially well in white patients by rubbing the forehead until a red line is formed and then observing the change of color in this red line. Another excellent method consists in pressing a glass slide against the everted lower lip. This capillary pulse is most commonly seen in aortic insufficiency, but is also present at times in patients with hyperthyroidism and with severe anemia.

BIBLIOGRAPHY

Boas, Ernest P., and Goldschmidt, Ernst F.: The Heart Rate. Springfield, Ill., Charles C Thomas, 1932.

von Bonsdorff, Bertel, and Wolf, Hans Julius: Weitere Erfahrungen mit der Registrierung absoluter Sphygmogramme der Arteria cubitalis. Ztschr. f. d. ges. exper. Med. 86:12, 1932.

Broadbent, W. H.: The Pulse. London, Cassell & Co., 1890.

Dock, G.: Dominic John Corrigan: His place in development of our knowledge of cardiac disease; water-hammer pulse. Ann. M. Hist. 6:381, 1934.

Floyer, Sir John: The Physician's Pulse-Watch. London, 1707.

Holman, Emile: The physiology of an arteriovenous fistula. Arch. Surg. 7:64, 1923.

Holman, Emile: Experimental studies in arteriovenous fistulas. Arch. Surg. 9:882, 1924.

Horine, Emmet Field: An epitome of ancient pulse lore. Bull. Hist. Med. 10:209, 1941.

MacCallum, William G.: The changes in the circulation in aortic insufficiency. Bull. Johns Hopkins Hosp. 22:197, 1911.

Mackenzie, James: The Study of the Pulse. Edinburgh and London, Young J. Pentland, 1902.

Major, Ralph H.: Raymond Vieussens and his treatise on the heart. Am. M. Hist. 4: 147, 1932.

Marey, E. J.: La Méthode Graphique. Paris, G. Masson, 1878.

Paulus Aegineta: Opus de re medica, apud Andream Arrivabenum, Venice, 1542.

Paulus Aegineta: Seven Books, transl. from the Greek by Francis Adams. London, 1844, Vol. 1.

Pease, E. A.: Voluntary control of the heart. Boston Med. & Surg. Jour. 120:525, 1889.

Rosenbloom, Jacob: The history of pulse timing with some remarks on Sir John Floyer and his physician's pulse watch. Ann. M. Hist. 4:97, 1922.

Sanctorii Sanctorii: Commentaria in Primam Fen Primi Libri Canonis Avicennae. Venice, 1625.

Stewart, Hugh A.: Experimental and clinical investigation of the pulse and blood pressure changes in aortic insufficiency. Arch. Int. Med. 1:102, 1908.

Vierordt, Karl: Die Lehre vom Arterienpuls in gesunden und kranken Zuständen. Brunswick, Friedrich Vieweg, 1855.

Vieussens, Raymond: Traité nouveau de la structure et des causes du movement naturel du coeur. Toulouse, Jean Guillemette, 1715.

West, Howard F., and Savage, William E.: Voluntary acceleration of the heart beat. Arch. Int. Med. 22:290, 1918.

Wilson, R. McNair: The Beloved Physician, Sir James Mackenzie. New York, The Macmillan Company, 1927.

Wolf, Hans Julius, and von Bonsdorff, Bertel: Blutige Messung des absoluten Sphygmogramms beim Menschen. Ztschr. f. d. ges. exper. Med. 79:567, 1931.

Wong, K. Chimin, and Wu, Lien-Teh: History of Chinese Medicine. Tientsin, 1932.

CHAPTER 12

BLOOD PRESSURE

THE DISCOVERY OF the blood pressure was made not by a physician, but by a clergyman, the Rev. Stephen Hales, the "perpetual" curate of Teddington. In the year 1708 he carried out some experiments on dogs and shortly afterward on horses. "I caused a *mare* to be tied down alive on her back; she was 14 hands high, and about 14 years of age, had a fistula on her withers, was neither very lean nor yet lusty: having laid open the crural artery about 3 inches from her belly, I inserted into it a brass pipe, whose bore was 1-6 of an inch in diameter; and to that, by means of another brass pipe which was fitly adapted to it, I fixed a glass tube, of nearly the same diameter, which was 9 feet in length: then untying the ligature in the artery, the blood rose in the tube 8 feet 3 inches perpendicular above the level of the left ventricle of the heart."

PALPATORY METHOD

Hales' discovery of the blood pressure was followed by numerous attempts to measure the blood pressure in man, since obviously the method used by Hales on animals could not be followed. The first accurate and practical instrument for the estimation of the blood pressure in patients was devised by

Samuel von Basch in 1880, one hundred and seventy-two years after the discovery of the blood pressure. This was a simple instrument consisting of a rubber ball filled with water with a mercury manometer attached above it.

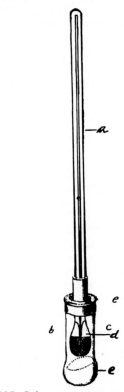

FIG. 337. Sphygmomanometer of von Basch.

212

The ball was pressed upon the pulse until the beat was obliterated, this point of disappearance being registered by the manometer (Fig. 337).

This instrument was improved by Potain, who attached a rubber tube with an aneroid manometer to a compressible bulb filled with air. The bulb was placed over the radial artery, pressure exerted until the pulse could no longer be felt at the wrist, and this pressure, which was registered by the manometer, taken as the systolic pressure (Fig. 338). This instrument, as Vaquez remarks, "for an entire medical generation was as useful in research as the clinical thermometer."

In 1896 Scipione Riva-Rocci demonstrated an instrument for the estimation of blood pressure. His apparatus consisted of a rubber bag surrounded by a cuff of inelastic material and connected with a mercury manometer and a rubber bulb (Fig. 339). In taking the blood pressure, the cuff with the rubber bag was placed around the arm, air pumped into the bag with the rubber bulb and the pressure raised until the radial pulse disappeared at the wrist. The air was then released, and, as the mercury fell in the manometer, the point on the scale was noted when the pulse reappeared at the wrist. This was the systolic pressure.

Riva-Rocci's method, however, gave only the systolic pressure. Accurate estimation of the diastolic pressure dates from the observations of Korotkoff.

AUSCULTATORY METHOD

Korotkoff in 1905 introduced the auscultatory method of estimating the blood pressure. This method has also gained universal acceptance, for with it one can estimate both the systolic and diastolic pressures.

In carrying out the auscultatory method the arm cuff is pumped up until the pulse disappears. The bell of the stethoscope is placed over the brachial artery at the bend of the elbow, and, on listening, nothing is heard—the period of

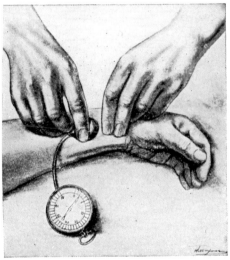

FIG. 338. Sphygmomanometer of Potain. (Vaquez.)

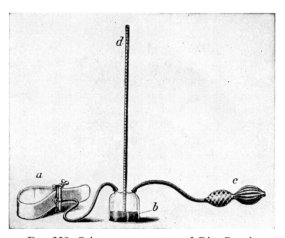

FIG. 339. Sphygmomanometer of Riva-Rocci.

silence. The pressure is now released, and as the mercury falls in the manometer, a point is reached when beats appear—this is the systolic pressure. As the mercury continues to fall, the sound of the beats becomes louder, then gradually diminishes until a point is reached where there is suddenly a marked diminution in intensity—at this point we have the diastolic pressure. The weakened beats are heard for a few moments and at a point 5 to 10 mm. lower disappear altogether (Fig. 340). *Not the point at which the sounds disappear, but the point at which the intensity suddenly diminishes is the diastolic pressure.* The dictum that the blood pressure is "from silence to silence" is incorrect.

Occasionally there is no disappearance of the sounds and the beats are heard to zero (Fig. 341). This phenomenon has given rise to numerous interesting but erroneous case reports

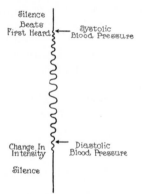

Fig. 340. Diagram of events in auscultatory method of estimating blood pressure.

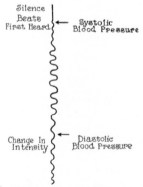

Fig. 341. Case of so-called "absence of diastolic pressure."

of patients who "have no diastolic pressure." Obviously, every patient having a systolic pressure also has a diastolic pressure. The error arises from failing to estimate the diastolic pressure at the point where the sudden change in intensity occurs. We have encountered this phenomenon in patients with aortic insufficiency, in hyperthyroidism and, occasionally, in persons apparently normal.

Comparison of the Palpatory and Auscultatory Methods. Many observers use the auscultatory method to the exclusion of the palpatory. This we believe to be a mistake. For the estimation of the systolic blood pressure, the reading at which we can first palpate the pulse is obviously the systolic pressure, regardless of what we hear. Usually there is little difference between the systolic pressure as determined by the palpatory or the auscultatory methods, although, on an average, the auscultatory method gives readings 10 to 15 mm. higher. Occasionally, however, we can palpate the pulse when the manometer reading is 200 mm., but can hear nothing until the manometer falls to 170 or 160 mm. Obviously, in such conditions, the systolic pressure is 200 mm., since the pulse appears at this level of pressure. Conversely, we occasionally hear the pulse sounds at 200 mm., but do not feel the pulse until 160 is reached. In

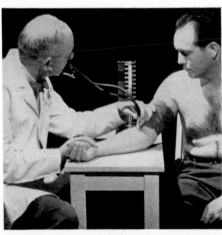

Fig. 342. Taking the blood pressure, employing both palpatory and auscultatory methods.

this case we hear the column of blood beating against the compressed artery which is somewhat relaxed, but not patent, the pressure in the cuff not being sufficiently low to allow the pulse wave to pass through.

Since errors in determining the systolic blood pressure by auscultation are more likely to occur, the palpatory method is more reliable. It requires, however, more practice to become adept in this method. A safe rule is to use both methods, but, in case of difference, to regard the palpatory findings as more reliable.

In the estimation of the diastolic pressure we have only the auscultatory method. Fortunately, numerous experiments have shown that it is nearly always reliable.

Accuracy of the Palpatory and Auscultatory Methods. These methods, like many methods used in clinical medicine, have only a relative accuracy. Estimations of the blood pressure by the direct method of introducing directly into the artery a needle connected with a sensitive recording apparatus show that the blood pressure taken by the Riva-Rocci apparatus has often an error of 10 to 20 mm., sometimes too high, at other times too low. This holds for both the palpatory and auscultatory methods and for systolic as well as for diastolic pressure. However, we know what the average normal blood pressure is when estimated by the Riva-Rocci apparatus, so that it is the variations from this normal

value that allow us to determine whether the blood pressure is normal, increased or decreased.

The resistance of the tissues in the arm which must be overcome by the arm band is a factor of error. This probably accounts for the fact that the blood pressure as estimated by the Riva-Rocci apparatus is usually too high, since the pressure applied to the cuff must overcome the resistance of the tissues before compressing the brachial artery. For this reason patients with abnormally fat arms often show readings grossly inaccurate and far too high.

OSCILLOMETRIC METHOD

The oscillometric methods of estimating the blood pressure are based on the oscillations of the arterial walls. The principle of the oscillometer depends upon the following phenomena: When the pressure outside a blood vessel is raised above the systolic blood pressure, there are no oscillations of the blood vessel wall. As the outside pressure is lowered, oscillations first appear at the point where the pressure inside the artery exceeds the pressure without. This is the systolic pressure. As we approach the minimal pressure, the oscillations become larger and then suddenly cease at the point where the pressure without the artery is less than the minimal pressure. This is the diastolic pressure.

The Pachon oscillometer is one of the best-known instruments of this type (Fig. 343). In this apparatus the oscil-

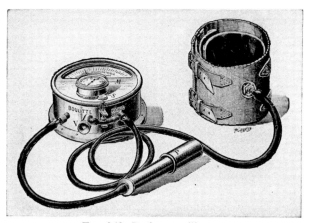

Fig. 343. Pachon oscillometer.

lations of the artery are transmitted through a special cuff which contains two rubber bags. The oscillations are observed by means of a needle which passes across the face of the indicator with each oscillation. There is a small aneroid manometer on the instrument which registers the pressure at which the oscillations appear and the pressure at which they disappear.

The oscillometer of Pachon is theoretically an ideal instrument, but practically has two serious disadvantages. The systolic blood pressure determinations are often too high, and frequently it is impossible to tell at what point the oscillations actually appear, particularly in arterial hypertension. The estimation of the diastolic pressure by this instrument is particularly accurate.

The Tycos recording sphygmomanometer is an oscillometer in which the appearance and disappearance of the oscillations are recorded by an ingenious writing device (Fig. 344). This instrument has the advantage of giving us a permanent record of the blood pressure with an exclusion of the personal factor in the recording. In the interpretation of the records, however, the personal factor may play a large role. This instrument has the disadvantages of all oscillometers, and, in our experience, many records are obtained in which, instead of a sudden appearance and disappearance of the oscillations which should indicate the systolic and diastolic pressures, the oscillatory waves appear so gradually that the systolic pressure cannot be determined and disappear so gradually and almost imperceptibly that the diastolic pressure also cannot be determined.

This instrument makes interesting tracings of cardiac irregularities, and a diagnosis can frequently be made from such a tracing (Fig. 345).

Kilgore in 1915 demonstrated the important role played by the personal factor in the interpretation of blood pressure determinations made by the oscillatory method. Kilgore sent 100 records of blood pressure taken with the Erlanger apparatus to nine competent observers and asked them to mark the systolic and diastolic pressures. On comparing these marks, Kilgore found the difference between the highest and lowest readings of the systolic pressure in one patient was 62 mm. of mercury, while the average variations were from 15 to 35 mm. The variations in the diastolic readings were essentially the same.

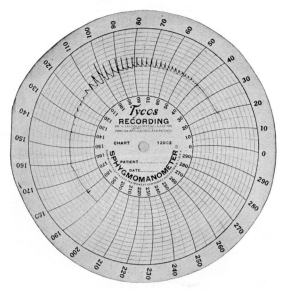

Fig. 344. Record of Tycos apparatus in normal case.

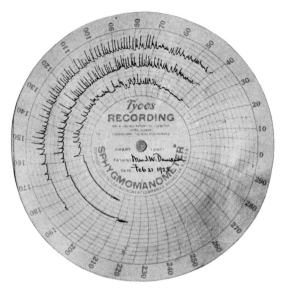

FIG. 345. Record of Tycos apparatus in patient with auricular fibrillation.

THE NORMAL BLOOD PRESSURE

In the average normal adult from twenty to forty years of age the systolic pressure is from 90 to 120, the diastolic pressure from 60 to 80 mm. of mercury. The pressure is often higher as the age increases, not because an increase in pressure is normal with an increase in age, but because hypertension is a disease of middle age and not of youth. The "rule" that the systolic blood pressure should be the age plus 100 is not a rule but a superstition. Many persons seventy or eighty years of age show a systolic blood pressure of 120 to 140. It is a safe rule to consider a systolic blood pressure above 140 and a diastolic above 100 as definitely elevated.

The blood pressure is not a constant factor. It changes from day to day, from hour to hour, and even from minute to minute. Although it does show such periodic changes in health, it does not rise above the normal limits.

The normal blood pressure shows climatic and racial variations. The inhabitants of torrid and tropical zones show a lower blood pressure than those living in temperate zones. Chinese, Japanese and Malays have a lower blood pressure than Europeans. The blood pressure falls during sleep and may be strikingly elevated by fright or excitement.

ELEVATION OF BLOOD PRESSURE —HYPERTENSION

The blood pressure is dependent upon three factors: the force of the heart beat, the amount of peripheral resistance, and the quantity and viscosity of the blood. An increase in any one of these factors may produce an elevation in blood pressure. In most instances the elevation is produced by an increase in the peripheral resistance, by a spasm of the capillaries and arterioles.

A moderate elevation in blood pressure is seen in mitral stenosis and in aortic insufficiency. In both these diseases the systolic blood pressure may be elevated 20 to 30 mm. In aortic insufficiency, however, the diastolic pressure is lower than normal, and it is this combination of high systolic and low diastolic pressures that produces the Corrigan pulse.

The most common causes of elevation of the blood pressure or arterial hypertension seen in the practice of medicine are:

1. **Essential Hypertension.** This condition, also called hyperpiesia or hypertensive vascular disease, is by far the

commonest cause of a pathologically elevated blood pressure. This disease is one of the most widely prevalent of all diseases, it shows a marked familial tendency, it appears most commonly in middle-aged persons, and its victims usually die as the result of cardiac failure, cerebral hemorrhage or chronic nephritis. It is one of the most common causes of cardiac hypertrophy and of cardiac disease.

The blood pressure in essential hypertension is usually extremely variable and labile, and changes rapidly with the emotions (Fig. 346). It is often impossible to obtain the same systolic and diastolic readings twice in succession (Fig. 347). The systolic pressure is usually much more labile than the diastolic pressure.

Both the systolic and diastolic pressures are elevated. A marked elevation of the diastolic pressure is a bad prognostic sign. Blankenhorn showed that some patients with essential hypertension have a marked fall in blood pressure, often to normal, during sleep, while others show no change. The prognosis is better in the first group.

2. **Chronic Nephritis.** This may follow essential hypertension or occur independently. Compared to essential hypertension, chronic nephritis is an uncommon disease.

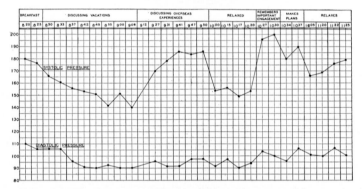

Fig. 346. Changes in blood pressure of hypertensive patient, caused by emotional states.

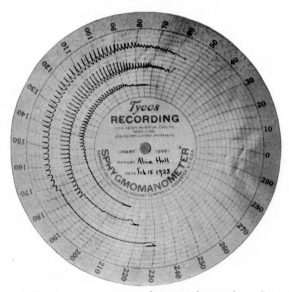

Fig. 347. Records of blood pressures on a hypertensive patient. Records made in rapid succession.

3. **Hyperthyroidism.** This disease may produce some elevation of the blood pressure, particularly the systolic pressure. The elevation is moderate compared to that seen in essential hypertension.

4. **Paroxysmal Hypertension.** This is a rare disease characterized by paroxysms of hypertension during which the systolic pressure may reach 250 or 300. These paroxysms may last a few hours or a few days, but afterwards the blood pressure falls to normal. Paroxysmal hypertension, in most cases, is due to a neoplasm of the adrenal gland.

5. **Cushing's Syndrome.** This syndrome, which is associated with basophilic adenomata of the pituitary gland, is characterized by obesity, hypertrichosis and hypertension (Fig. 348).

The idea that atherosclerosis produces hypertension has been abandoned by recent investigators. It may accompany hypertension, but its presence is incidental. Patients with extreme atherosclerosis often show normal blood pressures. Arteriolosclerosis, by contrast, is usually, if not invariably, present in essential hypertension.

In polycythemia vera (Vaquez-Osler disease) the blood pressure may be elevated when the blood count is high, and fall to normal when the blood count is reduced. Theoretically we should always expect an elevation of the blood pressure because of the increased viscosity of the blood. This, however, as Vaquez has pointed out, is not the case.

LOW BLOOD PRESSURE— HYPOTENSION

Since an elevation in blood pressure is due to an increased force of the heart beat, an increase in the volume and viscosity of the blood or an increased peripheral resistance, the reverse is true in low blood pressure. A weakening of the heart beat, a loss of blood or a marked anemia and peripheral vasomotor paralysis will cause a lowering of the blood pressure.

A sudden fall in blood pressure during or after a surgical operation, after heat prostration, in pericarditis with effusion, in cardiac disease, in hemorrhage or pneumonia is a serious sign. Indeed, all sudden falls in blood pressure indicate a collapse of either the heart or the vasomotor system, and should be regarded as a grave sign. In pericardial effusion the blood pressure falls as the amount of fluid increases. A marked fall in blood pressure is a sign of serious prognostic import in pericardial effusion and an indication for immediate drainage of the pericardium.

Chronic low blood pressure, both systolic and diastolic, is seen in tuberculosis, anemia and particularly in Addison's disease, in which it is a classic sign. It is often present in adult hypo-

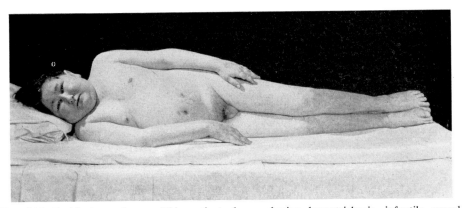

FIG. 348. Cushing's syndrome. This patient shows obesity, hypertrichosis, infantile sexual organs and a blood pressure of 200/130.

thyroidism, a possible diagnosis that should be kept in mind when hypotension is encountered in a patient. A low diastolic pressure is present in aortic insufficiency and in arteriovenous aneurysm.

In most persons, however, a low blood pressure produces no symptoms whatever. Several of the most energetic and healthy people of our acquaintance have persistent systolic pressures under 100. In youth or early adult life a low blood pressure carries with it a suspicion of tuberculosis, and the life insurance examiner is cautious. In later life it is a passport to ripe old age.

CARDIAC IRREGULARITIES

Cardiac irregularities of rate, caused by premature contractions and auricular fibrillation, are readily recognized when we use the auscultatory method of estimating the blood pressure. Mackenzie has pointed out that the sphygmomanometer is of great value in determining the presence of a cardiac irregularity of force, *pulsus alternans*.

If we inflate the arm cuff well above the systolic pressure in a case of *pulsus alternans* and allow the pressure to fall slowly, we presently hear the beats at the bend of the elbow coming through in a perfectly even and regular fashion, but at a rate one half that of the pulse rate. As the pressure continues to fall, these beats become louder, and presently another set of softer beats appear, each soft beat following a loud beat, the rate now being exactly the pulse rate. This alternation in strength of the beats is clearly heard, and the condition can be distinguished from a bigeminal pulse by the regularity with which the beats are spaced.

THE BLOOD PRESSURE IN COARCTATION OF THE AORTA

The blood pressure in coarctation of the aorta shows a higher systolic and diastolic blood pressure in the brachial arteries than in the femoral and the tibial arteries, since the brachial arteries take their origin above the stenosis and the tibial arteries below. In this connection the well-known physical law will be recalled that a partial obstruction to the flow of a fluid in a tube increases the pressure above the obstruction, but decreases it below. In coarctation of the aorta the patient may show a brachial systolic pressure of 200 mm. or over, while the femoral systolic pressure is 100 mm. or less.

The demonstration of a marked hypertension in a youthful person should always suggest the possibility of coarctation of the aorta, since the pressure is usually taken in the brachial artery.

BIBLIOGRAPHY

Blankenhorn, M. A.: The effect of sleep on normal and high blood-pressure. Tr. A. Am. Physicians *40*:87, 1925.

Fishberg, A. M.: Hypertension and Nephritis. Philadelphia, Lea & Febiger, 1930.

Janeway, Theodore C.: The Clinical Study of Blood Pressure. New York, Appleton, 1910.

Kilgore, Eugene S.: The large personal factor in blood pressure determinations by the oscillatory method. Arch. Int. Med. *16*: 893, 1915.

Kilgore, Eugene S., Berkley, Hugh K., Rowe, Albert H., and Stabler, W. H.: A quantitative determination of the personal factor in blood pressure measurements by the auscultatory method. Arch. Int. Med. *16*: 927, 1915.

Major, Ralph H.: The history of taking blood pressure. Ann. Med. Hist. *2*:47, 1930.

Stieglitz, E. J.: Arterial Hypertension. New York, Paul B. Hoeber, Inc., 1930.

CHAPTER 13

PHYSICAL FINDINGS IN CARDIOVASCULAR DISEASES

DISEASES OF THE HEART and of the blood vessels produce certain changes which can be recognized by inspection, palpation, percussion and auscultation. Sir James Mackenzie has said that "the main question in every examination of the heart is concerned with heart failure —whether it is present or foreshadowed." While this is quite true and while it is equally true that the diagnosis of pericarditis or of a valvular lesion does not always give the answer to this question, yet the recognition of pericardial, myocardial and valvular lesions is of fundamental importance to the physician. It not only establishes his diagnosis, but also directs his therapy and determines his prognosis. In this chapter the outstanding physical findings in the most important cardiovascular diseases will be considered.

PERICARDITIS

Pericarditis may be due to a variety of etiologic factors, the most important of which are rheumatic fever, tuberculosis, pneumonia, coronary occlusion and chronic nephritis. This varied etiology explains the fact that it may occur at any age, rheumatic pericarditis in a child, the pericarditis of coronary occlusion and of chronic nephritis in adults often of advanced age, and tubercular and pneumonic pericarditis at any age. Almost any infectious disease may be complicated by pericarditis, and it is occasionally seen in scarlet fever. Traumatic pericarditis may result from a blow, a stab wound or a shot.

Rheumatic fever is the most common cause of pericarditis, and recent studies show that the pericardium is commonly and often extensively involved in rheumatic fever. *Tubercular* pericarditis is usually the result of an extension of the tubercular process from the adjacent pleura, lung or mediastinal lymph glands. *Pneumonic* pericarditis is usually produced by an extension of the infection from an adjacent lobe of the lung, but may occasionally be due to a blood stream infection. The pericarditis of *coronary occlusion* may be important from the standpoint of diagnosis, since the presence of a small area over which a pericardial friction rub is heard may be the only physical finding present. The area of involvement is, however,

221

small, and as far as pericarditis is concerned the lesion is of little importance. Pericarditis in *chronic nephritis* is usually an accidental finding; the area of pericarditis is small, is painless and usually causes no symptoms or elevation of temperature. The pericarditis is unknown to the patient and unimportant as a complication of the disease.

Acute pericarditis may occur without or with effusion, this complication depending upon the character of the exudate. If the exudate is fibrinous, no effusion occurs; if it is serous, an effusion appears. Three types of pericarditis are observed clinically.

1. Acute Fibrinous Pericarditis

This is the most common and most benign form. The amount of exudate is usually small; the process may be localized to a small area or may be extensive. When the exudate is abundant, the fibrin may be in shreds, and the heart presents a shaggy or hairy appearance, the so-called *cor villosum*. The ancients considered such a heart a sign of great fortitude. According to Pliny, Aristomenes, the Greek hero, who single-handed put entire armies to flight, was found after death to have a heart "covered with hair."

Patients with acute fibrinous pericarditis usually have fever. The affection is painless unless the pleura or diaphragm is involved.

Inspection. This is usually negative.

Palpation. On palpation a fremitus due to the rubbing together of the pericardial surfaces is often felt.

Percussion. This reveals nothing abnormal.

Auscultation. The characteristic finding is the to-and-fro friction rub which corresponds to the systole and diastole of the heart, but is not synchronous with the heart sounds (Fig 349). It may be a soft, scratchy sound almost inaudible, or it may be loud and harsh, sounding like the creaking of new leather—*bruit de cuir neuf*. It may last only a few hours, then disappear and reappear a few hours later. This friction rub is most frequently heard over the right ventricle in the fourth and fifth left interspaces near the sternum, but is often heard at the base. Its intensity may be increased by pressure over the bell of the stethoscope. It disappears when the pericardial exudate completely separates the visceral from the parietal pericardium, but may persist in the presence of considerable effusion.

2. Pericarditis with Effusion

Pericarditis with effusion is the direct sequence of acute fibrinous pericarditis and is usually regarded as its second stage. The physical findings are distinctive.

Inspection. If the effusion is large, the patient may look anxious; the face is gray and cyanotic and covered with cold perspiration. Marked dyspnea may

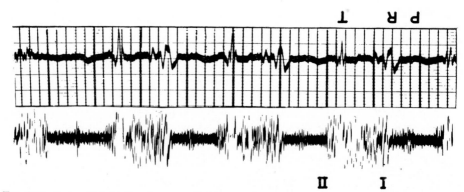

Fig. 349. Pericardial friction in acute fibrinous pericarditis. The friction rub is heard throughout systole, from the first sound I through the second sound II.

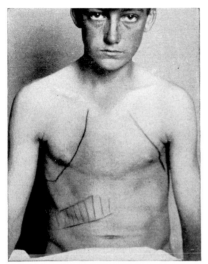

FIG. 350. Outline of dulness in pericardial effusion.

be present, the nostrils dilating with inspiration and the patient assuming a sitting posture for comfort. The superficial veins of the neck are engorged and distended.

The precordium often bulges, especially in children. The cardiac impulse may not be visible. The disappearance of this impulse in a patient with acute fibrinous pericarditis is a sign that a pericardial effusion is developing. The diaphragm and left lobe of the liver are pushed downward, causing a fulness in the epigastrium. This pressure on the diaphragm may produce hiccuping.

Palpation. In large effusions the apex impulse is not felt. Pericardial friction may be felt in moderate effusions, but disappears in large effusions. In some patients the friction is felt when the patient sits up, but disappears when he lies down.

Percussion. The area of cardiac dulness is definitely increased, particularly the absolute cardiac dulness. The outline of the cardiac dulness resembles that of a triangle with base down (Fig. 350). The relative cardiac dulness extends further to the right and left in the fourth interspaces when the patient sits up than when he lies down.

Shifting dulness at the base of the heart is a valuable diagnostic sign. This dulness in the first and second interspaces, elicited best by direct or immediate percussion, shows a narrowing when the patient sits up. This change is the reverse of the findings in the fourth interspaces.

Rotch's sign, an obtuse cardiohepatic angle, may be present (Fig. 278). The value of this sign is disputed by some observers.

Auscultation. The pericardial friction sound is usually audible with a moderate effusion, but disappears when the effusion is large. It may be heard in the erect but not in the recumbent position. As the pericardial effusion is absorbed, it usually reappears.

As the amount of pericardial fluid increases, the heart sounds become distant and feeble. The second pulmonic sound may be accentuated.

In massive effusions an accepted method of treatment is partial removal of the fluid followed by instillation of air. In such cases auscultation often reveals a slight splash with each systole, analogous to the classic Hippocratic succussion. The same auscultatory phenomenon is seen in traumatic pericardial effusion following wounds which admit air. This sign is called by the French "bruit de moulin."

Bamberger's or Ewart's sign is an area of dulness with bronchial breathing "at the left inner base, extending from the spine for varying distances outwards, usually not quite so far as the scapular angle line; commonly it does not extend higher than the level of the ninth or tenth rib" (Ewart). Christian found this sign present in 73.5 per cent of his cases of acute fibrinous or fibrinoserous pericarditis. The area over which the sign is heard may be "no larger than the bell of the stethoscope or may occupy the entire left base of the lung below the tip of the scapula and extend from the midline in the back out to the posterior axillary line" (Christian). It is most frequently seen in rheumatic pericarditis; indeed, Gevalt and Levine, in a study of 125 cases of pericardial effusion, found Ewart's sign present only in the rheumatic cases.

This sign was first noted by Bamberger and later studied more carefully by Ewart. Pins, in 1889, described a similar sign found only when the patient is lying down or seated leaning backwards, and disappearing when he bends forward or assumes the knee-chest position. This has been described as Pins' sign.

Pulse. The pulse is rapid and small, and may be irregular. A *pulsus paradoxus* may be present, a pulse which becomes weak or disappears during each inspiration. This *pulsus paradoxus* is, however, not always present, and is not pathognomonic of pericarditis with effusion.

The blood pressure is usually normal when the effusion is moderate, but falls as the amount of the effusion increases. A sudden fall in systolic pressure to 80 mm. is a danger signal.

3. Chronic Adhesive Pericarditis

Three types of chronic pericarditis are of clinical importance. In the first type there is complete but not dense adhesion between the visceral and parietal pericardial surfaces without firm adhesions to the chest wall, diaphragm or mediastinum. In such cases there is little interference with cardiac functions and no cardiac enlargement. No characteristic physical findings are present, and the diagnosis is often made only at autopsy. In the second type, *concretio cordis* (hardening of the heart), the pericardial adhesions are thick, solid or even calcified. In this variety, best designated as chronic constrictive pericarditis, the action of the heart is seriously impeded and the inflow of blood from the large veins is partially obstructed. Often the heart is also adherent to the diaphragm. The inelastic, thick pericardium encasing the heart prevents cardiac hypertrophy. In the third type of adhesive pericarditis the adhesions extend to the mediastinum, diaphragm and chest wall, causing much extra work for the heart and some enlargement of the heart. The third type, or a combination of the third and second types, is the variety under consideration.

Inspection. The most important physical findings in adhesive pericarditis are those of inspection. The precordium may bulge or may be flattened, and may be asymmetrical. The area of the cardiac impulse may be greatly increased, the apex is broad and heaving, and there is often a systolic retraction of the rib and interspaces in the region of the apex. In many cases, however, the heart is small and quiet. The apex is fixed and does not change its position when the patient is turned first on one side and then on the other.

A diastolic collapse of the veins in the neck may be observed.

Adhesions to the diaphragm may cause a marked systolic retraction of the eleventh and twelfth ribs in the back—the well-known Broadbent's sign, a sign, however, of limited value.

Palpation. Palpation of the apex beat confirms the observation that it is fixed and does not alter its position as the patient's position is changed.

The diastolic shock at the base of the heart when it follows the systolic retraction at the apex produces a see-saw sensation on palpation which is characteristic of adherent pericardium.

When systolic retraction, costal tugging and diastolic shock are all present, the surface of the heart never rests, and, to use the comparison of Morel-Lavèllae, "it seems to tremble like a mass of gelatin that has received a sudden sharp blow."

Percussion. On percussion there may be no change in some patients; in others, marked enlargement of the heart, the area of absolute dulness being increased relatively more than the area of relative cardiac dulness (Fig. 351). The extreme degree of hypertrophy seen in many of these cases has been attributed by some to the extra work thrown on the heart by the pull against the adhesions. Further study of such cases, however, has shown that these hearts of extraordinary size usually have

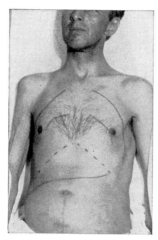

FIG. 351. Cardiac dulness in adhesive pericarditis.

valvular lesions or evidence of hypertension.

The area of cardiac dulness during deep inspiration is the same as during deep expiration.

Auscultation. On auscultation no signs of great value are made out. The heart sounds may be weakened, there may be coexisting valvular murmurs, and in some cases in which there is involvement of the pleura, pleural friction may be heard. In spite of these numerous characteristic physical signs, the diagnosis of adhesive pericarditis may be very difficult. It should always be suspected in a patient who has a markedly enlarged heart without evidence of valvular lesions or an elevation in blood pressure. When there is a history of a previous pericarditis, of rheumatic fever or tuberculosis, the probabilities are increased that the marked cardiac enlargement is due to adhesive pericarditis.

Pulse. The pulse may be regular. In some patients *pulsus paradoxus* may be noted, although the value of this physical sign has been greatly exaggerated.

Summary. In acute fibrinous pericarditis a fremitus is felt over the heart. This fremitus corresponds to the to-and-fro friction rub heard on auscultation. There is no change in the area of cardiac dulness and no alteration in the heart sounds.

In pericarditis with effusion the pre-cordium often bulges, and the cardiac impulse is usually neither visible nor felt. A pericardial friction is felt in a moderate effusion, but disappears when the effusion is large. The area of cardiac dulness, particularly the absolute dulness, is increased. Shifting dulness at the base of the heart and an obtuse cardiohepatic angle are important findings. On auscultation, the pericardial friction sound may be audible in the early stages of an effusion, but becomes fainter and disappears as the amount of effusion increases.

Chronic adhesive pericarditis may present no physical signs, or may be associated with marked cardiac enlargement. In the latter event the area of cardiac impulse is increased, the relative and absolute dulnesses are increased, and there is often systolic retraction of the ribs and interspaces at the left of the apex beat as well as retraction of the eleventh and twelfth ribs in the back. The apex beat is fixed and does not change its position when the patient turns from one side to the other.

Levine remarks: "The so-called signs of adhesive pericarditis are very numerous and bear the names of many prominent clinicians, but for the most part are unreliable diagnostically. Studies throughout the entire world tell the same tale, *i.e.,* that this condition is generally first recognized at the autopsy table. . . . The main difficulty is that most of the signs may be present when the heart is markedly enlarged and the pericardium is normal." In adhesive pericarditis the roentgen examination may be helpful.

CHRONIC VALVULAR HEART DISEASE

Rheumatic fever is the most common cause of chronic valvular lesions of the heart. Chorea, which may be regarded as a part of the rheumatic cycle, is also a frequent cause of valvular heart disease. Syphilis is the next most common etiologic factor, involving almost exclusively the aortic valves. Influenza and scarlet fever also produce endocarditis with a resulting valvular lesion. The gonococcus on rare occasions may produce an endocarditis, particularly of the tricuspid and of the pulmonary valves. In older persons arteriosclerosis is a common cause of valvular disease, particularly of the aortic valves.

Compiling statistics in more than 3000 cases, White found the mitral valve to be involved in 70 to 85 per cent, the aortic valve in 42 to 45 per cent, the tricuspid valve in 10 to 15 per cent, and the pulmonary valve in approximately 1 per cent. The mitral valve alone was diseased in 50 to 60 per cent, the aortic valve alone in from 10 to 20 per cent.

Mitral Insufficiency

Pure mitral insufficiency, once considered the most common of all valvular lesions, is probably not common if we exclude the cases in which there is also stenosis of the mitral valve. Cabot refers to pure mitral insufficiency as "that great rarity." Mitral insufficiency combined with mitral stenosis is, however, one of the most common of valvular lesions, and a pure mitral insufficiency may precede the development of mitral stenosis. Mitral insufficiency without mitral stenosis does not, however, cause death and for this reason is a rare lesion post mortem.

Inspection. The apex beat is to the left of the nipple in either the fifth or sixth interspace and sometimes may be seen in the anterior axillary line (Fig. 257).

Palpation. The principal value of palpation is to confirm the location of the point of maximum impulse. The beat when the heart is fully compensated is strong and forceful, but if a break in compensation has occurred, the apex beat may be feeble and wavy.

Percussion. Cardiac dulness is increased to the left and may also be increased to the right of the sternal margin.

Auscultation. A systolic murmur is heard, which is loudest at or just above the apex beat and is well transmitted to the axilla and frequently also to the inferior angle of the left scapula behind (Fig. 294).

Pulse. The pulse presents no characteristic changes.

Mitral Stenosis

Mitral stenosis is a lesion which demonstrates the serious after-effects of an attack of rheumatic fever or chorea in childhood. It may be regarded as the second stage of a mitral insufficiency, and ordinarily appears some five to ten years, occasionally within two or three years, after the attack of rheumatic endocarditis. The lesion is more common in females than in males.

Inspection. Patients commonly have flushed cheeks, many extremely attractive young women owing their high color to the presence of a mitral stenosis. The lower part of the sternum, the fifth or sixth left interspace and the intercostal cartilages are often prominent. The cardiac impulse is prominent, often diffuse, and frequently does not extend beyond the mammillary line. Pulsations in the third and fourth left intercostal spaces are occasionally seen.

Palpation. In many cases, palpation shows the characteristic *purring presystolic thrill* usually best felt at the apex or just inside it, the thrill having a definite crescendo quality and ending in a sharp sudden shock synchronous with the cardiac impulse. This thrill may be palpable only over a small area and may be present only after the patient has exercised and his heart rate has increased. It is one of the most distinctive findings in the field of physical diagnosis. From its presence alone the diagnosis of mitral stenosis can usually be made. There is also frequently a diastolic shock over the pulmonic area.

Percussion. As a rule, on percussion there is no significant increase in the size of the heart. Some increase in dulness at the right of the sternum and dulness at the left apex may be demonstrated in certain cases. The exact delineation of cardiac outlines, shown in Figure 352, cannot be determined

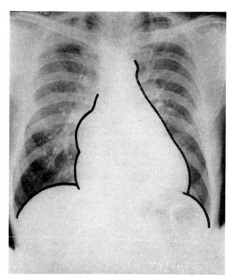

FIG. 352. X-ray of heart in mitral stenosis, showing convexity of left border and enlargement of the right auricle.

by percussion alone. While percussion reveals only cardiac enlargement to the right and to the left, an x-ray picture usually shows a characteristic contour (Fig. 352).

Auscultation. On auscultation at the apex a murmur is heard (Fig. 299) which carries the same auditory sensation as that felt on palpation. This murmur is presystolic in time, has a rough vibratory crescendo character, is often of brief duration, and usually terminates in a snapping first sound. In addition to this short presystolic or late diastolic murmur, there is also commonly present an early diastolic murmur which follows closely on the second heart sound and commonly lasts throughout the greater part of diastole. This murmur is the well-known diastolic murmur which often persists in auricular fibrillation, while the presystolic murmur usually disappears (Fig. 301).

Another characteristic finding on auscultation in mitral stenosis is an accentuation of the second pulmonic sound. A diastolic murmur at the pulmonic area, the Graham Steell murmur, is occasionally heard.

Mitral stenosis is usually combined with mitral insufficiency, and, in addi-

tion to a presystolic murmur, there is almost invariably a systolic murmur as well.

Pulse. The pulse in mitral stenosis is usually small. Auricular fibrillation, which is a common complication of mitral stenosis, produces a characteristic totally irregular pulse.

Aortic Insufficiency

Aortic insufficiency ranks second to mitral disease in frequency of occurrence and may be the result of a rheumatic fever, of syphilis or arteriosclerosis. The statistics regarding the relative frequency of rheumatic fever and syphilis as causative factors show certain variations in different parts of the country. The physical signs in aortic insufficiency are usually quite distinctive.

Inspection. The patient's face is usually sallow or pale, although examination of the blood shows that there is no anemia. This pallor of aortic insufficiency is frequently in marked contrast to the flushed cheeks of mitral stenosis. On observing the head, it is often seen to jerk slightly with each heart beat—*de Musset's sign.* Inspection of the neck shows marked throbbing of both carotid arteries, one of the most distinctive signs of aortic insufficiency. The capillary pulse of Quincke is usually present. The alternate flush and pallor of the capillary bed may be brought out by exerting gentle pressure at the tips of the fingernails. It may also be readily seen if one produces a narrow band of hyperemia in the center of the forehead by rubbing vigorously with the eraser of a lead pencil.

Inspection of the chest shows the cardiac impulse to be usually displaced downward as well as outward (Fig. 257), the impulse being markedly heaving in character and often lifting the entire anterior chest wall. The slow vigorous lifting of the interspace, the so-called "dome shaped heave," is often very striking.

Palpation. On palpation a diastolic thrill is occasionally felt. More common

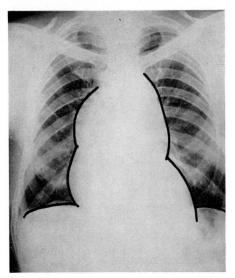

FIG. 353. X-ray of heart in aortic insufficiency. Roentgenogram shows marked enlargement of heart, also aneurysmal dilatation of the aorta.

is a systolic thrill when the valve segments are united or calcified.

Percussion. Percussion demonstrates a great increase in cardiac dulness to the left, the increase being outward and downward (Fig. 353).

Auscultation. Auscultation shows the characteristic diastolic murmur heard at the aortic area, often at the apex, but usually loudest along the left sternal border. It is often heard best after deep expiration. The murmur is usually soft and blowing and, as Hope noted, sounds "like whispering the word *awe* during inspiration." It begins directly with the second sound or replaces it. At the apex a presystolic rumble (the Flint murmur) is sometimes heard, which is described in detail on page 186. Thayer found the Flint murmur present in approximately 50 per cent of his cases of uncomplicated aortic insufficiency.

The first sound may be clear at the base, and frequently there is a soft systolic murmur following it. When the valve segments are fused or calcified, the systolic murmur may be harsh and rasping. Over the femoral arteries a to-and-fro murmur may be heard— *Duroziez's sign* and the *"pistol shot" sound.*

Pulse. The most striking feature on palpation is the character of the pulse— the *collapsing, water-hammer* or *Corrigan pulse,* which is rarely met with in any other condition. This is a forceful pulse; it rises sharply and falls quickly. Blood pressure determinations show that the pulse pressure is high, the systolic pressure being elevated and the diastolic being lowered.

Rupture of the aortic valve may produce an abrupt decline and disappearance of the diastolic arterial blood pressure, as pointed out by Bean and Schmidt.

Aortic Stenosis

Aortic stenosis is a comparatively uncommon lesion, but, when present, presents striking and characteristic physical findings.

Inspection. On inspection the point of maximum impulse of the heart may be displaced downward in some patients, while in other patients the cardiac impulse is not seen at all.

Palpation. A systolic thrill felt over the heart with maximum intensity in the aortic region is a characteristic and pathognomonic finding. This thrill may often be felt as far upward as the clavicle. When the thrill is present, we are safe in diagnosing aortic stenosis, although the absence of such a thrill does not invalidate this diagnosis. Frequently the thrill is felt only at the end of a deep expiration.

Percussion. Percussion may show nothing pathologic, but, in some patients, enlargement of the left ventricle can be demonstrated.

Auscultation. On auscultation a rough systolic murmur is heard in the second right intercostal space (Fig. 307). This murmur diminishes as we pass downward toward the xiphoid cartilage, but is well heard on passing upward toward the clavicle. It is usually well heard over the carotid arteries as well as over the brachial arteries (Fig. 306). This murmur is usually harsh, but may become soft and distant when cardiac compensation fails. There is usually

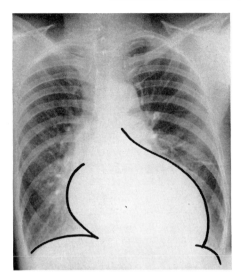

FIG. 354. X-ray of heart in aortic stenosis. Marked enlargement of left ventricle.

The most important physical findings are a systolic thrill perceptible in the second left intercostal space which is stronger when the patient turns to his left side or lies on his stomach, and a corresponding systolic murmur which is usually loud and rasping. This murmur is transmitted toward the clavicle and often around to the back.

Pulmonary Insufficiency

Relative pulmonary insufficiency is seen, particularly in advanced mitral stenosis, and produces the Graham Steell murmur. Organic pulmonary insufficiency is a rare lesion. The most important sign is a soft diastolic murmur heard along the left border of the sternum, usually being more intense during deep inspiration.

Triscuspid Insufficiency

Relative tricuspid insufficiency is an extremely common lesion and one which is more frequently overlooked than correctly diagnosed. Organic tricuspid insufficiency is relatively uncommon. The physical findings in well-marked tricuspid insufficiency are striking and characteristic.

Inspection. The patient usually shows a high degree of cyanosis. The veins in the neck are markedly engorged and, in advanced cases, show marked pulsation. The liver is usually enlarged and shows a marked systolic pulsation. This positive venous pulse and the enlarged pulsating liver are characteristic. There is commonly ascites and marked edema of the legs.

Palpation. Palpation confirms the striking systolic expansile pulsation of the liver. Pressure on the liver elicits pain. Accurate differentiation between the true pulsating liver and the transmitted impulse of the expanding subdiaphragmatic aorta may be difficult. If it is possible to actually grasp the liver within the hands recognition is easy. The expansile pulsation resulting from tricuspid insufficiency occurs late in systole, while transmitted pulsations

a diminution in intensity of the second sound in the aortic area, this sound at times being entirely absent. This latter finding is important in the diagnosis of aortic stenosis.

Pulse. The pulse in aortic stenosis is characteristic. A tracing of such a pulse is shown in Figure 310. It is usually small and slow, rises gradually and tardily, and falls away slowly. It is the classic *pulsus rarus, parvus et tardus*. Aortic stenosis, however, is often complicated by aortic insufficiency with a corresponding variation in the character of the pulse. The "classic" pulse is more frequently absent than present.

The slow pulse rate in aortic stenosis is a striking finding. The rate may be under sixty or seventy even with congestive heart failure, a phenomenon seen also in patients who have been digitalized or have heart block.

Patients with aortic stenosis are subject to attacks of faintness or actual syncope. Sudden death is not uncommon.

Pulmonary Stenosis

Pulmonary stenosis is a rare lesion usually of congenital origin. Although rare, it is one of the most common of congenital heart diseases.

from the aorta or the left ventricle occur simultaneously with systole. Verification of this has been made by simultaneous aortic and hepatic vein pressure tracings.

Percussion. Percussion shows enlargement of the heart both to the right and to the left, and downward. Occasionally there is a cardiac dulness in the second and third right interspaces, owing to dilatation of the right auricle.

Auscultation. The characteristic murmur of tricuspid insufficiency is a systolic murmur of maximum intensity over the lower part of the sternum. This murmur is frequently mistaken for a mitral systolic murmur and on auscultation alone may not be distinguishable from it. The second pulmonic sound is not accentuated.

Pulse. The pulse in tricuspid insufficiency presents no pathognomonic characteristics.

Tricuspid Stenosis

Tricuspid stenosis is exceedingly rare and usually is complicated by mitral stenosis. Cyanosis is usually marked and ascites common. The patient shows marked enlargement of the right side of the heart and a diastolic murmur with the point of maximum intensity over the lower area of the sternum. There is a snapping first sound in the tricuspid area, and a presystolic thrill is occasionally felt. The murmurs are similar to those heard in mitral stenosis, but are well heard over the lower part of the sternum and to the right of the midline. The pulse shows nothing characteristic, although fibrillation is common.

Summary

Mitral insufficiency usually causes an increase in the cardiac dulness, and at the apex there is a systolic murmur which is well transmitted to the axilla.

Mitral stenosis produces less enlargement of the heart to the left than does mitral insufficiency. A presystolic thrill, usually felt at the apex or just inside it, is a pathognomonic finding. Ausculta-

tion reveals a presystolic murmur coincident with the thrill and ending in a loud and snapping first sound. An early diastolic murmur is also frequently present. The second pulmonic sound is accentuated, and a diastolic murmur is often heard at the pulmonic area (*Graham Steell murmur*). The pulse is usually small. Mitral stenosis is often complicated by auricular fibrillation.

Aortic insufficiency can often be diagnosed on inspection alone. The throbbing carotids and the jerking of the head with each systole are characteristic. The capillary pulse can usually be demonstrated. The heart is markedly enlarged to the left and downward. The point of maximum impulse often shows the characteristic "dome-shaped heave." On auscultation there is a diastolic murmur heard over the aortic area at the apex of the heart, but usually best heard along the left sternal border. A presystolic rumble (Flint murmur) is often heard near the apex. The water-hammer or collapsing pulse is characteristic.

Aortic stenosis is diagnosed by the presence in the aortic area of a systolic thrill synchronous with a harsh systolic murmur. This murmur is usually well heard over the carotid arteries and over the brachial arteries. The pulse in aortic stenosis is pathognomonic. It is the *pulsus rarus, parvus et tardus.*

Pulmonary stenosis is diagnosed by the presence of a systolic thrill in the second left intercostal space and a corresponding systolic murmur.

Pulmonary insufficiency shows a soft diastolic murmur along the left border of the sternum.

Tricuspid insufficiency causes a high degree of cyanosis, marked engorgement of the veins of the neck and enlargement of the liver. Marked pulsation of the liver is commonly seen and may be confirmed by palpation. Auscultation shows a systolic murmur with maximum intensity over the lower part of the sternum.

Tricuspid stenosis shows a diastolic murmur with its maximum intensity over the lower part of the sternum.

ENDOCARDITIS

The type of endocarditis most commonly seen, aside from the rheumatic variety, is subacute infectious endocarditis, which is usually due to the *Streptococcus viridans*. In this disease the patient may have fever and evidence of embolism before the findings in the heart become distinctive. Cardiac findings depend upon the valve involvement, the most frequent involvement being that of the mitral and aortic valves. This type of endocarditis shows a predilection for the surface of a heart valve previously damaged by rheumatic fever. Congenital heart disease is also a frequent precursor of subacute endocarditis. The earliest known illustration of valvular endocarditis published by Sandifort in 1777 was in a patient suffering from Fallot's syndrome.

The signs of embolism are usually decisive in establishing the diagnosis. The most common locations of such emboli are the conjunctiva of the eyelid (Fig. 355), the finger tips and under the fingernails—"splinter hemorrhages" (Fig. 356). Hemorrhages are often seen in the retina on ophthalmoscopic examination. When the pulmonary or tricuspid valve is involved, the emboli are carried to the lungs and produce small pulmonary infarctions. Such infarctions cause pain in the chest and occasional

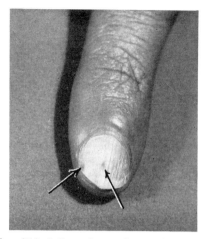

FIG. 356. Splinter hemorrhage of left index finger. Two hemorrhages at tips of arrows.

expectoration of blood-tinged sputum, and the patients show frequently a pleural friction rub over the site of the pain. If the endocarditis is confined to the pulmonary valve, no petechiae occur.

Painful subcutaneous nodes, often slightly red in color, may appear early, especially in the pulp of the fingers and toes—"Osler's nodes."

As the disease progresses, anemia and cachexia appear, petechiae become more numerous and the heart gradually becomes enlarged. The spleen is often palpable in the early stages of the disease and later may show considerable enlargement. Clubbing of the fingers is not uncommon.

CONGENITAL HEART DISEASE

Interest in congenital heart disease has increased greatly during the past few years largely because of the increased skill in diagnosis as well as phenomenal advances in cardiac surgery. For years, many varieties of congenital heart lesions were diagnosed only by the pathologist after death. Today, however, with the aid of x-ray studies, angiocardiograms, and cardiac catheterization, which makes possible an estimation of the oxygen content of the blood in the auricles and ventricles, the physician can diagnose with accuracy a large variety of congenital lesions.

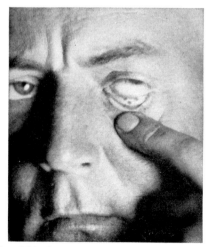

FIG. 355. Conjunctival petechial hemorrhages in subacute infectious endocarditis.

These advances have not made physical diagnosis obsolete but have proved that certain physical signs are pathognomonic of certain lesions, while other signs are incompatible.

For clinical diagnosis, congenital heart disease may be divided into two groups. The first group is the *cyanotic group*. These patients show a marked cyanosis, polycythemia (from 5,500,000 to 10,000,000 red blood corpuscles per cubic millimeter) with clubbing of the fingers and toes. This group has long been described under the term of *morbus caeruleus,* the blue disease, this term being at one time regarded as synonymous with congenital heart disease. Indeed, according to Osler, cyanosis appears in more than 90 per cent of patients with congenital heart disease. This group is represented chiefly by pulmonary stenosis. Such patients are usually poorly developed, do not attain normal height and from time to time may suffer from suffocative attacks.

The most characteristic physical findings are a loud systolic murmur with maximum intensity at the second or third left interspace, the murmur being often transmitted to the level of the clavicle, a palpable systolic thrill in the same area, and enlargement of the heart to the right.

The *tetralogy of Fallot,* as previously mentioned, consists of ventricular septum defect, pulmonary stenosis, dextroposition of the aorta, and hypertrophy of the right ventricle.

The tetralogy of Fallot was first described by Nicolas Steno in an embryo in 1673. In 1777, Eduard Sandifort reported a second case, describing not only the pathologic findings but also the clinical course of the patient. His patient, a boy of 13, also showed at autopsy an endocarditis of the pulmonary valve. Fallot in 1888 published an analysis of 55 cases of cyanotic congenital heart disease and found that 74 per cent suffered from a combination of four lesions—ventricular septum defect, pulmonary stenosis, dextroposition of the aorta, and hypertrophy of the right

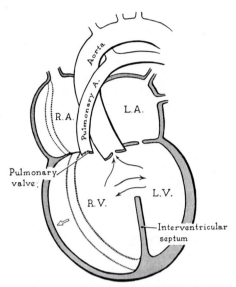

Fig. 357. Tetralogy of Fallot. Ventricular septal defect, pulmonary stenosis, dextroposition of the aorta, and hypertrophy of the right ventricle.

ventricle. This combination of the four abnormalities has since been known as the *tetralogy of Fallot* (Figs. 357, 358). These patients usually show marked cyanosis, a systolic murmur over the pulmonary area, and often a systolic murmur with a thrill at the third left interspace and at the P. M. I. They often have severe aching in the legs and dyspnea when standing but are immediately relieved when they assume a squatting position.

Eisenmenger's complex is an anomaly with a large defect of the interventricular septum, dextroposition of the aorta and a normal or dilated pulmonary artery. It has sometimes been described as a variation of *Fallot's tetralogy,* but this is obviously inaccurate since in *Eisenmenger's complex* a distinguishing feature is the normal or dilated pulmonary artery in marked contrast to the stenosis or atresia of this vessel in *Fallot's tetralogy.* In *Eisenmenger's complex,* there is a harsh systolic murmur usually accompanied by a thrill over the base of the heart and a diastolic murmur at the pulmonary area.

In the second, *acyanotic group,* cyanosis is either absent or transient. The

I ↓ II

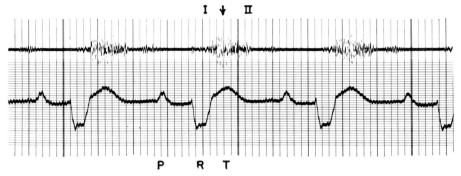

P   R   T

FIG. 358. Blowing systolic murmur at left sternal border in Fallot's tetralogy. Ventricular septal defect has also produced a bundle branch block shown in the electrocardiogram.

I ↓ II

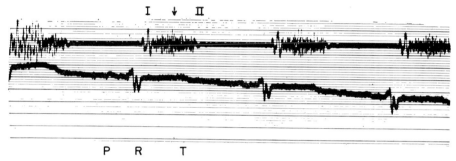

P   R   T

FIG. 359. Roger's murmur in interventricular septal defect. Murmur lasts through systole, marked with arrow.

most common heart lesions in this group are defects of the interventricular septum, patent foramen ovale and patent ductus arteriosus. In defects of the interventricular septum a thrill and a harsh systolic murmur are present over the third and fourth left interspaces to the left of the sternum. The murmur is transmitted leftward directly toward the axilla. It is exactly systolic and usually persists throughout systole (Fig. 359). This murmur is known as *Roger's murmur,* and uncomplicated interventricular septum defect has been called Roger's disease. This murmur is unaccompanied by other murmurs, is best heard in the midline at the left sternal border, and from this central point diminishes in intensity uniformly as one moves to either side.

The characteristic findings in *patent ductus arteriosus (Botalli)* is a continuous loud murmur, accentuated in systole, best heard at the second rib on the left and in the second left intercostal space at the sternal margin. It is usually limited to this area and is not heard in the neck. This murmur is commonly spoken of as a "machinery murmur" and is almost invariably harsh (Fig. 360). A similar harsh machinery-like murmur has been described in rupture of an aortic aneurysm into the pulmonary artery. A palpable thrill may be felt synchronous with the murmur. Ligation of the patent ductus was first successfully performed by Gross and Hubbard in 1939. In 1947, records of more than 500 successful operations were published.

There is a high incidence of subacute bacterial endocarditis in ventricular septal defects (57%) and in patent ductus arteriosus (28%). Five per cent of all cases of bacterial endocarditis occur in patients with congenital heart lesions.

Coarctation of the aorta may for years cause no symptoms and few physical signs. In well developed cases there is often marked pulsation in the neck,

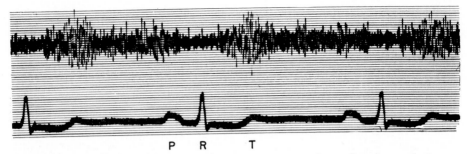

P   R   T

FIG. 360. Harsh "machinery murmur" of patent ductus arteriosus. Sound record at second left intercostal space.

in the scapular region, and in the intercostal spaces. Pulsation in the femoral artery is feeble or absent. A systolic murmur may be heard to the right of the sternum and is especially loud over the back, over the scapulae, and often along both sides of the vertebral column. The blood pressure is elevated in the brachial artery, low in the femoral artery. Surgical operations for the relief or cure of coarctation have been performed with increasing frequency since the first successful operation reported by Crafoord and Nylin in 1945.

CONGESTIVE HEART FAILURE

Congestive heart failure usually results from valvular lesions, chronic arterial hypertension, or myocardial infarction from coronary thrombosis. Less common causes are rheumatic carditis, thyrotoxicosis, congenital heart lesions, severe anemia or long-continued and uncontrolled tachycardia, as in auricular fibrillation, auricular flutter and paroxysmal tachycardia.

Congestive heart failure may be due to failure of the left ventricle, the right ventricle, or both. Failure of the left ventricle is more common, but often leads to failure of the right ventricle as well.

The earliest and chief symptom of left ventricular failure is dyspnea while at rest or when carrying out some physical activity which previously caused no discomfort. Dyspnea at rest is especially marked when the patient lies down (orthopnea) and may be relieved when he sits up. The onset of congestive heart failure in many patients coincides with the time when they begin to find it necessary to sleep sitting up in a chair instead of lying down in bed.

One striking type of dyspnea seen in left ventricular failure is acute paroxysmal dyspnea. This may be accompanied by signs of pulmonary edema, particularly in patients suffering from mitral stenosis. Acute paroxysmal dyspnea with pulmonary engorgement, when associated with an asthmatic type of breathing, is called *cardiac asthma,* and resembles bronchial asthma so closely that a differential diagnosis may be difficult. The history of the attacks, the age of the patient, the presence of accompanying signs of cardiac disease, which are conspicuously lacking in most patients with bronchial asthma, aid in establishing the correct diagnosis.

Cheyne-Stokes respiration is commonly seen in the early stages of congestive heart failure, especially during sleep. If present during waking hours, it is a serious sign of circulatory failure.

The most marked signs of right ventricular failure are those of cyanosis, and congestion of the liver. The patient is cyanotic, and the neck veins are markedly engorged and pulsate forcibly. There is a generalized edema or anasarca, and the ankles pit on pressure. The liver is tender and enlarged and, on palpation, is found to extend below the costal margin. Ascites is often present, and a fluid wave can be detected in the abdomen. The pleural cavity shows an accumulation of fluid which is readily detected by percussion. Auscultation over the lungs shows numerous moist rales.

Physical examination of the heart during congestive heart failure always shows evident cardiac enlargement, often marked, sometimes acute, due to dilation, and may show the sudden appearance of auricular fibrillation, of premature contractions or of a gallop rhythm. Heart murmurs may increase in intensity or may, in extreme cardiac dilatation, disappear completely. The pulse rate is usually increased, and a *pulsus alternans* is common.

As the condition of congestive heart failure persists, the cyanosis becomes more marked, the dyspnea more distressing, the edema more obvious and more burdensome. The pulse rate increases, the pulse itself is often feeble and easily compressed, and the blood pressure falls. In patients with arterial hypertension, the blood pressure often rises still higher at the onset of congestive heart failure. Later, however, with increasing heart failure, it falls, often to a normal or even a subnormal level. This fall in blood pressure may be associated with partial or total suppression of urine.

There is an increasing amount of evidence which shows that the congestive heart failure is not due entirely to ventricular failure with an increased venous pressure, the so-called "backward failure," but may also be due to a "forward failure" because of the inability of the kidneys to secrete salt and water in a normal manner.

COR PULMONALE

The term *cor pulmonale* has been used with increasing frequency during the past few years to designate a cardiac condition produced primarily by disease of the pulmonary vessels or of the parenchyma of the lung. Primary arteriosclerosis of the pulmonary artery and its branches may cause cor pulmonale. More frequent causes are bronchiectasis, pulmonary tuberculosis, emphysema, asthma and silicosis. These conditions produce an increased resistance to the

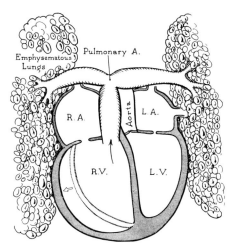

Fig. 361. Diagram of cor pulmonale produced by emphysema of the lungs. Increased resistance to the blood flow through the lungs dilates the pulmonary artery and the right ventricle.

blood flow through the lungs, and an increased strain thrown on the right ventricle with a resultant dilatation and hypertrophy of the ventricle. Later, cardiac decompensation appears.

The chief symptoms are dyspnea, vertigo and precordial pain. Cyanosis appears and, when it is extreme and associated with polycythemia, the condition is known as Ayerza's disease.

Clubbed fingers may develop, the veins of the neck are often distended, and the patient may show hemoptysis. The cardiac dulness may be diminished because of the overlying distended lungs. The breath sounds are often feeble and the heart sounds at the apex distant. The pulmonic second sound may be loud. The roentgenogram and electrocardiogram are of great value in the diagnosis of this condition.

CHEST DEFORMITIES AS A CAUSE OF MYOCARDIAL INSUFFICIENCY

When the thoracic cage is markedly deformed through kyphosis, scoliosis, or a combination of the two as a result of early poliomyelitis or tuberculosis of the spine, a serious myocardial insufficiency may result. A marked displacement of the heart may produce dilatation and hypertrophy of the cardiac

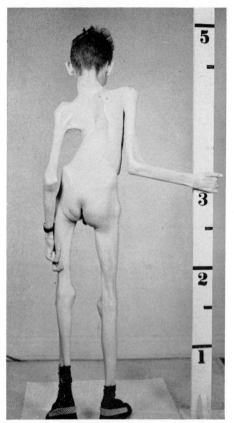

FIG. 362. Marked chest deformity in a boy of 15 who had an attack of poliomyelitis at the age of 9. Patient has cor pulmonale with myocardial insufficiency.

chambers with congestive heart failure. Pressure on the lungs may impede the pulmonary circulation and produce a true cor pulmonale.

This condition was recognized by Traube in 1878 and has been studied by numerous observers since that time. White notes, "In badly deformed individuals survival to old age is frequently prevented by the cardiovascular strain as well as by pulmonary complications." The patient shown in Figure 362 as the result of marked scoliokyphosis resulting from poliomyelitis has cor pulmonale with marked myocardial insufficiency.

ANGINA PECTORIS AND CORONARY OCCLUSION

Angina pectoris has been recognized as a disease entity since the classic description of William Heberden in 1768.

It is diagnosed either from the history given by the patient or from the evidences of pain and distress observed during a typical attack. The disease may be readily feigned or simulated, and the physician may find it difficult or impossible to determine whether a person is suffering from an attack or is only a malingerer. It is also often difficult to determine whether a patient is suffering from a "true" angina pectoris or a "false" angina. Heberden was familiar with this "false" angina and observed that "the breast is often the seat of pains, which are distressing, sometimes even from their vehemence, oftener from their duration, as they have continued to tease the patient for six, for eight, for nine, and for fourteen years. . . . There has appeared no reason to judge that they proceed from any cause of much importance to health, or that they lead to any dangerous consequences; and if the patient were not uneasy with what he feels, he needs never to be so on account of anything which he has to fear."

Heberden continued, "But there is a disorder of the breast marked with strong and peculiar symptoms, considerable for the kind of danger belonging to it, and not extremely rare, which deserves to be mentioned more at length. The seat of it, and sense of strangling, and anxiety with which it is attended, may make it not improperly be called angina pectoris."

They who are afflicted with it, are seized while they are walking (more especially if it be uphill, and soon after eating) with a painful and most disagreeable sensation in the breast, which seems as if it would extinguish life, if it were to increase or continue; but the moment they stand still, all this uneasiness vanishes.

In all other respects, the patients are, at the beginning of this disorder, perfectly well, and in particular have no shortness of breath, from which it is totally different. The pain is sometimes situated in the upper part, sometimes in the middle, sometimes at the bottom of the os sterni, and often more inclined to the left than to the right side. It likewise very frequently extends from the breast to the middle of the left arm. The pulse is, at least sometimes, not disturbed by this pain, as I have had opportunities of observing by feeling the pulse during the paroxysm. Males are most liable to that disease, especially such as have passed their fiftieth year.

After it has continued a year or more, it will not cease so instantaneously upon standing still; and it will come on not only when the persons are walking, but when they are lying down, especially if they lie on their left side.

Heberden notes further, and this point has been corroborated by numerous successors, that the attacks could be brought on by "any disturbance of mind." John Hunter, who died during an attack of angina pectoris provoked by anger, had remarked for years that his "life was in the hands of any rascal who chose to worry him."

During a severe attack of angina pectoris the patient usually looks pale and anxious, drops of sweat appear on his face, his pulse is rapid and thready, and he remains thus awaiting the death which he thinks must surely come. Percussion and auscultation carried out during such a paroxysm rarely yield information of any value. The pulse is usually increased in rate and may be irregular. The blood pressure may be high or low, and commonly falls after an attack. The heart sounds may be muffled.

To many patients the diagnosis of angina pectoris is terrifying. In spite of its serious import it should not be forgotten that it may not for years cause much impairment in the activities of some patients. Heberden in his initial report described a patient who lived for fifteen years after the diagnosis was established and died at the age of seventy-five. John Hunter lived for twenty years after the onset of his cardiac pains.

The pain of angina pectoris and of coronary occlusion has been ascribed by most observers to cardiac anoxemia. The actual method of the production of pain has been ascribed to stimulation of the pain receptors in the walls of the coronary arteries. This stimulation has been usually attributed to chemical substances resulting from the anoxemia, to tension, compression, or from some other mechanical cause. There is increasing evidence of the importance of mechanical stimulation of the pain points especially in coronary occlusion, where the appearance of severe pain coincides almost exactly with the plugging of the vessel. Allbutt believed it to be due to disease of the aorta, but the weight of opinion today is that it is due to poor blood supply to the myocardium and that it is usually, if not invariably, associated with sclerosis of the coronary arteries. Patients may completely recover from the attacks, in which event the condition is often called later "pseudo angina." Some patients have repeated attacks of typical angina pectoris for years and then suffer from a typical attack of coronary occlusion. The pathologic findings in typical angina pectoris are inconclusive. Heberden noted in one of his cases that "a very skillful anatomist could discover no fault in the heart, in the valves, in the arteries or neighboring veins," and successive generations of pathologists have reported the same findings. The coronary arteries may, as in the case of John Hunter, be "in a state of bony tubes, which were with difficulty divided by the knife" or may show no more sclerosis than those of any person of the same age.

Coronary occlusion, although recognized much later as a disease entity, is today better understood than angina pectoris. The first case of coronary occlusion, described by Adam Hammer in 1878, was in a patient thirty-four years of age and was not accompanied by pain. The great majority of cases are, however, in older persons and are accompanied by intense pain.

The appearance of a patient during an attack of coronary occlusion may resemble that of a patient suffering from a severe attack of angina pectoris. The onset of pain in the precordium is usually accompanied by profound shock, the patient's face has an ashen-gray color, and there is frequently a drenching perspiration, an irregular pulse and a marked fall in blood pressure. The patient's color may become normal and the perspiration may disappear with the subsidence of severe pain. The pain is frequently felt only in the abdomen and may simulate gallbladder disease.

Auscultation of the heart commonly shows some acceleration of the rate. Premature contractions are common and gallop rhythm is frequently heard. The cardiac tones usually sound distinct, but faint and poorly differentiated. A pericardial friction rub is occasionally heard and, when present, is conclusive evidence of infarction of the myocardium. Heart block and auricular fibrillation may follow immediately the attack of coronary occlusion and may persist after recovery from the acute attack.

This picture of coronary occlusion is produced by practically no other disease, and the diagnosis may be made with a fair degree of accuracy. In addition, the patient usually has an elevation of temperature and a moderate leukocytosis and shows a characteristic electrocardiogram. Occasionally there is no pain at all, and the only symptoms are fainting, dyspnea, syncope and sweating.

The first attack of coronary occlusion may prove fatal, or the patient may recover from the first attack and live for several or many years before succumbing to a second or third attack, or may recover completely and have no further attacks. It is noteworthy that coronary occlusion often occurs when the patient is at rest or even asleep, while the initial attacks of angina pectoris almost invariably occur during exercise. The pathologic findings of coronary occlusion are as clear and distinctive as those of angina pectoris are obscure and confused. In coronary occlusion, examination of the coronary arteries shows occlusion by a thrombus.

Later pathologic studies indicate that, with improved methods of study, occlusion of the coronary can be demonstrated in most patients dying from what had been previously diagnosed as angina pectoris. This does not, however, prove the identity of angina pectoris and coronary occlusion, since angina pectoris may occur in hyperthyroidism and in normal youthful persons who have thrown great strain on their vascular systems. The pain of angina pectoris, as Mackenzie pointed out, resembles the pains in the legs in intermittent claudication and has the same cause—anoxemia of the muscles. Levine remarks, "Coronary thrombosis is related to angina pectoris in much the same way as an occlusion of a vessel of the leg with gangrene is related to intermittent claudication. The anginal state may be regarded as a transitory one leaving the heart in practically the same condition after an attack as before. . . . Sometime during the life of those suffering from angina a thrombosis of a coronary artery is apt to occur."

MYOCARDITIS AND MYOCARDIAL DISEASE

Myocarditis was at one time a common diagnosis. Heart disease was considered to be valvular or myocardial. If the patient had dyspnea, cyanosis, edema and other signs of cardiac disease, and had no evidence of valvular lesions, the diagnosis of myocarditis was made. The later demonstration of the important role played by coronary occlusion and bundle branch block in cardiac pathology aroused much skepticism regarding the correctness of such diagnosis and regarding the frequency of myocarditis. In some clinics myocarditis is considered a rare affection. Scherf and Boyd state categorically that "myocarditis is a common disease and quite often remains unrecognized." The correctness of this statement is borne out by extensive electrocardiographic studies.

Myocarditis is of infectious origin. Rheumatic fever, typhoid fever, septicemia, pyemia, syphilis, pneumonia, scarlet fever, diphtheria and influenza are common causes. In practically every case of rheumatic endocarditis there is also present myocarditis. In lobar pneumonia, the rapid cardiac failure is often due to myocarditis. Foci of infection in the teeth or tonsils may cause myocarditis. Dental therapy or tonsillectomy in such cases often produces striking therapeutic results.

Myocardial degeneration is not a primary disease. The heart muscle degenerates only from some external cause. Severe anemia, cachexia as the result of long-continued malignant or metabolic disease, poisoning from phosphorus or alcohol are important causative factors. Diphtheria and Graves' disease may cause acute and extensive myocardial degeneration. The "fatty" heart, so dreaded by the layman, is a form of fatty degeneration of the heart which is rare and usually of little clinical import.

Chronic myocardial disease may be due to chronic myocarditis representing a chronic stage of an acute myocarditis due to infection, but is more commonly due to myocardial degeneration, also called myocardial fibrosis, or myocardosis. A common cause of myocardial fibrosis is an infarction of the myocardium, the size of the area depending upon that of the vessel occluded.

The subjective symptoms of myocarditis may be slight or intense. Pain in the precordium and palpitation are common; weakness, fever and headache are usually present.

The cardiac findings are often minimal. Tachycardia may be present, but is sometimes absent. The heart sounds may be enfeebled, a tic-tac rhythm may be present, or as often happens, there may be no appreciable alterations in the heart sounds. Before deciding that the heart sounds are weakened, we should, if possible, have a previous examination as a basis of comparison, since in some normal persons the heart sounds seem feeble when compared with those of other normal persons.

The pulse is commonly small in myocardial disease, and the blood pressure low.

In chronic myocardial disease the patient often shows Cheyne-Stokes respiration, which is frequently unnoticed by the patient himself. Palpation of the pulse may show a *pulsus alternans,* and auscultation of the heart may reveal a gallop rhythm. Cheyne-Stokes respiration, *pulsus alternans* and gallop rhythm are common and characteristic of severe myocardial disease. These three findings constitute the myocardial triad.

The electrocardiograph, which has demonstrated conclusively to skeptics the frequency of myocarditis, is often absolutely necessary for the diagnosis. In many cases of myocarditis the diagnosis rests on the electrocardiogram alone.

ANEURYSM

Most of the aneurysms seen clinically are of syphilitic origin. Arteriosclerotic aneurysms, congenital aneurysms, mycotic aneurysms and traumatic aneurysms are occasionally seen, but they are greatly outnumbered by the cases due to *Treponema pallidum.*

Aneurysm of Thoracic Aorta

Broadbent classified aneurysms as "aneurysms of signs" and "aneurysms of symptoms." Aneurysms of signs are those occurring in the ascending part of the arch of the aorta, while the aneurysms of symptoms are located in the transverse and descending arch of the aorta. This second group may call forth distressing symptoms, but the diagnosis may be possible only after use of the x-ray. Aneurysm of the ascending arch usually gives characteristic physical findings.

Inspection. The pathognomonic sign of aneurysm of the ascending arch is a heaving, expansile pulsation in the upper part of the right chest at the level of the third rib to the right of the sternum (Fig. 363). It sometimes extends over the manubrium, may involve the right sternoclavicular joint or may be seen in the second left interspace. A good light is absolutely essential for the demonstration of such pulsations. The expansile character can often be brought out better by drawing with a skin pencil a small hatched area over the pulsation.

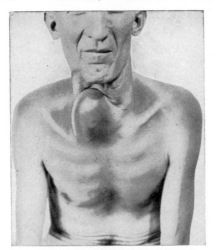

FIG. 363. Aneurysm of the ascending aorta.

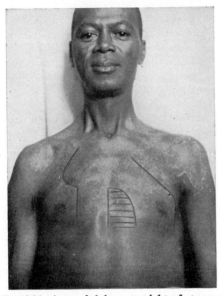

FIG. 364. Area of dulness to right of sternum in the second and third costal interspace due to aneurysm of the ascending arch of the aorta.

As the aneurysm enlarges, it may extend forward, and sometimes produces a swelling larger than a coconut.

The pupil of the patient's eye may be dilated or contracted on one side.

Palpation. Palpation of the larynx may elicit a tracheal tug, as noted first by Oliver. Palpation over the area of pulsation may disclose a diastolic shock, often intense, which is an important sign of aneurysm. A systolic thrill is sometimes felt.

Percussion. Dulness can usually be made out to the right of the sternum and may be extensive even when pulsation is minimal (Fig. 364). The percussion note over an aneurysm is flat.

Auscultation. A systolic murmur is commonly present, and, since the disease is frequently associated with aortic insufficiency, a diastolic murmur may also be heard. A continuous "humming-top" murmur is usually present when there is a communication between the aneurysm and the vena cava or the pulmonary artery.

Pulse. Palpation of the pulse may show marked difference between the pulse in the right and left radial arteries, one pulse being small and showing a definite lag in the time of its appearance as compared with the other.

Aneurysm of the Abdominal Aorta

On inspection of the epigastrium, there is a marked pulsation, sometimes a definite tumor. A thrill is occasionally felt. The pulsation is forceful and expansile. On auscultation a systolic murmur is usually audible.

Marked pulsation of the epigastrium is extremely common in thin, nervous patients, especially in those with a marked anemia. The diagnosis of an abdominal aneurysm should not be made by palpation alone unless the observer feels definitely in his hand a tumor with an expansile pulsation.

Dissecting Aneurysm

Dissecting aneurysm of the aorta is relatively rare, although noted by Morgagni as early as 1760. Pain is one of the most common findings, usually severe; it may, however, occasionally be slight or even absent altogether. The location of the pain depends upon the location of the part of the aorta undergoing dissection, whether in the chest, interscapular region, lumbar region, in the abdomen, in the sacral region or in the hips. Weakness of the lower extremities, paresis of the legs, urinary retention, syncope, convulsions, coma and hemiplegia may occur. A diastolic aortic murmur, due to dilatation of the aorta, may appear. Logue and Sikes have pointed out the diagnostic significance of pulsation of the sternoclavicular joint in dissecting aneurysm of the aorta.

Arteriovenous Aneurysm

Arteriovenous aneurysm, arteriovenous fistula or an abnormal communication between an artery and an adjacent vein, is usually the result of a wound, occasionally of an ulceration. Such aneurysms are found most commonly in the extremities and present a characteristic picture. The affected limb is larger, often has a definite cyanotic hue, and the skin temperature is elevated in the neighborhood of the aneurysm. In young people the leg or arm, the seat of the aneurysm, may grow longer, and develop more hair than the corresponding side. A systolic thrill can be felt over the aneurysm and a continuous murmur with a systolic accentuation heard (Fig. 365). Pressure over the aneurysm, closing the fistula, causes a sharp drop in the pulse rate (Branham's sign). The sign was first reported by Branham in 1890 in a case of arteriovenous aneurysm of the femoral vessels. He noted: "The most mysterious phenomenon connected with the case, one which I have not been able to explain to myself, or to obtain a satisfactory reason for from others, was slowing of the heart's beat, when compression of the common femoral was employed. . . . This symptom became more marked until pressure of the artery above the wound caused the heart's beat to fall from 80 to 35 or 40 per minute

and so to remain until pressure was relieved. Compression of the artery of the sound limb would produce no such effect."

Accompanying the decrease in the pulse rate there is usually an elevation of both systolic and the diastolic blood pressure. This bradycardia which is apparently of vagal origin, is abolished by the use of atropine. Holman believes that closure of the fistula increases the aortic pressure, causing a stimulation of the depressor fibers of the vagus in the arch of the aorta and a resultant slowing of the heart. An arteriovenous aneurysm in the extremities leads to cardiac hypertrophy and later to myocardial insufficiency.

Arteriovenous aneurysms of the vessels of the head or neck often cause great annoyance to the patient because of the constant whirring sound which is heard. A fistula between the thoracic aorta and the vena cava produces intense cyanosis of the upper part of the body, similar to that caused by crushing injuries of the chest.

Summary

Aneurysms of the ascending thoracic aorta, called "aneurysms of signs," show a heaving, expansile pulsation, a diastolic shock over the pulsation, a flat percussion note, and a systolic murmur on auscultation. A tracheal tug is often present. The radial pulse often shows marked differences on the two sides.

Aneurysms of the descending arch of the aorta, "aneurysms of symptoms," although producing distressing dyspnea

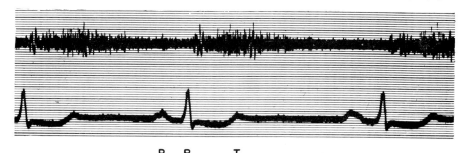

P   R   T

Fig. 365. Arteriovenous aneurysm. Tracing taken in antecubital fossa.

and pain, are often recognized only after roentgen-ray examination.

Aneurysms of the abdominal aorta produce a marked epigastric pulsation. The diagnosis, however, should not be made unless the examiner can definitely feel an expansile, pulsating tumor under his hand.

Arteriovenous aneurysms are commonly suspected from the history. A systolic thrill is felt and a systolic *murmur heard* over the aneurysm. Pressure causes a sharp fall in pulse rate. The increase in temperature of the leg or arm involved is readily appreciated and significant.

THE ELECTROCARDIOGRAM

In this book we have purposely omitted extensive discussion of the electrocardiogram. Electrocardiography is a science in itself. Though some of the most striking abnormalities in the electrocardiogram are obvious to the beginner, more subtle and often extremely important pathologic alterations are appreciated and understood only after extensive experience. As an adjunct to physical diagnosis it is often of equal or even of greater value than the roentgen ray in the study of cardiac disease. Electrocardiography often also gives us conclusive and decisive information which can be obtained by no other method of examination. The medical student should avail himself of every opportunity to become familiar with the technic of electrocardiograms.

The history of electrocardiography began with the discovery of Kölliker and Müller in 1856 that each beat of the frog's heart was accompanied by the production of an electric current. In 1887 Waller showed that this current could be demonstrated in animals and in man, by attaching electrodes to the front and back of the chest and connecting them with a capillary electrometer. Figure 1 in this article, the first published electrocardiogram, is essentially the chest lead reintroduced in recent years as lead 4 (Fig. 366). Willem Einthoven in 1903 substituted for the capillary electrometer a string galvanometer of his own design, and introduced the electrocardiograph as a clinical instrument.

The string galvanometer consists of a minute quartz filament suspended between the poles of a powerful electromagnet. The feeble current accompanying each cardiac contraction is led away from the body by the arm and leg and, passing through the quartz string in the magnetic field, causes a movement of the string with each heart beat. This movement is photographed upon a moving film, producing a record or tracing. This record shows a wave corresponding to auricular contraction P, while the QRS complex is recorded during ventricular systole.

For many years the three so-called standard leads were used—No. 1 between right arm and left arm, No. 2 between right arm and left leg, and No. 3 between left arm and left leg. The introduction of multiple precordial leads

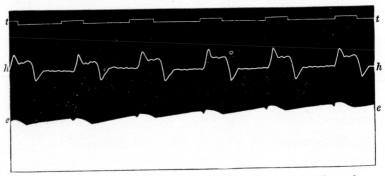

FIG. 366. First electrocardiogram published. *e.e,* electrometer; *h.h,* cardiograph; *t.t,* time in seconds.

has increased greatly the precision and accuracy of electrocardiographic diagnosis.

The electrocardiograph has gradually displaced the polygraph in the clinic. The electrocardiograph in the beginning was considered only of value in the study of cardiac irregularities, and the statement was made on the highest authority that the polygraph of the Mackenzie type gave precisely the same and as much information as the electrocardiograph. Later experience has shown that the electrocardiogram gives far more information concerning the heart. In addition to furnishing accurate information regarding cardiac irregularities, the electrocardiogram gives data regarding the fundamental properties of heart muscle—stimulus production, rhythmicity, irritability, and conductivity, as well as information regarding the muscle mass of the heart and lesions of the heart muscle.

In cardiac irregularities the electrocardiogram differentiates clearly premature contractions, demonstrating whether they are auricular, ventricular or nodal in origin and showing in which ventricle they originate. In auricular fibrillation and in auricular flutter the tracings are characteristic, the absence of the normal P wave being very evident.

In paroxysmal tachycardia the electrocardiogram shows whether the beats originate in the auricle, in the ventricle or in the auriculoventricular node.

In disturbances of conduction, such as heart block, the electrocardiogram demonstrates that the electric impulse fails to pass regularly from the auricle to the ventricle, and that the auricles and ventricles beat at different rates. In bundle branch block the electrocardiogram indicates in which branch of the auriculoventricular bundle (bundle of His) the block occurs. This is an important bit of information, since the prognosis of left bundle branch block is poor, while in right bundle branch block many patients continue in good health for a great many years (Levine).

In coronary occlusion with infarction,

a characteristic electrocardiogram is seen, and usually it is possible to determine in which coronary artery the occlusion has taken place. In this condition the electrocardiogram is of great service in estimating the probable rate of recovery and the ultimate prognosis.

In valvular heart disease the electrocardiogram aids in the diagnosis by showing a preponderance of the right or left ventricle during contraction due to increased work and hypertrophy. In mitral stenosis there is right ventricular preponderance, while in aortic insufficiency there is preponderance of the left ventricle. In pulmonary stenosis there is right ventricular preponderance, in aortic stenosis left ventricular preponderance.

In myocarditis the electrocardiogram may vary greatly from day to day as new foci of inflammation light up and then disappear. The most important of these changes are disturbances in conduction, broadened QRS complexes, abnormal T waves and S-T segment changes.

In arterial hypertension of long standing with cardiac hypertrophy, the electrocardiogram shows a left ventricular preponderance.

In cor pulmonale the electrocardiogram often shows a right ventricular preponderance.

The electrocardiogram gives valuable information regarding the intensity of the heart beat. A feebly acting heart usually shows a low electromotive force with waves of low voltage, while a powerfully beating heart shows waves of high voltage.

The electrocardiogram frequently gives suggestive or conclusive confirmatory evidence of hyperthyroidism, myxedema, potassium intoxication, calcium depletion, dextrocardia, congenital heart disease, acute fibrinous pericarditis, pericarditis with effusion, infarction of the heart and multiple abscesses of the heart.

This brief review of the achievements of the electrocardiogram in the field of diagnosis demonstrates the necessity of an extensive study of and familiarity with electrocardiography. It is a great error, however, to assume that this new method of study has made other methods of physical examination of the heart obsolete. As Levine, who has done outstanding work in the field remarks: "An able clinician who knows nothing about the string galvanometer can still do better work than an expert in electrocardiography who has limited bedside experience and inadequate clinical judgment."

The electrocardiogram has certain definite limitations. It does not diagnose valvular disease; it does not furnish a definite prognosis; it does not indicate cardiac reserve. Such decisions are made by the physician on the basis of all available data. Furthermore, while it may show definite deviations from the normal, it often fails to explain the abnormality; hence the frequent expression "consistent with" as "there is evidence of right ventricular strain, consistent with mitral stenosis."

THE ROENTGEN RAY IN THE DIAGNOSIS OF CARDIAC DISEASE

The roentgen ray is of great assistance in the diagnosis of cardiac disease. Although in this book we have avoided any extended discussion of x-ray findings, a few of the outstanding contributions of roentgenology to cardiac diagnosis should be mentioned.

First of all, the roentgenogram shows us the position, location and size of the heart. Dextrocardia is obvious in an x-ray plate, and a dislocation of the heart to either side is apparent.

An increase in the size of the heart can easily be seen. The transverse diameter of the normal heart does not exceed one half of the transverse diameter of the thorax. An increase in size, due to hypertrophy and dilatation, may be general, or it may affect particularly one of the auricles or ventricles. The hypertrophy of one auricle or ventricle affects the shape of the heart in the roentgenogram, producing a contour which is pathognomonic of certain lesions.

Pericarditis. Pericarditis with effusion produces a characteristic roentgenogram. The cardiopericardial shadow is much increased in size and shows an excessive increase in the horizontal diameter as compared with the vertical. The shadow is broad at the base, is often pear-shaped or like a water bottle, and when the patient sits up, its outline may suggest that of a triangle. Under the fluoroscope the outlines alter materially when the patient changes from a recumbent to an erect position. There may be an obvious diminution in the amplitude of the cardiac pulsations as determined at the contours of the shadow.

In adhesive pericarditis the roentgenogram and fluoroscope demonstrate an enlarged heart. The heart may fail to descend with deep inspiration or to alter its position with change in posture. Tugging of the diaphragm or pleura may be seen with each systole of the heart. Adhesions may be visible, and occasionally calcification of the pericardium.

Mitral Insufficiency. Pure mitral insufficiency may show enlargement of the left ventricle. When there is a complicating mitral stenosis, the picture is that of the latter.

Mitral Stenosis. A roentgenogram of the patient taken in the anteroposterior position may show no enlargement of the left ventricle, but marked enlargement to the right of the sternum—enlargement of the right auricle. The upper left heart border shows frequently a characteristic convexity due to enlargement of the left auricle with rotation of the heart, thus making a silhouette of the pulmonary conus (Fig. 352). A plate in the right oblique position shows enlargement of the left auricle, which may also produce a definite angulation of the esophagus or push it to the right, changes readily visible during the act of swallowing a barium meal.

Aortic Insufficiency. In aortic insufficiency the shadow of the heart is greatly elongated downward, and there is increase in the shadow to the left because of hypertrophy of the left ventricle (Fig. 353). Calcified aortic heart valves may be visible under the fluoroscope.

Aortic Stenosis. A roentgenogram or fluoroscopic examination of a patient with aortic stenosis shows marked enlargement of the left ventricle, which has a slow, somewhat leisurely, but forceful movement (Fig. 354). This slow movement of the left ventricle is so characteristic that an experienced roentgenologist, on observing it, can make the diagnosis of aortic stenosis.

Calcification of the aortic valve may be seen on fluoroscopic examination and confirmed by the flat plate.

Pulmonary Stenosis. In this disease the roentgenogram shows a striking picture. The apex of the heart is pushed outward and elevated, the tip of the right ventricle is rounded, and the right ventricle is pushed downward and also extends far to the right of the sternum. The horizontal diameter of the heart is greatly increased. This outline of the heart has been called the "sabot" heart from its resemblance to the sabot or wooden shoe worn by French peasants. This "sabot" heart is seen most frequently in Fallot's tetralogy, which comprises, not only pulmonary stenosis, but also interventricular septum defect and dextroposition of the aorta.

Congenital Heart Disease. In these patients, the roentgenogram or fluoroscopic examination is of the greatest assistance in diagnosis. Dilatation of the pulmonary artery, which causes an increased convexity or bulging of the middle arc of the left cardiac border, is seen in patent ductus arteriosus, aortic septal defect, pulmonary stenosis with a closed ventricular septum, *Eisenmenger's complex,* and interauricular septal defects.

Fallot's tetralogy shows the "sabot" heart in about 50 per cent of the cases. Increased translucency of the lung fields is often seen in this condition. Dextrocardia can be positively diagnosed by x-ray.

Angiocardiography is of much assistance in the diagnosis of certain cases of congenital heart disease. By this method, the pulmonary artery may be readily identified and the auricular and ventricular septa visualized. In interventricular septal defect, both ventricles fill simultaneously, and, in *Fallot's tetralogy,* both aorta and pulmonary artery may be filled at the same time. In severe stenosis or atresia of the pulmonary artery, there may be delay in filling of this vessel. However, there is a certain danger in the employment of angiocardiography, and fatalities occasionally occur.

In *coarctation of the aorta,* as previously mentioned, erosion of the ribs is commonly present, and the condition may be first diagnosed by the roentgenologist. The roentgenogram in cor pulmonale shows a marked dilatation of the right ventricle.

The roentgen ray aids also in the diagnosis of *cardiac arrhythmias.* Examining the heart under the fluoroscope, one readily sees extrasystoles, the delirious irregularity of auricular fibrillation, and in heart block one may actually see the auricles beating more rapidly than the ventricles.

The roentgen ray is invaluable in the diagnosis of *aortic aneurysms.* The aneurysmal sac usually casts a clear shadow in the x-ray plate, and under the fluoroscope is seen as a dark mass pulsating with each beat of the heart. At times, however, it is difficult for the roentgenologist to differentiate between an aneurysm and a mediastinal tumor.

Arteriosclerosis, dilatation and tortuosity of the aorta are clearly demonstrable by x-ray examination.

BIBLIOGRAPHY

Allbutt, Sir Clifford: Diseases of the Arteries Including Angina Pectoris. New York, The Macmillan Company, 1915.

Bamberger, H.: Beiträge zur Physiologie und Pathologie des Herzens. Virchows Arch. f. path. Anat. *9:*328, 523, 1856.

Bean, W. B., and Schmidt, M. D.: Rupture of the aortic valve. J.A.M.A. *153:*214, 1953.

Bishop, Louis Faugeres: A Key to the Electrocardiogram. New York, Wm. Wood & Co., 1923.

Blumgart, H. D., Schlesinger, M. J., and Zoll, P. M.: Angina pectoris, coronary failure and acute myocardial infarction. J.A.M.A. *116:*91, 1941.

Branham, Harris H.: Aneurysmal varix of the femoral artery and vein following a gunshot wound. Int. J. Surg., New York 3:250, 1890.

Brown, James W.: Congenital Heart Disease. New York, Staples Press, 1950.

Cabot, Richard C.: Facts on the Heart. Philadelphia, W. B. Saunders Co., 1926.

Delp, Mahlon H., and Maxwell, Robert: Rupture of an aortic aneurysm into the pulmonary artery. J.A.M.A. 110:1647, 1938.

DeVeer, J. Arnold: A mechanical explanation of sudden death in aortic stenosis. Am. Heart J. 15:243, 1938.

Dimond, E. Grey: Electrocardiography. St. Louis, C. V. Mosby Co., 1954.

Ewart, William: Practical aids in the diagnosis of pericardial effusion. Brit. M. J. 1: 717, 1896.

Gevalt, Frederick C., Jr., and Levine, Samuel A.: The significance of Ewart's sign. New Internat. Clin. 4:1, 1940.

Gross, R. E., and Hubbard, J. P.: Surgical ligation of a patent ductus arteriosus: report of first successful case. J.A.M.A. 112: 729, 1939.

Hollman, Emile: Arteriovenous aneurysm Ann. Surg. 80:801, 1924.

Kölliker, A., and Müller, H.: Nachweis der negativen Schwankung des Muskelstroms am natürlich sich contrahierenden Muskel. Verh. der physikal-medicin. Gesellsch. in Würzburg. 6:528, 1856.

Leaman, William G., Jr.: The history of electrocardiography. Ann. M. Hist. 8:113, 1936.

Levine, Samuel A.: Clinical Heart Disease. 4th ed. Philadelphia, W. B. Saunders Co., 1951.

Levine, Samuel A., and Harvey, W. Proctor: Clinical Auscultation of the Heart. Philadelphia, W. B. Saunders Co., 1949.

Lewis, Sir Thomas: Clinical Electrocardiography. 3rd ed. London, Shaw & Sons, Ltd., 1924.

Lewis, Sir Thomas: Diseases of the Heart. New York, The Macmillan Company, 1933.

Lewis, Sir Thomas: The Mechanism and Graphic Registration of the Heart Beat. 3rd ed. London, Shaw & Sons, Ltd., 1925.

Lewis, Sir Thomas: Pain in muscular ischemia. Arch. Int. Med. 49:713, 1932.

Logue, R. Bruce, and Sikes, Clayton: A new sign in dissecting aneurysm of the aorta. J.A.M.A. 148:1209, 1952.

Martin, S. J., and Gorham, L. W.: Cardiac pain. Arch. Int. Med. 52:840, 1938.

Matas, Rudolph: On the systemic or cardiovascular effects of arteriovenous fistulae. Internat. Clin. Ser. 35, 2:58, 1925.

Merrill, A. J.: Edema and decreased renal blood flow in patients with chronic congestive heart failure. J. Clin. Investigation 25:389, 1946.

Mote, Clayton D., and Carr, Jesse L.: Dissecting aneurysm of the aorta. Am. Heart J. 24:69, 1942.

Neuhof, Selian: The Heart. Philadelphia, P. Blakiston's Sons & Co., 1923.

Pardee, Harold E. B.: Clinical Aspects of the Electrocardiogram. 2d ed. New York, Paul B. Hoeber, Inc., 1928.

Pins, E.: Ein neues Symptom der Pericarditis. Wien. med. Wchnschr. 39:210, 1889.

Pullen, Roscoe L.: Medical Diagnosis, Applied Physical Diagnosis. 2d ed., Philadelphia, W. B. Saunders Co., 1950.

Reich, Nathaniel E.: The Uncommon Heart Diseases. Springfield, Charles C Thomas, 1954.

Roth, Irving R.: Cardiac Arrhythmias. New York, Paul B. Hoeber, Inc., 1927.

Sancetta, S. M.: Clinical detection of "pulsating" liver. J.A.M.A. 158:922, 1955.

Sandifort, Eduard: Observationes anatomico-pathologicae. Leyden, Eyk and Vygh, 1777–1781.

Scherf, David, and Boyd, Linn J.: Cardiovascular Diseases, Their Diagnosis and Treatment. St. Louis, C. V. Mosby Co., 1939.

Schnitker, Maurice A.: Congenital Anomalies of the Heart and Great Vessels. New York, Oxford University Press, 1952.

Smith, Samuel Calvin: Heart Records: Their Interpretation and Preparation. Philadelphia, F. A. Davis Co., 1923.

Tice, G. M.: Radiographic evidence of cardio-vascular disease. Bull. Univ. Kansas School of Med. 5:8 (June), 1934.

Traube, L.: Gesammelte Beiträge zur Pathologie und Physiologie. Berlin, Hirschwald, 1878.

Vaquez, H., and Bordet, E.: The Heart and the Aorta, transl. from the second French edition by James A. Honeij and John Macy. New Haven, Yale University Press, 1920.

Waller, Augustus D.: A demonstration on man of electromotive changes accompanying the heart's beat. J. Physiol. 8:229, 1887.

Warren, James V., and Stead, Eugene, A., Jr.: Fluid dynamics in chronic congestive heart failure. Arch. Int. Med. 73:138, 1944.

White, Paul D.: Heart Disease. 4th ed. New York, The Macmillan Company, 1951.

Wiggers, Carl J.: Principles and Practice of Electrocardiography. St. Louis, C. V. Mosby Co., 1929.

Willius, Fredrick A.: Clinical Electrocardiography. Philadelphia, W. B. Saunders Co., 1922.

CHAPTER 14

ABDOMEN AND GENITALIA

THE PHYSICAL EXAMINATION of the abdomen is a procedure less exact than that of the chest. Because of this fact there is a tendency for students and physicians to slight this part of the physical examination. This tendency cannot be condemned too severely. Although the physician is often helpless in the diagnosis of abdominal conditions without the use of the x-ray and of certain laboratory procedures, the diagnosis in many cases can be established by the physical examination alone, and in many other cases the proper interpretation of x-ray and laboratory findings can be made only in the light of the physical findings.

In an examination of the abdomen we chiefly use inspection, palpation and percussion. Auscultation is rarely of much assistance.

ABDOMEN

Topographical Anatomy

For the purpose of describing and localizing lesions in various parts of the abdomen it is customary to divide the abdomen into various regions. Two vertical lines are drawn on either side from the middle of Poupart's ligament upward and two lines horizontally, one across the lower margin of the tenth costal cartilage, the other joining the

crest of the ilium on either side (Fig. 367). This divides the abdomen into nine regions. In the middle are the epigastric region, the umbilical region and the hypogastric region. On the sides are the right and left hypochondria, the

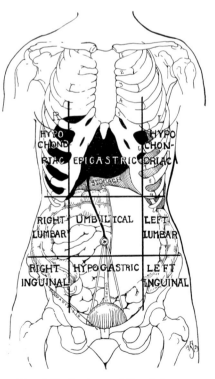

FIG. 367. Regions of the abdomen.

247

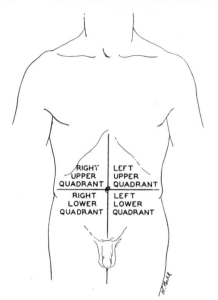

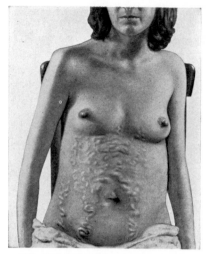

FIG. 369. Dilated abdominal veins in obstruction of vena cava.

FIG. 368. Division of abdomen into quadrants.

right and left lumbar regions and the right and left inguinal regions. The relationship of these areas to the important organs underneath is seen in the illustration.

Another division of the abdominal areas which is much used is that of dividing the abdomen into four quadrants, drawing a horizontal and a vertical line through the umbilicus (Fig. 368).

In the examination of the abdomen the same sequence of procedure is followed as elsewhere in the physical examination.

Inspection of the Abdomen

Skin. The skin of the abdomen shows the same lesions of various diseases as seen elsewhere. Petechiae, and the eruptions of measles, scarlet fever, smallpox and syphilis are well marked over the abdomen. In icterus the skin of the abdomen is yellow as elsewhere. The rose spots of typhoid are often visible only over the abdomen (Fig. 64).

Dilated veins appear on the surface of the abdomen when there is venous obstruction (Fig. 388). In obstruction of the inferior vena cava there is often marked distention of the superficial ab-

dominal veins (Fig. 369). Marked ascites, a large intra-abdominal tumor or a greatly enlarged spleen may cause a similar dilatation of the superficial veins (Fig. 382).

In cases of obstruction to the portal circulation the so-called *caput medusae,* a cluster of dilated veins radiating out from the umbilicus, may appear. Our experience coincides with that of Cabot, that the caput medusae is "commonly found in textbooks, but rarely in cirrhosis of the liver."

The *striae of pregnancy* are seen in pregnant women and in women who have borne children. In pregnant women they are pinkish or slightly bluish depressed lines over the lower abdomen and hips, parallel to the long axis of the body. In women who have borne children they are glistening, silvery-white in color. They are produced by rupture and are frequently observed in nonpregnant women or even men, when there has been a rapid increase in size of the abdomen as the result of abdominal tumors or obesity.

Movements. The respiratory movements in health are regular and free over the abdomen. In inflammatory diseases of the abdomen there is often a marked limitation of the respiratory movements. Singultus, or hiccuping, caused by spasmodic contractions of the diaphragm, produces similar spasmodic movements of the abdominal wall.

Umbilicus. The umbilicus may be the seat of hernias or neoplasms. In small hernias a slight protrusion may be produced by coughing or by an increased intra-abdominal tension. Figure 370 shows a patient with a small umbilical hernia resulting from ascites. In some patients the hernia may be so large and the protrusion so striking that it is the first abnormality noticeable on examination of the abdomen (Fig. 371).

When the umbilicus is the seat of a carcinoma, either primary or secondary, there is a hard, protruding, small mass which later becomes ulcerated (Fig. 372).

Nutrition. The nutrition of a patient is well reflected in his abdomen. A fat person usually has a large, protruding abdomen along with other evidences of excessive subcutaneous deposit of fat (Fig. 373). In patients with pituitary obesity the contour of the abdomen is often flattened and the fat hangs in folds like an apron, as seen in Figure 374. This patient, although of enormous girth, has little excess adipose tissue on the forearms, wrists, hands, legs, ankles or feet. The fat is centrally and not peripherally distributed.

In emaciated persons the abdomen is concave and the pulsations of the abdominal aorta are clearly seen. The patient shown in Figure 375 was somewhat emaciated and suffered from in-

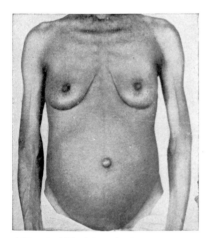

FIG. 370. Umbilical hernia in patient suffering from ascites.

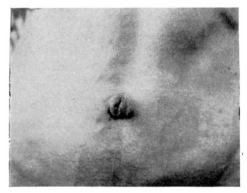

FIG. 372. Carcinoma of umbilicus.

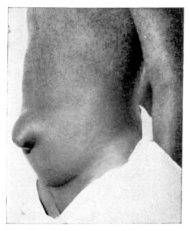

FIG. 371. Umbilical hernia.

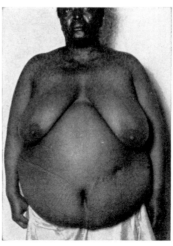

FIG. 373. Obesity.

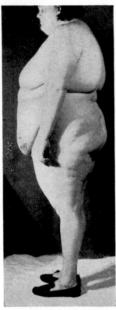

FIG. 374. Obesity in hypopituitarism.

testinal obstruction due to a carcinoma of the intestine. The outlines of the distended intestinal loops are clearly visible, and peristalsis could be clearly seen. The patient shown in Figure 376 shows extreme emaciation, a scaphoid abdomen and, in addition, a large mass in the epigastric region, which proved to be a carcinoma of the stomach.

In Hirschsprung's disease the dilated large intestine often produces what appears to be a marked generalized distention of the abdomen (Fig 377). In emaciated patients the dilated large intestine is often visible, as in Figure 378.

Shape and Size of the Abdomen. The shape and size of the abdomen are profoundly changed by the presence of free fluid (ascites) in the peritoneal cavity and by masses in the abdomen. Two of the most common causes of

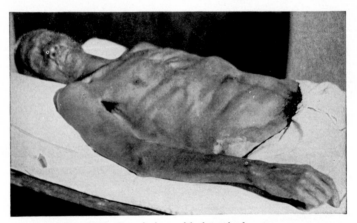

FIG. 375. Emaciation with intestinal patterns.

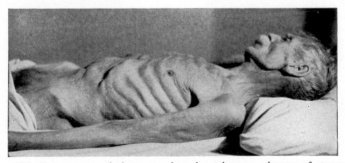

FIG. 376. Extreme emaciation, mass in epigastrium, carcinoma of stomach.

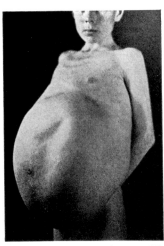

FIG. 377. Hirschsprung's disease. (Courtesy of Frederic M. Hanes.)

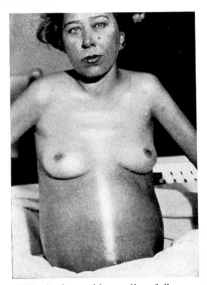

FIG. 379. Ascites with cardiac failure; note dark shade of lips due to cyanosis.

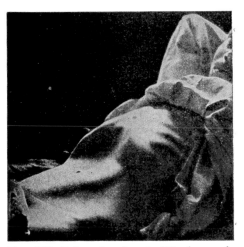

FIG. 378. Enlarged colon in Hirschsprung's disease. (Külbs.)

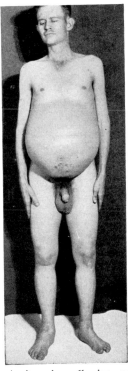

FIG. 380. Ascites in adhesive pericarditis; note marks of old paracenteses below umbilicus.

generalized abdominal enlargements are ascites and ovarian cysts.

Ascites (from ἀσκός = a bag). Patients with cardiac failure often show marked ascites. A typical example is seen in Figure 379. This patient, in addition to a tense, shiny abdomen, shows a marked cyanosis of the lips and nose, and is obviously dyspneic. The diagnosis in such cases is aided by the presence of an enlarged, tender liver and of a cardiac enlargement with murmurs. Chronic adhesive pericarditis often causes intense recurring ascites. The patient shown in Figure 380 had this disease, and the marks left by several abdominal tappings are visible in the suprapubic region.

Cirrhosis of the liver is a classic cause of ascites. The patient shown in Figure

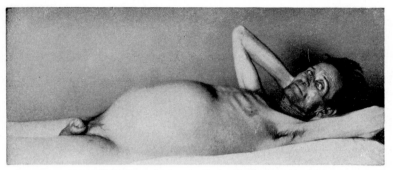

FIG. 381. Ascites in cirrhosis of liver.

381 had a marked distention of the abdomen with atrophy and emaciation of the subcutaneous tissue of the chest and arms, neither of which was present in the two patients shown in Figures 379 and 380. He also had the sharp, pinched features with a sallow, yellowish tint of the skin of the face which has been described as hepatic facies. Banti's disease shows, in its later stages, a marked ascites associated with splenomegaly and cirrhosis of the liver (Fig. 382).

Tuberculosis of the peritoneum usually produces ascites (Fig. 383). The diagnosis in such cases is established by the presence of other evidence of tu-

berculosis and especially by injecting a small quantity of the fluid into a guinea pig, causing the subsequent development of tuberculosis in the animal.

Ascites occurs often in nephritis and especially in the nephrosis of children, being associated here with a generalized edema (Fig. 384).

Ascites occurs frequently with malignant tumors of the abdominal organs, especially when there are peritoneal implantations and metastases. Figure 385 shows a patient with a malignant papilloma of the ovary and ascites. Part

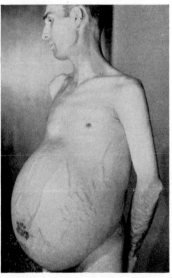

FIG. 382. Ascites associated with Banti's disease. Note marked distention of abdominal veins, also marks of recent tappings about the umbilicus.

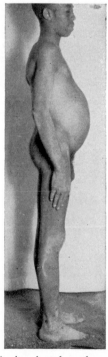

FIG. 383. Ascites in tuberculous peritonitis.

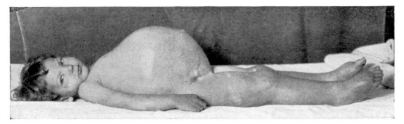

FIG. 384. Ascites in nephrosis.

of the tumor mass is seen protruding at the umbilicus. The patient shown in Figure 386 had a marked ascites associated with carcinoma of the gallbladder.

A pathognomonic sign of ascites is the presence of a fluid wave, which will be discussed under palpation.

Tympanites. "The Dropsie called Tympanites," according to Riverius in the quaint translation of Nicholas Culpepper, "hath its name from *tympanum,* a drum, because the abdomen is stretched out like a Drum, and if you strike it with your hand, it sounds like it. This stretching comes from wind shut up in the Cavity of the Abdomen. But sometimes this wind is in the Cavity of the Guts."

Tympanites is present after perforation of the stomach or intestines when the air escapes into the abdominal cavity. More commonly this condition is seen in intestinal obstruction and in typhoid fever, the air in both instances being within and producing a marked distention of the intestines.

Ovarian Cysts. Ovarian cysts are a common cause of marked enlargement of the abdomen in women (Fig. 387). The cysts at times may attain such size that, after removal, the cyst itself weighs as much as or more than the patient. Here the sex, age and history aid in the diagnosis.

Ascites and ovarian cysts are the most common causes of general abdominal enlargement, but tumors of the liver, spleen and ovaries may at times attain such size that the enlargement of the abdomen is general as well as local. The patient shown in Figure 388 at first

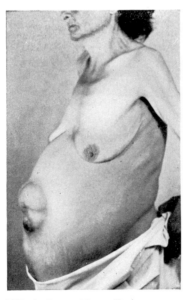

FIG. 385. Ascites with malignant tumor of ovaries.

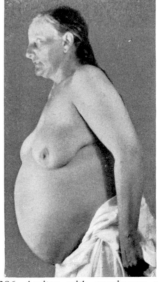

FIG. 386. Ascites with carcinoma of gallbladder.

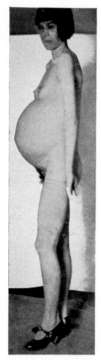

FIG. 387. Ovarian cyst.

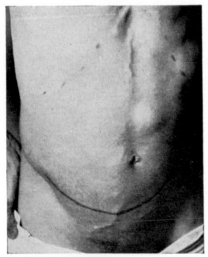

FIG. 388. Nodule above umbilicus which was part of enlarged spleen. Note enlarged veins on abdomen.

glance displays a small mass above the umbilicus. Further examination showed the abdomen to be filled with a huge mass extending down to the iliac crests which proved to be the enlarged spleen of splenomyelogenous leukemia. The

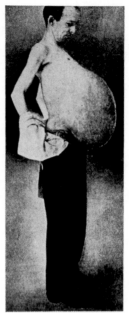

FIG. 389. Hemangioma of liver.

small nodule was an irregularity of the surface of the huge spleen.

Tumors and cysts arising in the liver, spleen, ovaries, kidneys or mesentery may at times attain such dimensions that they alter the entire configuration of the abdomen. The patient shown in Figure 389 had a huge hemangioma of the liver.

There is a marked enlargement of the abdomen in women in pseudocyesis or pseudopregnancy. In this interesting condition the abdomen enlarges until the patient imagines herself pregnant and may almost convince her physician that she is, even if her menstruation has not ceased. Under anesthesia this abdominal tumor disappears. The cause of pseudocyesis has never been fully explained, but it is apparently a psychoneurotic condition, probably best classified as hysteria.

Epigastrium. A marked pulsation of the epigastrium is seen in aneurysm of the abdominal aorta. Far more commonly, however, this pulsation is seen in nervous, anemic persons with thin abdominal walls and a shallow abdomen.

In some persons, especially women who have borne children, the recti muscles become separated in the midline and cause a condition known as diastasis recti (Fig. 390). When such a patient lies down and flexes the head toward the chest, a part of the intra-abdominal contents bulges out between the recti, producing a picture resembling that of an abdominal tumor.

Enlargements in the epigastric region usually have their origin in the stomach, the great majority of them being produced by carcinoma. In some patients they are seen best in profile view of the abdomen (Fig. 391). The patient shown in Figure 392 has a carcinoma of the stomach which has produced a marked protrusion of the epigastric region. In Figure 376 the patient is markedly emaciated, and the concavity of the abdomen makes the stomach tumor obvious.

Marked enlargement of the epigastrium occurs in acute dilatation of the stomach. At times such an acute dilatation occurs through the patient's swallowing air. In a patient seen recently the distention of the stomach was extreme and even alarming. Such tumors disappear immediately on introduction of the stomach tube.

Right Hypochondrium. Enlargements in this area are usually due to hepatic disease. In an emaciated person the margin of an enlarged liver may be clearly seen, descending on inspiration and rising on expiration. An enlargement of the gallbladder is visible at times. In tricuspid insufficiency the pulsations of an enlarged liver may be seen.

Tumors of the liver may produce visible enlargements. The patient shown in Figure 393 had a cystic tumor of the liver.

Left Hypochondrium. Enlargements of the left hypochondrium are usually synonymous with enlargements of the spleen. The most common causes of

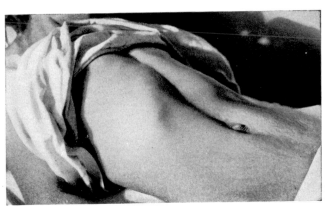

FIG. 390. Diastasis recti.

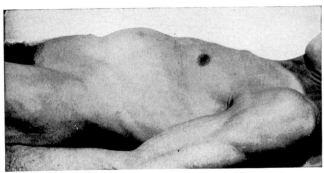

FIG. 391. Carcinoma of stomach, mass in epigastrium.

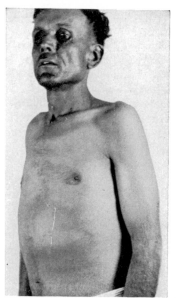

FIG. 392. Carcinoma of stomach, mass in epigastrium.

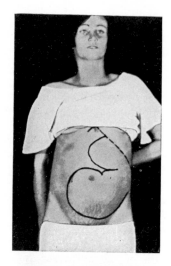

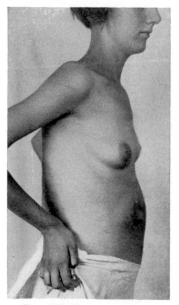

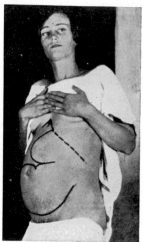

FIG. 394. Enlarged spleen in leukemia.

FIG. 393. Tumor of liver.

such enlargements are: malaria, typhoid fever, Banti's disease, splenomyelogenous leukemia. This last condition produces the largest spleens encountered in clinical medicine, and practically the only ones obvious on inspection. The patient seen in Figure 394 shows a marked enlargement of the left hypo-

chondrium and the left side of the abdomen. On palpation the outlines of a large mass were clearly felt and marked out.

Lumbar Region. Enlargement in the lumbar regions is associated particularly with malformations of the kidneys, such as hydronephrosis, cysts and tumors. Figure 395 shows a huge hypernephroma arising from the left kidney and projecting forward and downward. Figure 396 shows a tumor of the right kidney which is clearly visible when brought forward by pressure with the hand.

Pubic Region. A distended bladder (Fig. 397) may produce a large tumor

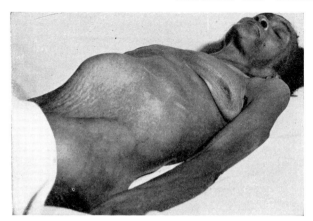

FIG. 395. Hypernephroma of kidney.

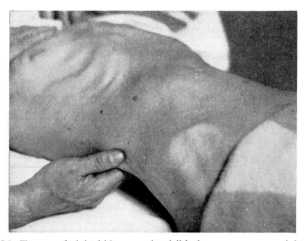

FIG. 396. Tumor of right kidney made visible by pressure over right back.

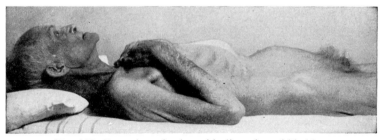

FIG. 397. Retention of urine with distention of bladder.

in the pubic region which disappears after catheterization. Such enlargements are usually diagnosed without difficulty. In the presence of an ascites a distended bladder may not be recognized, and has occasionally been tapped in an abdominal paracentesis. For this reason, it is an axiom with physicians that the patient should void or be catheterized before the abdominal trochar is introduced.

Tumors of the bladder may cause enlargement in this area. In women, neoplasms of the uterus and adnexa are frequent causes.

Inguinal Region. Frequent causes of swelling in the inguinal regions are herniae. The patient shown in Figure

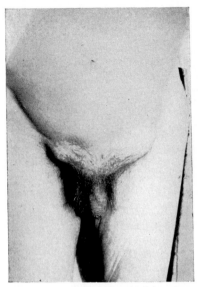

FIG. 398. Bilateral inguinal herniae.

398 had bilateral inguinal herniae. Such swellings increase in size on coughing.

Palpation of the Abdomen

Palpation is in many respects the most important procedure in the physical examination of the abdomen. It requires attention, practice and experience. Usually the patient should lie perfectly flat, better without a pillow. In some conditions, however, when there is an enlargement or tumor of the abdominal viscera, palpation is more instructive if carried out with the patient standing.

The position of the hand in palpation of the abdomen is important. It should be held parallel to the surface of the abdomen and never at right angles (Fig. 399). When held at right angles the tips of the fingers cause muscular resistance which blocks successful palpation. Palpation should be at first soft, gentle and superficial; then, as the tenseness of the muscles relaxes, deeper palpation may be attempted.

Palpation of the liver (Fig. 400) is best accomplished with the patient supine, his head and shoulders slightly elevated by pillows, the thighs slightly flexed. The patient is instructed to breathe regularly, preferably through the mouth. The examiner should stand or, preferably, sit at the patient's right side, placing the right hand gently but firmly upon the abdominal wall. The examiner may find it desirable and advantageous to place the left hand under the patient's right flank, pressing gently upward in an effort to elevate the bulk of the liver into a more easily accessible location. The positioned right hand is then moved downward and slightly upward just as the patient takes a deep breath. The descent of the diaphragm during deep inspiration carries the liver down, and its margin as well as an enlarged gallbladder may be palpated by the fingers of the examining hand.

The procedure for palpating the kidneys is similar to that used in palpating the liver. With deep inspiration the

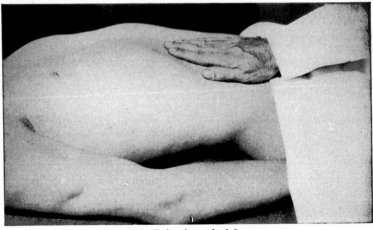

FIG. 399. Palpation of abdomen.

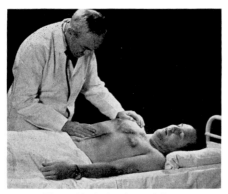

FIG. 400. Palpation of liver.

kidneys descend, and in certain cases, particularly in thin persons, the lower poles of the kidneys may be felt.

Palpation of the spleen should be carried out by the following method: With the patient lying on his back, the examiner stands at the patient's right side and places his right hand flat with the abdominal wall just at the costal margin in the anterior mammillary line. The patient is directed to inspire deeply, the spleen descends with the diaphragm and, if enlarged, touches the tips of the fingers of the examining hand. This procedure is further assisted by placing the left hand under the spleen and gently pushing upward (Fig. 401). At times the spleen, although not felt when the patient lies on his back, is readily palpable if the patient lies on his right side.

In most instances palpation of the abdomen is carried out most satisfactorily when the examiner is seated by the patient's bedside rather than leaning over. Such a position favors a deliberate, careful and exhaustive examination.

One of the important features of palpation is to confirm and amplify the findings of inspection. A mass, for instance, which is visible on inspection may be firm or soft, smooth or irregular, fixed or movable. Frequently a mass which is not visible is easily felt on palpation.

Palpation is of especial value in determining the outlines of the liver, spleen, kidneys and bladder when these organs are enlarged, and in determining the outlines and extent of masses in the abdomen.

Palpation of the Normal Abdomen. Palpation of the abdomen in well-nourished or obese normal persons yields nothing tangible. In thin persons we may feel the abdominal aorta and spinal column at or below the umbilicus, a part of the liver where it leaves the costal margin and passes to the left, and the lower pole of the right kidney. The normal intestine, appendix, stomach, spleen, pancreas, left kidney, bladder and pelvic organs cannot be recognized as such on palpation of the abdomen.

Abdominal Reflex. This reflex may

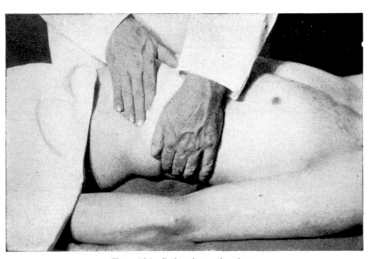

FIG. 401. Palpation of spleen.

be obtained by stroking the skin of the abdomen on either side parallel to the costal margin or to Poupart's ligament. This stroking causes a contraction of the rectus muscle which is obvious.

The abdominal reflex does not appear until several months after birth. It is often absent in acute appendicitis, in typhoid fever and in hemiplegia. The absence of the abdominal reflex in a young person may, when it is associated with other signs, suggest multiple sclerosis.

The abdominal reflex may be exaggerated in the gastric crises of tabes dorsalis.

Palpation of the Abdominal Wall. The wall of the abdomen in health with the patient relaxed is soft and gives when the examining hand presses it. Usually there is some muscular resistance to this procedure, but after a few minutes the resistance disappears. The degree of softness of the abdominal wall varies in different persons.

The "feel" of the individual abdominal wall is an important thing to acquire in patients with typhoid fever. In this disease the abdomen should be palpated at least once a day. A slight but definite increase in the resistance of the abdominal wall may point to a deep ulceration or an early perforation. The amount of resistance which is normal for one patient may be abnormal in another. This emphasizes the need of becoming familiar with the "feel" of the individual abdomen.

Spasm of the Abdominal Wall. Spasm of the abdominal wall may be local or general. Spasticity and tenderness of the abdominal wall over McBurney's point are pathognomonic of acute appendicitis. McBurney's point is located "between an inch and a half and two inches from the anterior spinous process of the ilium in a straight line drawn from that process to the umbilicus" (Fig. 402). This increase in spasticity is often on the entire right side of the abdomen. It is best appreciated by comparing the two sides and by palpating the left side of the abdomen first.

Spasm of the right hypochondrium is extremely suggestive of acute cholecystitis, for in this disease pressure usually elicits acute pain in this region.

A generalized spasticity of the abdomen occurs in general peritonitis. Since this condition is often the result of perforation of the stomach, appendix or intestines, air enters the peritoneal cavity and, combined with the exudation

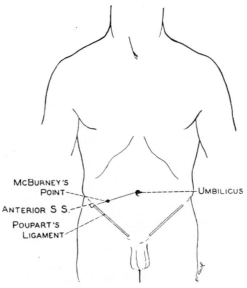

FIG. 402. McBurney's point.

of fluid, produces marked abdominal distention.

Subcutaneous emphysema is readily diagnosed when the examiner notes that palpation of the skin produces a crackling sensation which the examining fingers feel quite clearly. Subcutaneous emphysema appears, not only over the abdomen, but over the thorax and extremities as well. It indicates the presence of gas or air under the skin and is seen in gas bacillus infections, and after thoracentesis, where it is localized about the site of the puncture, and occasionally after abdominal operations when it is located about the operative wound. In gas bacillus infections it is of grave prognostic import; after thoracentesis and abdominal operations it indicates only the escape of air into the subcutaneous tissues and is of interest, but not of importance.

Fluid Wave. In ascites, whether the result of cardiac disease, of cirrhosis of the liver or of general peritonitis, a fluid wave is pathognomonic of free fluid in the abdominal cavity. In eliciting a fluid wave, it is important to exclude a wave which may be produced in the subcutaneous tissue. For this reason an assistant is necessary who holds his hand in the midline with the ulnar margin pressed gently but firmly against the surface of the abdomen. The examiner places the fingers of one hand against the lateral wall of the abdomen and taps firmly with the other hand. This procedure produces a wave in the fluid which is transmitted to the hand upon the other side of the abdomen and is felt as a shock (Fig. 403). The wave is sometimes better felt when the patient stands up than when he is lying down. A fluid wave may also be felt in ovarian cysts, in mesenteric cysts and in huge myxomatous tumors within the peritoneal cavity. The two last conditions are rare.

This fluid wave may often be seen. Celsus more than nine hundred years ago observed that "the fluid often collects within the abdomen so that if it be shaken by any movement of the body the fluctuation of the fluid can be seen."

Epigastrium. *Aneurysm of the Abdominal Aorta.* Many patients, especially thin, anemic, nervous persons, show on inspection a marked throbbing of the epigastrium. On palpation the violently throbbing abdominal aorta can be felt in this region, and the examiner suspects an aneurysm. This diagnosis, however, should never be made unless a definite, enlarged mass can be felt which has an expansile pulsation.

Palpation of the epigastrium may show a small hernia in the abdominal wall which was not visible on inspection. Such small herniae frequently produce pain in the epigastrium which is falsely believed to be due to disease of the stomach.

Diastasis or separation of the recti, when present, is readily recognized on palpation.

Tumors of the stomach and pancreas

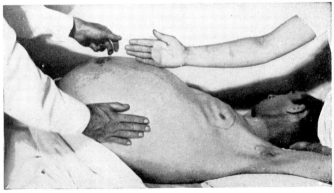

Fig. 403. Examination for fluid wave.

are often readily palpable when not seen on inspection.

Right Hypochondrium. An enlarged liver due to chronic passive congestion, alcoholic or syphilitic cirrhosis, carcinoma, abscess or hepatitis is readily palpable in the right hypochondrium (Fig. 404). Such enlargements of the liver frequently extend downward into the right lumbar region. The irregularities and bosses on the surface of the liver with carcinoma or syphilitic cirrhosis are readily felt. In tricuspid insufficiency a pulsating liver may be palpated.

An enlarged gallbladder can often be palpated and its outlines made out.

"The most characteristic and constant sign of gallbladder hypersensitiveness," wrote John B. Murphy, "is the inability of the patient to take a full, deep inspiration, when the physician's fingers are hooked up deep beneath the right costal arch below the hepatic margin. The diaphragm forces the liver down until the sensitive gallbladder reaches the examining fingers, when the inspiration suddenly ceases as though it had been shut off. I have never found this sign absent in a calculous or in-

fectious case of gallbladder, or duct disease." Murphy's sign is an important indication of gallbladder disease. It occurs also in inflammation of the liver.

Right Lumbar Region. Tumors of the right kidney may be felt in this region. A thickened colon or cecum due to carcinoma, tuberculosis or actinomycosis can often be palpated in the right lumbar region extending down to the inguinal region. Appendicular abscess and regional ileitis often occur in this region.

Left Hypochondrium. In this region a slightly or moderately enlarged spleen may be felt. The character of the spleen is often important. In typhoid fever it feels soft, in malaria hard and firm. In Vaquez's disease the spleen is enlarged, hard, smooth and painless.

The enlarged spleen of leukemia is felt first in this region, but as it enlarges it extends downward and to the right, at times seeming to occupy a large part of the abdomen (Fig. 405). The outlines of such a huge spleen can be readily felt, the presence of the splenic notch being characteristic of this organ (Fig. 406). Pulsation of the spleen is a rare phenomenon, although noted as far back as 1652 by Nicholas

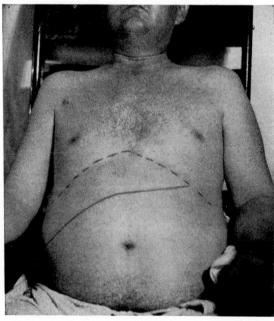

Fig. 404. Enlargement of liver due to chronic passive congestion in cardiac failure.

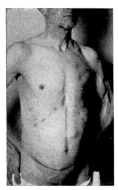

FIG. 405. Marked enlargement of spleen in leukemia.

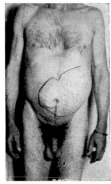

FIG. 406. Enlargement of spleen in leukemia with notch.

Tulp. It has been described in patients with aortic insufficiency who had splenic enlargement, usually due to malaria or typhoid fever. It occasionally occurs in combined mitral and tricuspid diseases.

Left Lumbar Region. An enlarged kidney, the result of tumor growth or of hydronephrosis, is readily palpable in this region.

Diseases of the tubes and ovaries produce enlargements which may be palpable in the lumbar regions.

Pubic Region. A distended bladder may be felt here. In women, tumors of the uterus, especially myomata, can often be felt.

Percussion of the Abdomen

Percussion of the abdomen has its value mainly in confirming the findings of inspection and palpation. An enlarged liver, gallbladder or spleen, which can be felt on palpation, gives a dull note on percussion. The outlines made out on percussion are usually smaller than those obtained on palpation.

Normally the percussion note is tympanitic over the abdomen, except for the area of liver dulness. Complete absence of liver dulness indicates the presence of air in the abdominal cavity and is most commonly the result of a perforated peptic ulcer.

Shifting Dulness. When there is free fluid in the abdomen, the fluid gravitates to the flanks and the intestines float upward when the patient lies on his back. Under such conditions the percussion note is tympanitic over the anterior surface of the abdomen and dull in the flanks. The crucial test, however, is to turn the patient on one side. If there is free fluid in the abdomen, the dulness shifts; the percussion note on the side which is uppermost becomes tympanitic, while the note on the lower side is dull.

The following procedure is of value in differentiating splenic enlargement from that of the kidney. If a rectal tube is inserted into the rectum and air pumped in with a hand bulb, the percussion note over the mass becomes more tympanitic if the mass is kidney, since the colon over the kidney is distended. If the mass is the spleen, distention of the colon pushes the spleen forward and the percussion note becomes less tympanitic (Fig. 407). This procedure often fails to give clear-cut results because the colon is displaced downward by the enlarged spleen.

The Roentgen Ray in the Diagnosis of Diseases of the Abdomen

The field of abdominal diagnosis has been revolutionized by the roentgen ray and by its more modern refinements. The use of opaque media in the gastrointestinal and urinary tracts and of the substances which have a selective affinity for certain organs and cast a shadow in the roentgen plate greatly increases the value of the roentgen ray. As the result of these methods we can now visualize

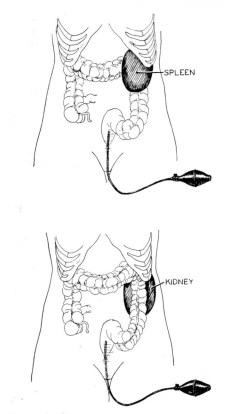

FIG. 407. Distention of colon with air forces enlarged spleen forward, enlarged kidney backward.

the stomach, intestines, liver, gall-bladder, kidneys and spleen on the x-ray plate. A brief summary of these methods indicates their value in the diagnosis of diseases of the abdomen.

Stomach. The size and outlines of the stomach can be accurately determined under the fluoroscope or in the x-ray plate after the ingestion of a meal containing barium sulfate. This information cannot be obtained with any degree of accuracy by either palpation or percussion. The presence of a diverticulum of the esophagus or a herniation of the stomach through the diaphragm can be clearly seen in the x-ray picture and cannot be diagnosed by any other method of examination.

Carcinoma of the esophagus or stomach, when the condition is advanced, produces a change in the outline of these organs which is pathog-

nomonic. In the stomach the carcinomatous mass growing into the lumen changes the normal contour of the stomach, producing a characteristic "filling defect." In scirrhous carcinoma of the stomach, which produces a condition known as "linitis plastica," or "leather bottle stomach," the stomach is visualized as a long, narrow organ and the normal rugae of the mucosa are absent. Polyps of the stomach or esophagus produce characteristic deformities in the x-ray plate.

In cardiospasm the constriction of the lower end of the esophagus closes the aperture of the stomach and causes the barium meal to accumulate and to distend the esophagus, a process which is readily seen under the fluoroscope. The obstruction due to cardiospasm can be differentiated from that caused by carcinoma of the esophagus, since the cardiospasm can be relieved by the administration of amyl nitrite. A pylorospasm causing a failure of the stomach to discharge its contents is readily visible under the fluoroscope.

In gastric or duodenal ulcer, fluoroscopic examination may show a greatly increased peristalsis of the stomach. Roentgen-ray plates show an irregular surface produced by the ulcer of the stomach and a distortion of the duodenal bulb produced by a duodenal ulcer. In some instances an area of spasm appears in the stomach opposite the ulcer, causing a marked indentation or incisura. Organic hour-glass constriction of the stomach is most commonly due to scarring produced by a girdle ulcer and is obvious in a roentgen plate. It is occasionally seen as a result of gastrospasm, in which condition, however, the hour-glass constriction is only temporary or even momentary.

Liver. Marked enlargement of the liver is often seen in the x-ray plate, the mass of liver throwing a darker shadow than the remainder of the intestinal contents. An enlarged liver or a subdiaphragmatic abscess may cause marked elevation of the diaphragm on the right side (Fig. 408). This elevation

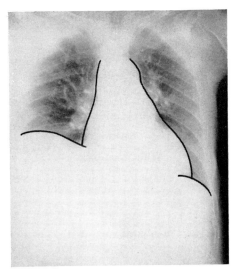

Fig. 408. X-ray of chest in a patient with carcinoma of the liver. Note marked elevation of the diaphragm on the right produced by the enlarged liver.

produces a difference between the lower level of pulmonic resonance on the two sides, a difference which can be demonstrated by percussion. By the use of a new contrast medium, Thorotrast, the outlines of the liver can be clearly shown in every instance. The shrunken liver of cirrhosis, the enlarged and nodular liver in carcinoma, and solitary liver abscess are all obvious. This contrast medium is, however, according to some workers, not without danger.

X-ray plates of the gallbladder region often demonstrate gallstones in cholelithiasis, although it has been known for many years that certain types of gallstones cast no shadows. By the use of tetraiodophenolphthalein, a compound which is secreted in the bile and concentrated by the gallbladder and is opaque to the roentgen rays, the gallbladder itself can be visualized as a light shadow, the stones, if present, appearing as darker areas. This method of cholecystography also gives us accurate knowledge regarding the shape and the size of the gallbladder as well as its filling and emptying time. This information is of great value in the diagnosis of inflammations, malformations and tumors

of the gallbladder. Indeed, the greatest value of cholecystography is in determining whether a gallbladder is functioning or nonfunctioning. If the gallbladder does not function, there is a 70 per cent possibility that gallstones are present and about a 95 per cent probability that the gallbladder is diseased.

Intestines. By the use of a barium meal and barium enema information of great value can be obtained from the intestinal tract. The presence of intestinal spasm, of abnormal dilatation, and of distortions or constrictions due to pressure or tumors are all readily made out. Dilated small intestine in intestinal obstruction and peritonitis is obvious. Diverticuli and polyps of the intestine, as well as abnormal communications, are readily seen.

Spleen. An enlarged spleen is usually visible in an x-ray plate which has been taken with the proper precautions. The use of Thorotrast visualizes the spleen as clearly as the liver. The size, shape and outline of such a visualized spleen are well seen.

Genitourinary Tract. *Kidneys.* In many roentgenograms the outlines of both kidneys are seen. After the use of an intravenous contrast medium, Diodrast, the outlines are seen with great distinctness if the kidney function is good. If an advanced hydronephrosis or nephritis is present, the kidney may excrete the dye so slowly that no shadow appears. The excretion of this contrast medium is to a certain extent an index of renal function. Marked enlargement, irregularity or distortion of the kidneys produced by hypernephroma, congenital cysts, or hydronephrosis may be visible if the kidney function is fairly normal.

Kidney stones, whether located in the mass of the kidney or in the pelvis, are usually demonstrated by a roentgenogram. The pelvis of the kidney and the ureters can be clearly visualized by the use of contrast media injected through the ureters. This procedure demonstrates distortions or malformations of the pelvis as well as distortions or constrictions of the ureters. Outlines of the pelvis and ureters may also be demonstrated by the use of an intravenous contrast medium.

The appearance in the x-ray plate of the area surrounding the kidney may be significant. In perirenal abscess the outlines of the psoas muscle, which are generally sharp, may be very obscure or entirely absent.

Bladder. The presence of stones in the bladder is readily detected by the x-rays. The outline of the bladder may be clearly demonstrated by the injection of a contrast medium, and the presence of a diverticulum may be shown by the same procedure.

The roentgen ray will clearly show the presence of a fetus in the fourth or fifth month of pregnancy, and often explains the cause of marked abdominal enlargement. Occasionally calcification of a uterine fibromyoma and of the adrenal is demonstrated in the x-ray picture. Dermoid tumors of the ovary may be visible in the x-ray picture. Erosion of the vertebra and aneurysm of the abdominal aorta may be obvious and explain obscure abdominal pain.

The presence of free air in the abdominal cavity is demonstrable under the diaphragm with the patient in the sitting position. Similarly, the presence of a subdiaphragmatic abscess may be diagnosed by the high position of the diaphragm on the affected side.

The x-ray also demonstrates in many instances the displacement of an organ from its normal position. Frequently it shows also that a mass felt in the left side of the abdomen is not the spleen, because the spleen itself is visible in its normal position. Ovarian cysts may displace the intestines upward, a change obvious in the x-ray plate.

This brief summary indicates how indispensable the x-ray has become in the diagnosis of many diseases of the abdomen. Physical examination of the abdomen has not, however, been displaced by these methods; it has rather been supplemented by them. Many diseases of the abdomen must be diagnosed by the eye, the finger and the ear,

where the x-ray, from the nature of the condition, is of little assistance.

GENITALIA

An exhaustive study of the genito-urinary organs is a science in itself, but no physical examination is complete without at least inspection and palpation of the external genitalia.

Male Genitalia

Deviations from the normal in the size of the genitalia immediately attract our attention. *Infantilism,* which is usually due to hypopituitarism, is characterized by extremely small genitalia. The patient shown in Figure 409 is seventeen years of age, but the genitalia are extremely small, the size of the genitalia of a small child. This lad, who is suffering from Fröhlich's syndrome, is fat, has no pubic hair and no sexual desire whatever.

Virilism is the opposite condition. The genitalia shown in Figure 410 belong, not to a man, but to a lad of five (Figure 411). This condition is due to hyperadrenalism, usually associated with an adrenal tumor, or it may occur

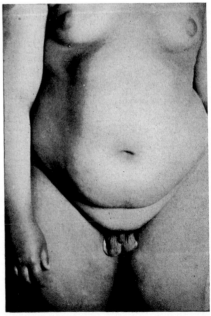

FIG. 409. Genitalia in boy of seventeen suffering from infantilism.

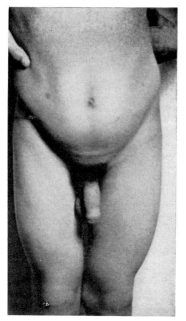

FIG. 410. Genitalia in boy of five suffering from virilism.

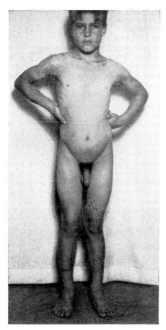

FIG. 411. Genitalia in boy of five suffering from virilism.

in precocious puberty. The boy shown in Figure 411 was seen later when fourteen years of age, was quite normal, and his penis was no longer abnormally large for his age.

Elephantiasis of the penis and scrotum is a relatively common condition in the tropics and also seen occasionally in temperate zones (Fig. 412). This condition is due to inflammation and obstruction of the lymphatics causing hypertrophy of the skin and subcutaneous tissues. In the tropics the obstruction of the lymphatics is commonly produced by the *Filaria sanguinis hominis* (*Wuchereria bancrofti*). In temperate zones the cause of the obstruction of the lymphatics is not usually apparent.

Phimosis is a condition in which the prepuce cannot be retracted over the glans penis. It is sometimes congenital, but more commonly is inflammatory in origin and is a complication of chancroid and gonorrhea. An attempt to retract the prepuce in phimosis may lead to paraphimosis, in which the prepuce is caught behind the gland and cannot be drawn forward. Paraphimosis produces marked edema and discomfort in the penis.

Balanitis, or inflammation of the glans penis, may follow filth or lack of cleanliness, but is most commonly the result of gonorrhea. In balanitis the mucosa of the glans is swollen and reddened, the surface shows irregular areas of desquamation, and there is often a purulent secretion at the corona.

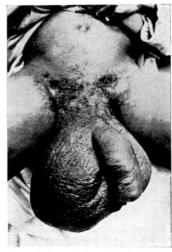

FIG. 412. Elephantiasis of penis and scrotum.

The penis and scrotum may show marked *edema* in ascites (Fig. 413), in cardiac disease with cardiac failure and in nephritis. In such cases the penis may be swollen to twice its normal size, and urination may be difficult.

A marked collection of fluid in the tunica vaginalis of the testis produces *hydrocele* (Fig. 414). Acute hydrocele is always secondary to inflammation of the testis or epididymis, commonly gonorrheal or syphilitic. Chronic hydrocele is most common between the ages of forty and sixty. It usually develops slowly and insidiously and may attain considerable size before causing any dis-

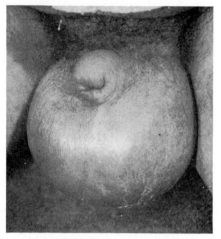

FIG. 413. Marked edema of scrotum in ascites.

comfort. Although most examples have been described as chronic idiopathic hydrocele, further examination usually discloses disease of the epididymis. In hydrocele the swelling is painless and fluctuates, and the skin is tense, shiny and somewhat reddened and has a translucent appearance. A light held behind and against the scrotum will transillumine the hydrocele sac.

Urethritis, usually of gonorrheal origin, may be instantly diagnosed on seeing a drop of pus exudate from the meatus. In many patients, however, it may be necessary to milk the urethra in order to obtain pus. A mild urethritis is occasionally seen as the result of injecting irritating antiseptic solutions to prevent venereal infection. A stained smear is sufficient for establishing the correct diagnosis.

Scabies not infrequently attacks the penis. The lesions consist of minute multiple elevations with burrows in the center; they itch intensely and are associated with similar lesions elsewhere, especially between the fingers.

Herpes of the penis is common and is sometimes confused with a chancre. The lesion consists of small vesicles, usually on the glans, but also on the prepuce, causing some pain or itching. They usually disappear in a few days, leaving no scars.

"Venereal warts," verrucae or *condylomata acuminata* (Fig. 415), are some-

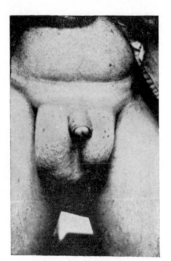

FIG. 414. Hydrocele.

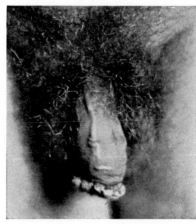

FIG. 415. Venereal warts in male.

times mistaken by the layman for chancres. They have nothing in common with chancres, except that venereal warts, like other warts, may be mildly contagious and sometimes are apparently transmitted by sexual intercourse. The most important factor in their production is not venereal exposure, but irritation, uncleanliness and a long or tight prepuce. They may occur in gonorrhea and occasionally ulcerate or even suppurate.

Chancroid is, with gonorrhea and syphilis, one of the three most important venereal diseases. It is commonly referred to as a soft chancre in contrast to the hard chancre of syphilis. Chancroids are commonly associated with filth and lack of cleanliness. Chancroids are more common than hard chancres in dispensary practice, while in private practice the hard chancre of syphilis is the more common. Chancroid is due to the Ducrey bacillus and is transmitted by sexual contact.

The simple chancroid appears as a number of small, superficial punched-out ulcers located about the corona. If this lesion does not heal, through lack of cleanliness or continued irritation, the ulcers become larger, and edema of the prepuce appears and, with it, phimosis. A bubo or inguinal lymphadenitis appears so commonly in chancroid that it is classed as part of the disease picture. These enlarged inguinal lymph glands frequently break down and suppurate.

Chancre, the primary lesion of syphilis, is almost always located on the penis, just behind the glans penis or on the prepuce (Fig. 416). John Hunter, it may be recalled, inoculated himself on the penis with some pus from the urethra of a gonorrheal patient. Unfortunately, the patient had syphilis as well, and a chancre developed. Since this memorable experiment in 1767 it has been common practice to speak of a hunterian sore or a hunterian chancre. It is even more common to call it a hard sore or hard chancre.

The chancre appears as a rule in a

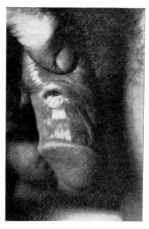

FIG. 416. Chancre in male.

month after exposure as a small red papule, which slowly enlarges and then breaks, forming a small ulcer. The small ulcer is often partially covered by a grayish membrane, and the tissue about it becomes indurated and soon has a hard, cartilaginous consistence. This cartilaginous thickening is characteristic of a true syphilitic chancre. It is also noteworthy that it is practically painless.

Chancres are usually single and are not autoinoculable, so that a chancre of the penis in contact with the scrotum will not produce a chancre on the scrotum. Chancroids are usually multiple, are autoinoculable and commonly associated with suppurating inguinal buboes. In spite of these clinical differences chancres and chancroids are frequently indistinguishable, and, before making a positive diagnosis, a smear from the lesion should be examined under the dark field and a Wassermann test carried out.

Granuloma inguinale is found almost exclusively in Negroes. The lesion begins as a small papule which later ulcerates and persists as an indolent, eroding ulcer with a shallow crater, the base of which is covered by granulation tissue. The edges of the ulcer are often redundant and seem to overlap the healthy skin margins. The lesions are not painful or sensitive, are commonly extensive, usually multiple, and are most commonly seen in the groins, on the pre-

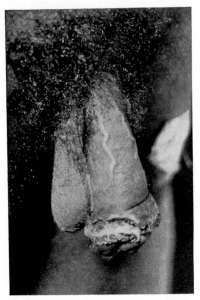

FIG. 417. Carcinoma of penis.

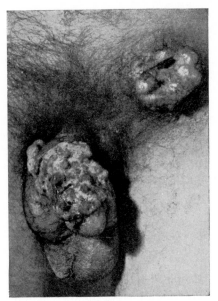

FIG. 418. Carcinoma of penis; note metastases in inguinal lymph glands.

puce, glans, uvula, perineum, buttocks and anus.

Carcinoma of the penis is usually located on the glans, less commonly on the prepuce. It is always an epithelioma and is the second most common of all skin cancers. Two types of carcinomata are observed—one a papillary, cauliflower-like type (Fig. 417), the other an indurated ulcer. The lesion, which at first appears as either a small ulcer or a wart, grows slowly, and causes no pain or untoward symptoms. Later, after attaining some size, it causes pain for which the patient seeks medical attention. It sometimes grows to considerable proportions, becomes a large bleeding mass and even develops metastases (Fig. 418) before the patient consults a physician.

Varicocele consists in a dilatation and engorgement of the veins of the pampiniform plexus. It usually occurs in a mild form, is present on the left side and causes no serious physical inconvenience. It is a common complaint of sexual neurasthenics and a source of income to many genitourinary quacks. Impotence never results from varicocele, and marriage, with satisfactory sexual relations, cures most cases.

The testis on one or on both sides may not have descended. *Undescended testicles* may be associated with infantilism. Occasionally an undescended testis may give rise to a malignant tumor.

The testis and epididymis may be enlarged and painful as the result of inflammatory processes or tumors. The most common cause of acute orchitis is mumps. During World War I one out of every seven cases of mumps developed orchitis. Syphilis may cause an acute orchitis and a chronic orchitis as well. Gonorrhea and tuberculosis rarely cause orchitis, but are among the commonest causes of epididymitis. In distinguishing between lesions of the testis and of the epididymis one should palpate gently and carefully, remembering the anatomical position of each.

Tumors of the testis are uncommon, of the epididymis rare. The most commonly described ones have been sarcomata.

Female Genitalia

Deviations from the normal, in the size of the female genitalia, attract our

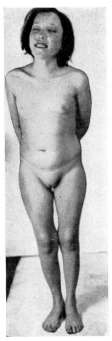

Fig. 419. External genitalia in girl of twenty with infantilism.

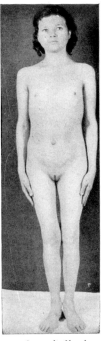

Fig. 420. External genitalia in girl of nineteen with infantilism.

attention just as they do in the male. *Infantilism* in the female is quite as striking as in the male. The patients seen in Figures 419 and 420 are two young ladies aged twenty and nineteen, respectively. Neither has pubic or axillary hair and neither has menstruated. In appearance and mentality, both patients resemble girls of ten or eleven. The patient shown in Figure 419 developed pubic and axillary hair and menstruated after treatment with antuitrin G and theelin. The patient shown in Figure 420 showed no response to this

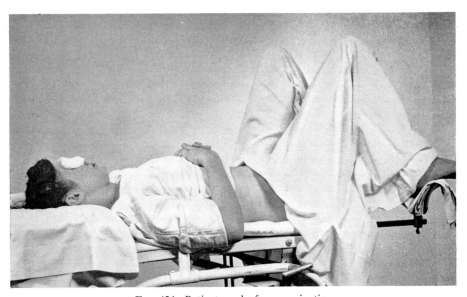

Fig. 421. Patient ready for examination.

therapy and was later found to have an ovarian tumor.

Precocious sexual maturity in the female leads to the appearance of pubic and axillary hair sometimes as early as

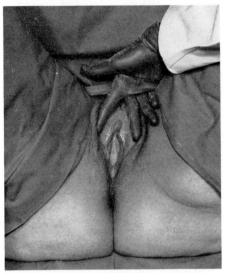

FIG. 422. Examination of the external genitalia.

the age of five. *Hypertrophy of the clitoris,* with a tendency to masculinity, is occasionally due to adrenal tumors. *Elephantiasis of the labia and clitoris* is the analogue of elephantiasis of the scrotum and penis in the male and is due to lymphatic obstruction. *Edema of the vulva* may occur in patients with nephritis or cardiac disease, but more commonly it is the result of vulvitis or vaginitis.

In the examination of the female genitalia it is advisable, as in all other examinations, to place the patient in a comfortable relaxed position. This is best attained by placing the patient on a comfortable well-padded table with the knees drawn up and widely separated, the so-called lithotomy position (Fig. 421). The examiner first proceeds with the gloved fingers to separate the labia which permits a clearer view of the clitoris, urethra and labia minora (Fig. 422). A finger inserted into the vagina and pressed forward under the urethra (Fig. 423) performs the well

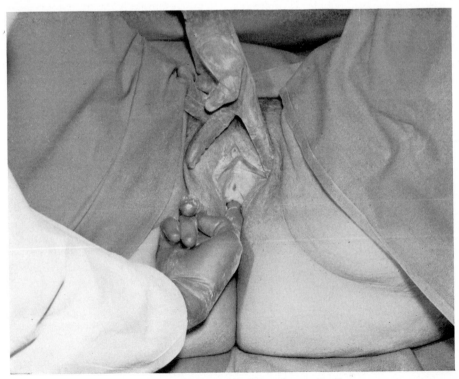

FIG. 423. Procedure of "milking the urethra."

known procedure of "milking the urethra" which will express pus in a patient suffering from urethritis, the usual finding in gonorrheal infection.

A relatively common genital lesion is a Bartholin's cyst, described on page 277, and palpated most readily by the method illustrated in Figure 424. Lesions in the floor of the vagina or in the rectum can be best palpated by inserting one finger in the vagina, the other in the rectum and then drawing the two fingers together (Fig. 425). Examination of the vaginal wall and cervix of the uterus is carried out best with a vaginal speculum. Incidentally this instrument was well known to classical antiquity and numerous examples almost identical with those employed today, can be seen in the museums of Naples and Athens. Figure 426 illustrates the method of introducing the instrument with the blades closed, from the left side while the right forefinger presses down on the floor of the vagina. After introduction (Fig. 427) the spec-

ulum is straightened and the blades opened, a maneuver which spreads apart the walls of the vagina and permits a good view of the cervix of the uterus (Fig. 428). The procedure of bimanual palpation of the uterus described on page 278 is illustrated by Figs. 429 and 430.

Herpes, erysipelas and eczema of the vulva are seen occasionally. In herpes there are numerous small blisters or vesicles which resemble herpetic eruptions elsewhere in the body. Erysipelas of the vulva is a rapidly spreading inflammation accompanied by fever and often ushered in with a chill. The external genitalia are markedly swollen and reddened, and the patient complains of throbbing and burning.

Trichophytosis or ringworm of the vulva resembles the well-known "athlete's foot" and causes a dermatitis of the vulva and adjacent skin of the thighs. *Scabies* may also attack the vulva.

Pruritus vulvae, accompanied by

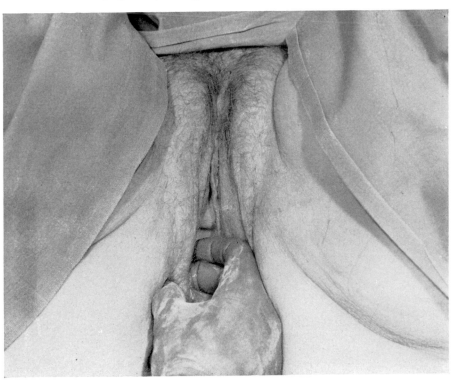

FIG. 424. Palpation of Bartholin's gland.

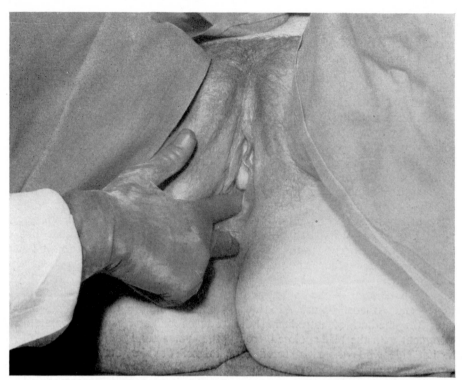

FIG. 425. Bidigital palpation with one finger in the vagina and the other in the rectum.

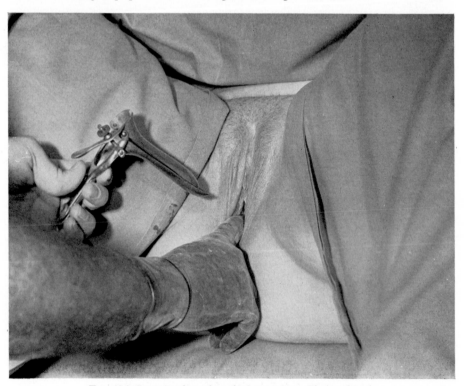

FIG. 426. Introduction of vaginal speculum. Blades closed.

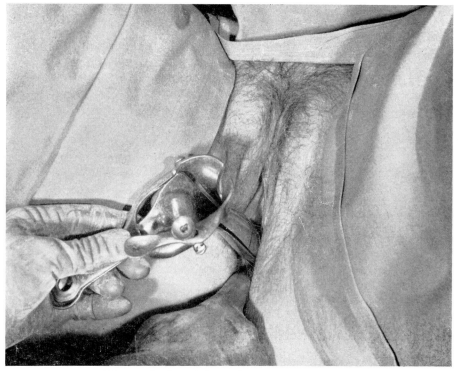

FIG. 427. Introduction of the vaginal speculum. Blades closed.

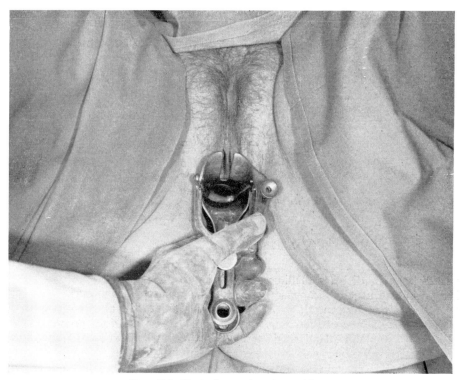

FIG. 428. Vaginal speculum in position.

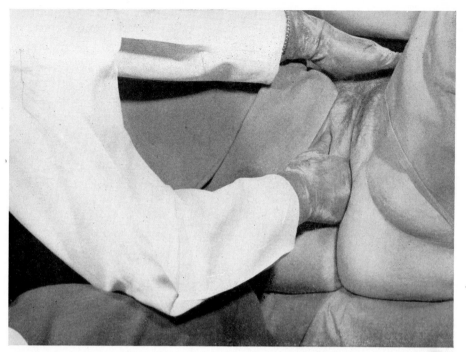

FIG. 429. Bimanual palpation of the uterus.

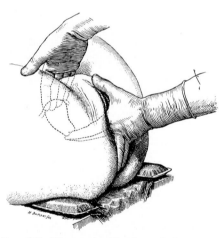

FIG. 430. Bimanual palpation of the uterus. (Modified after Hermann Becker.)

marked reddening of the vulva, is frequently seen in diabetes mellitus. The intense itching usually disappears when the diabetes is under control.

Leukorrhea is one of the commonest of female complaints. Under this term are included all abnormal discharges from the female genital tract which are not bloody. The most common cause of leukorrhea in women who have not been pregnant is gonorrhea. In patients who have borne children, lacerations and local infections may later cause leukorrhea. It may also be due to Monilia infections and to cancer of the cervix. Most types of vaginitis are associated with leukorrhea.

Vaginitis in its most severe form is usually caused by a gonorrheal infection. Gonorrhea commonly produces an inflammation of the vulva, the vagina and the urethra. The vulva is red, swollen and painful. There is a yellowish discharge from the vagina and from the urethra. On digital examination with the gloved finger the vaginal walls are roughened, hot and tender, and pressure on the urethra brings forth some drops of pus. A stained smear from the pus shows numerous gonococci.

Vaginitis may also be due to the *Trichomonas vaginalis* and to *Corynebacterium diphtheriae*. In the former condition the *Trichomonas* may be demonstrated in a hanging-drop preparation. In diphtheritic vaginitis there is usually a false membrane on the vaginal wall, and the patient shows marked systemic symptoms.

Atrophic or *senile vaginitis* is seen in patients usually at or past the menopause and is associated with a mild inflammation and denudation accompanied by a small amount of discharge and burning or itching.

Condylomata or *venereal warts* occur on the vulva. Three types have been described: the common wart (verruca vulgaris), the pointed condyloma (condyloma acuminatum), and the flat condyloma (condyloma latum) (Fig. 431). The common wart is like a simple wart elsewhere on the body. The pointed condyloma or moist wart occurs on the moist parts of the vulva. This wart is produced by an irritating discharge from the vagina, most commonly, but not always, a gonorrheal discharge. The flat condyloma is the characteristic vulvar lesion of syphilis. They are a secondary manifestation of syphilis, are multiple and, when small, are often referred to as "mucous patches of the vulva." Frequently the top of the condyloma sloughs off, leaving an ulcer beneath.

Chancroid is frequently seen on the vulva, and the lesions present the same characteristics as those on the male genitalia. The lesions are commonly multiple, show no cartilaginous induration and are often accompanied by painful or suppurating buboes.

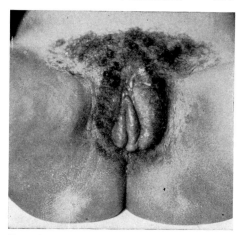

FIG. 432. Chancre in female; chancre not obvious, edema very apparent.

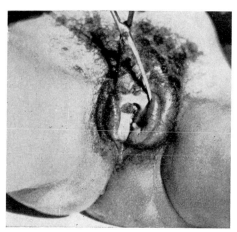

FIG. 433. Chancre in female; obvious on separating labia.

Chancres of the vulva resemble chancres of the penis. The lesion is single and indurated and may not be seen on a casual inspection (Fig. 432). On separating the labia, it is obvious (Fig. 433).

Cysts of Bartholin's glands are usually but not always caused by gonorrheal infection. They are readily recognized as small reddish swellings, tender on palpation and causing swelling of the vaginal wall.

In *prolapse of the uterus* the uterus escapes from the pelvic cavity and protrudes from the vagina (Fig. 434). The prolapse may be partial or complete: when partial, it is called *descensus;*

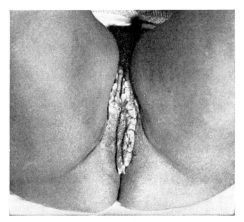

FIG. 431. Condyloma latum.

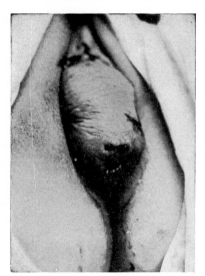

F<small>IG</small>. 434. Prolapse of the uterus. The cervix is seen at the lower surface of the mass.

when complete, *procidentia*. It may appear at the time of childbirth or may only become noticeable later when the prolapse is marked. *Cystocele* is a hernia of the bladder which causes a marked sagging or bulging of the anterior vaginal wall. It is also commonly the result of injuries sustained at childbirth.

Carcinoma of the vulva is by no means uncommon, and occurs usually on the labia, perineum and prepuce of the clitoris. The usual tumor is an epithelioma, similar to epitheliomata elsewhere—an ulcerating, fetid, cauliflower-like growth. Leukoplakia of the vulva and tertiary syphilitic lesions are frequent forerunners. Carcinoma of the vulva is a disease of older women.

Inspection of the cervix of the uterus should be carried out with a uterine speculum aided by a light which can be thrown directly upon the part examined. *Palpation of the cervix* is best carried out with the index finger. While the examiner should usually wear a glove, many gynecologists advise the use of the naked, more sensitive finger in testing the induration or friability of a suspicious lesion.

Carcinoma of the cervix is the most common carcinoma seen, with the pos-

sible exception of carcinoma of the female breast. It occurs occasionally in young women, is rare before the age of thirty and uncommon before the age of forty. Carcinoma of the cervix causes three cardinal symptoms: a watery discharge, often foul in odor; bleeding, at first scant, but later more abundant; and pain. Inspection, which should be carried out with a speculum, reveals an ulcerated area or a bleeding, fungating mass which projects into the wall of the vagina. On palpation the mass, although hard, is irregular and friable on the surface and bleeds easily.

Cervical polyps, soft pedunculated tumors arising from the mucous membrane of the cervix, usually project outside the os uteri and are readily seen on inspection. They are usually freely movable and cause slight bleeding.

Bimanual palpation is often necessary for a satisfactory examination of the genital organs. The patient lies on her back with her knees flexed and wide apart. The examiner introduces his gloved forefinger, which is well lubricated with soap or petroleum jelly, into the vagina, while the other hand is placed over the lower part of the abdomen. By pressure downwards over the abdomen, the uterus and adnexa are forced down to the examining finger. By this method the examiner can feel the uterus, determine its size, its relative position and its movability in a normal state, but cannot palpate the tubes. In disease conditions he can palpate a prolapsed or cystic ovary, enlarged tender tubes, the seat of salpingitis, ovarian tumors, chronic pelvic inflammatory disease with adhesions and a tubal pregnancy. By this method he readily palpates and outlines fibromyomata of the uterus, the most common of all uterine new growths.

In *palpating the uterus* the examiner should note six points—position, size, shape, consistency, tenderness, and mobility. In retroversion the uterus as a whole is turned backwards, while in retroflexion the upper part of the uterus is bent back. The size, shape and consistency of the uterus are profoundly changed by neoplasms and by pregnancy. The uterus may be tender in inflammatory conditions. The mobility of the uterus is markedly affected by the presence of tumors in the uterus or adhesions due to inflammation. In the condition called "frozen pelvis," usually the result of puerperal cellulitis, the uterus is fixed and immovable, so that the examiner has the impression that he is examining an anatomical model. This sensation has given rise to another name for the condition—"plaster-of-Paris pelvis."

RECTUM

A rectal examination should be carried out in every case. A wag once remarked, with considerable truth, that a consultant is a doctor who makes a rectal examination.

Inspection of the rectum is best carried out with the patient in the knee-chest position, or standing, with the legs wide apart and the body bent forward. A good light is essential and a head mirror extremely useful. When examination of the rectum beyond the anal margin is indicated, a rectal speculum should be inserted with the patient in the knee-chest position. No examination of the rectum is complete without palpation carried out by inserting the gloved finger into the rectum. The most common lesions seen are hemorrhoids, anal fissures, ischiorectal abscess, condylomata and cancer of the rectum.

Hemorrhoids are dilatations of the hemorrhoidal veins, which contain blood and bleed easily. External hemorrhoids are readily seen on inspection, while internal hemorrhoids are visible only after inserting a rectal speculum, dilating the rectum slightly and throwing a light into it. Hemorrhoids may lead to extremely severe secondary anemia with hemoglobin as low as 12 per cent, due to bleeding over a long period of time.

Anal fissures are small cracks in the mucosa at the margin of the anus. They may cause considerable pain during defecation and lead to the formation of ulcers. An *ischiorectal abscess* causes a swelling at the margin of the anus, which is red, hot and painful. It presently ruptures, forming a fistula in ano, a sinus which empties into the rectum or just outside it. A fistula is often tortuous and usually tuberculous in origin.

Condylomata of the rectum are seen especially in females and have the same significance as condylomata of the vulva. They may, however, occur in males, as in Figure 432. The most common variety are the flat condylomata of syphilis.

Cancer of the rectum usually develops at the anal margin or at the junction of the rectum and sigmoid. It usually causes bleeding and pain and at first may be mistaken for hemorrhoids. When it is at the anal margin it can be readily seen, but more commonly is seen with a speculum or palpated by the finger as a hard, ulcerating mass in the rectum.

The *prostate* and *seminal vesicles* are readily palpated with the patient in the standing position. By firm pressure downward on the prostate, the prostate may be "milked" and prostatic fluid obtained for examination. The enlarged prostate may be readily determined, in many cases, by rectal examination alone. It should be remembered, however, that in prostatic enlargement the prostate may grow forward into the bladder; then the enlargement cannot be

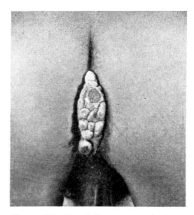

FIG. 435. Condyloma acuminatum.

made out by rectal examination alone. In such cases a determination of the residual urine after voiding or a cystoscopic examination may be necessary. Carcinoma of the prostate produces a stone-like enlargement of the prostate.

A *prostatic abscess,* usually of gonorrheal origin, may be readily palpated by rectal examination. The demonstration of a large, boggy, tender prostate may explain the sudden appearance of chills and fever in a patient suffering from gonorrhea.

Rectal polyps, similar to cervical polyps, may produce much bleeding. Strictures of the rectum are usually located 2 to 3 inches inside the anal margin and are often syphilitic in origin. In most cases, however, they are probably due to lymphogranuloma venereum.

By rectal examination the position of the uterus and adnexa in females can be readily made out. Malformations of the uterus or adnexa, inflammatory masses, tumors of the uterus, ovaries or tubes can be palpated. In children and in virgins rectal examination should be used instead of vaginal examination.

BIBLIOGRAPHY

Bivin, George D., and Klinger, M. P.: Pseudocyesis Principia. Bloomington, 1937.

Curtis, Arthur H., and Huffman, J. W.: A Textbook of Gynecology, 6th ed. Philadelphia, W. B. Saunders Co., 1950.

Eisendrath, D. N., and Rolnick, H. C.: Textbook of Urology. 4th ed. Philadelphia, J. B. Lippincott Co., 1938.

Graves, William P.: Gynecology. 4th ed. Philadelphia, W. B. Saunders Co., 1928.

Major, Ralph H., and Black, Donald R.: A huge hemangioma of the liver associated with hemangiomata of the skull and bilateral cystic adrenals. Am. J. M. Sc. *156:* 469, 1938.

Murphy, John B.: The diagnosis of gall stones. Med. News *82:*825, 1903.

Osler, William: Lectures on the diagnosis of abdominal tumors. New York M. J. *49:*129, 161, 193, 260, 385, 417, 481, 545, 477; *50:*65, 97, 1894.

Pullen, Roscoe L.: Medical Diagnosis, Applied Physical Diagnosis. 2nd ed. Philadelphia, W. B. Saunders Co., 1950.

Sailer, Joseph: Pulsating spleen in aortic insufficiency. Am. Heart J. *3:*447, 1928.

Sutton, Don C., and Rawson, Vance: A case of pulsating spleen in mitral and tricuspid disease. Am. Heart J. *10:*1096, 1935.

Weiss, Samuel: Diseases of the Liver, Gall Bladder, Ducts and Pancreas, Their Diagnosis and Treatment. New York, Paul B. Hoeber, Inc., 1935.

CHAPTER 15

THE EXTREMITIES

IN THE EXAMINATION of the extremities we rely mainly upon inspection and palpation, both percussion and auscultation playing a minor role. This is due to obvious physical reasons. The value of percussion depends largely upon the differentiation between resonant, dull and tympanitic tones. Naturally, the differentiation is impossible in the extremities, since they are not air-containing organs. The value of auscultation depends upon the phenomena produced in the lungs by respiration, and in the heart by the heart beat, and no such analogous phenomena occur in the extremities, with the exception of pulsation of the blood vessels.

In the description of the physical findings in the extremities, inspection and palpation will be considered together, since the two methods of procedure are intimately related, and palpation is generally used to confirm the findings of inspection.

HANDS

Size and Shape. In examining the hands, we note first the *size* and *shape*. In acromegaly the hands are large; the stubby, broadened fingers and the widened palm giving the appearance of the typical "spade hand" (Fig. 436) characteristic of this condition.

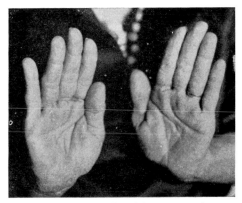

FIG. 436. Spade hand in acromegaly.

Some people have small, though long hands, hands with long, tapering fingers. Such long hands with tapering fingers are seen in association with abnormally long arms and legs in the Lorain type of pituitary insufficiency (Fig. 437).

The size of the two hands should be compared. Edema of the arm usually causes swelling of the hand on the same side and a marked increase in size as compared with the other hand (Fig. 438). Such swelling may be the result of nephritis, local phlebitis, or obstruction to the blood or lymph flow. In congestive heart failure it often occurs in the arm on the side on which the patient lies. The patient shown in Figure 439 was suffering from a mediastinal

281

tumor. Women, after breast amputa-
tions, often have edema of the arm and
hand on the side of the operation, the
result of interference with the lymphatics which drain the arm.

Color and Temperature. We next
note the color of the hands, whether
normal, pale, blue or mottled. The hand
of a Negro seen in Figure 440 shows
irregular white patches—the characteristic appearance in vitiligo or acquired
leukoderma. Vitiligo is a condition in
which there are circumscribed patches

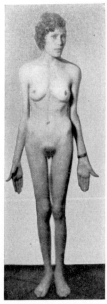

Fig. 437. Long hands of pituitary insufficiency; note abnormally long arms and legs
of Lorain type.

which are smooth, lacking in pigment,
and milky-white, and usually surrounded by areas of increased pigmentation.
The hair on these white areas may retain or lose its normal pigment. It occurs in the Caucasian as well as in the
Negro race. These areas, where there is
a loss of pigment, usually gradually increase in extent. The cause of vitiligo
is unknown.

A comparison of the color of the
palms of the patient's hands with those
of a normal person is of great value. In
xanthosis, a condition common in diabetes mellitus, the palms have a yellowish-orange color; in anemia they
may be pale; while in plethora and polycythemia they are usually reddish or
purple.

In pellagra the skin lesions are often
so characteristic that a diagnosis can be
made from examination of the hands
alone. The lesions are on the backs of
the hands, beginning first with redness
like an ordinary sunburn. The skin then
becomes darker, desquamates and
shows numerous cracks (Fig. 441).
Later, vesicles, or bullae, may form and
the skin becomes thickened.

The hands should next be palpated
and their temperature and texture noted.
In Graves' disease the hands are warm
and moist, in myxedema cold and harsh.
Many nervous persons have warm,
moist palms.

Movements. The movements of the
hands should be noted. In Graves' dis-

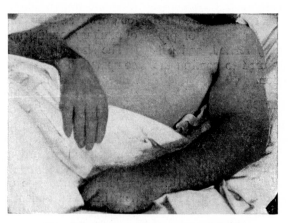

Fig. 438. Edema of left arm in nephritis.

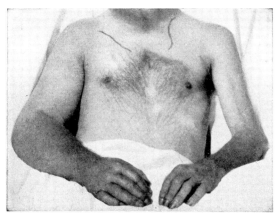

Fig. 439. Edema of right arm in mediastinal tumor.

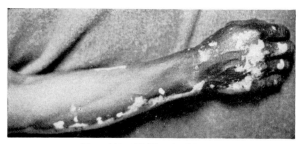

Fig. 440. Vitiligo in Negro.

ease we note a fine tremor which is well brought out by placing a white card over the back of the hand or fingers, and noting its rapid movements. In paralysis agitans the patient's hand is in constant motion, but ceases to tremble when he makes a voluntary movement. In multiple sclerosis we see the reverse: at rest the hand is quiet, but when the patient moves it—for instance, toward his mouth—a tremor appears— the *intention tremor*. The three findings in multiple sclerosis—intention tremor, with scanning speech and nystagmus— are often referred to as Charcot's triad.

In severe fevers, delirious patients, as Hippocrates noted, "pick the wool from their blankets." This picking at the bed clothes is called *carphologia* (κάρφος, karphos = chaff + λέγειν, legein = collect). *Subsultus tendinum* is a twitching of the tendons and muscles, especially of the wrist. Carphologia and *subsultus tendinum* are seen especially in typhoid fever.

In some cases of lead poisoning there is a *wrist drop* due to paralysis of the radial nerve. A similar paralysis involving the radial nerve may occur in other types of neuritis. The hand remains flexed on the wrist and cannot be raised (Fig. 442).

In tetany the hand is commonly flexed and the fingers drawn together at the tips, resembling the position of the physicians' hand when making a vaginal examination. For this reason it has been referred to as the *obstetrical position*. This position is assumed by the patient during a tetanic spasm (Fig. 443), but during the intervals can be produced by exerting pressure around the forearm. Pressure can be conveniently applied with the arm cuff of a sphygmomanometer. This convulsive drawing together of the fingers after pressure is applied to the arm is called *Trousseau's sign*. Tetany was formerly not uncommon after removal of the thyroid gland, when the surgeon inadvertently removed the

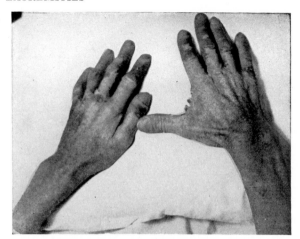

FIG. 441. Pellagra.

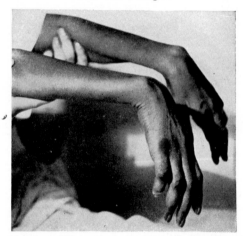

FIG. 442. Wrist drop in radial paralysis. Patient suffering from multiple neuritis.

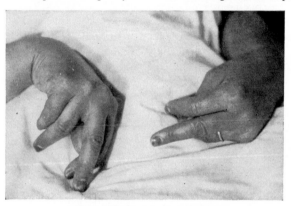

FIG. 443. Hands in tetany.

parathyroid glands as well. It is also seen from time to time in children (Fig. 444).

Deformities. Various types of new growths may appear in the hand, pro-

ducing deformities which vary in size and location. A common example of a benign new growth is the fibroma of the palmar fascia which causes tension of the flexor tendons and flexes the

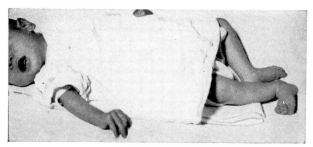

FIG. 444. Child in tetanic convulsion. Note position of hand.

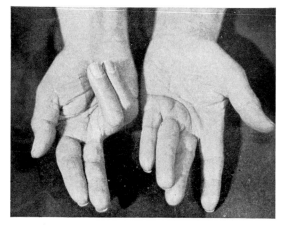

FIG. 445. Dupuytren's contracture, more marked in the right than in the left hand.

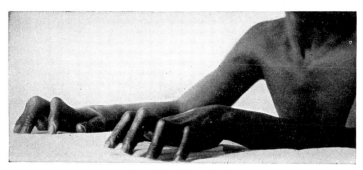

FIG. 446. Claw hand.

fingers on the palm, especially the ring and little fingers. This has caused it to be referred to as the "position of the Papal benediction" (Fig. 445). This condition usually appears in elderly patients and has long been known as *Dupuytren's contracture*. It is usually bilateral, although commonly more marked in one hand than in the other, and it may appear on one hand some years before the other is involved.

Another type of deformity which is very striking is the "claw hand" caused by hyperextension of the metacarpal joints and flexion of the phalanges. It is seen most frequently in progressive muscular atrophy and in leprosy. The patient shown in Figure 446 suffers from an unusual congenital variety which is present in several members of his family and which he has had since birth. Chronic arthritis of the wrist may pro-

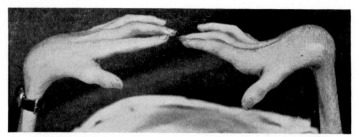

Fig. 447. Chronic arthritis; atrophy of the interossei muscles.

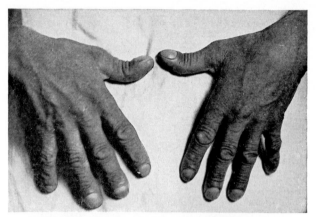

Fig. 448. Hippocratic fingers in bronchiectasis.

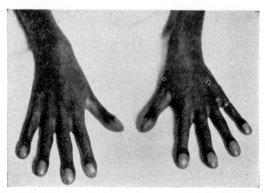

Fig. 449. Hippocratic fingers in congenital heart disease.

duce marked atrophy of the interossei muscles with hyperextension of the fingers (Fig. 447).

FINGERS

Hippocratic Fingers. Clubbed or drumstick fingers were first described by Hippocrates in empyema of the chest and have since been called "Hippocratic fingers." Figure 448 shows this characteristic appearance in a patient suffering

from bronchiectasis. These fingers have an appearance that suggests drumsticks, the tips of the fingers being enlarged, the fingernails unusually broad and curved slightly over the tips of the fingers. Clubbed fingers are also a characteristic finding in congenital heart disease (Fig. 449). They are seen also in empyema, pulmonary neoplasms (Fig. 450), subacute bacterial endocarditis, chronic diarrhea and pulmonary tuber-

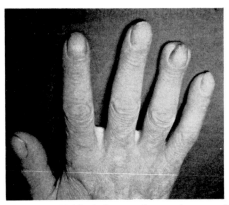

FIG. 450. Clubbed fingers in carcinoma of lung.

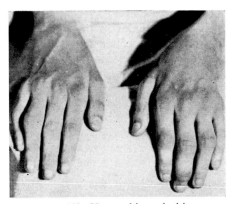

FIG. 452. Haygarth's nodosities.

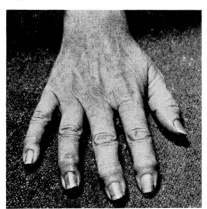

FIG. 451. Heberden's nodes.

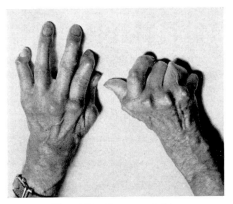

FIG. 453. Gouty arthritis.

culosis. A congenital and familial form has also been observed. Unilateral Hippocratic fingers have been described, usually the result of an aneurysm of the subclavian artery on the same side.

Heberden's Nodes. "What are those little hard knobs," wrote William Heberden, "about the size of a small pea, which are frequently seen upon the fingers, particularly a little below the top near the joint? They have no connection with gout, being found in persons who never had it; they continue for life."

These nodes are small bony outgrowths at the terminal phalangeal joints. They are often the first manifestation of osteoarthritis, but patients who show them rarely have severe involvement of the larger joints. They are more common in women than in men (Fig. 451) and are often seen in persons whose general health is excellent.

Haygarth's Nodosities. This is the term sometimes applied to joint swellings seen in arthritis (Fig. 452). These swellings, as seen in the illustration, frequently involve all the fingers and are usually associated with similar arthritic changes elsewhere. The joints are tender, and there is commonly redness with local elevation of temperature. Haygarth's description suggests that these joint changes were observed in both atrophic and hypertrophic arthritis.

Gouty arthritis often produces marked distortion of the hands due to the deposits in the joints (Fig. 453). In a patient once studied by the authors, the patient had a large tophus on the knuckle. The tophus had eroded the skin, projected from the joint, and the patient amused his friends by writing with it on the blackboard as if it were a piece of chalk.

Osler's Nodes. Osler's nodes are small painful nodes in the pulp of the fingertips, often better felt by the patient himself than by the examiner. They are present in subacute infectious endocarditis.

Raynaud's Disease. Maurice Raynaud in 1862 described an "asphyxia" of the fingers as a disease entity which has since been known by his name. His first patient was a woman who "under the influence of cold . . . saw the fingers become exsanguinated, completely insensible and of a yellowish white color. This phenomenon appeared often without reason, lasted a very little time and terminated with a period of reaction which was very painful, during which the circulation became established little by little and returned to the normal state." His second patient complained of "dead fingers" which "became in an instant the seat of coldness, pallor, and absolute insensibility."

Raynaud's disease, according to most authorities, is a vascular change without organic disease of the vessels and is due to vasomotor instability. Most of its victims are women. An attack can usually be produced by immersing the fingers in cold water. The toes as well as the fingers may be involved in this disease.

Scleroderma. The word "scleroderma" means hard skin ($\sigma\kappa\lambda\eta\rho\acute{o}s$ = hard + $\delta\acute{e}\rho\mu\alpha$, derma = skin), but the term "tight skin" would often be more descriptive. In the early stages of this disease the skin over the hand, and particularly over the fingers, looks tight and glistening as though it were too small and was stretched by the hand (Fig. 454). In the later stages the phalanges become gangrenous, and the gangrenous part falls off or must be amputated (Fig. 455).

Tumors. Tumors of the hands and fingers, though not seen so frequently as tumors elsewhere in the body, are encountered from time to time. Figure 456 shows an osteoma of the terminal phalanx of the forefinger.

Miscellaneous Conditions. Chancres of the finger are seen occasionally. They show the characteristics of chancre elsewhere, slowly developing ulcerations showing marked induration and a serous discharge. Spirochaeta can usually be demonstrated in the exudate.

The fingernails at times give valuable clues. The patient whose hands are shown in Figure 457 was a nervous woman who had the habit, common

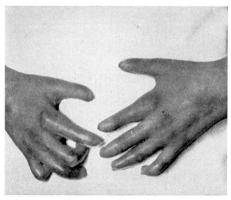

FIG. 454. Scleroderma.

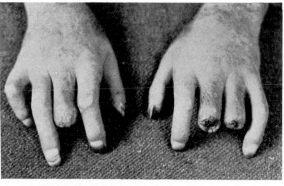

FIG. 455. Scleroderma, advanced stage.

among neurotics, of biting her finger-nails. The effects of this habit are obvious.

The effects of chronic infectious diseases, wasting diseases and anemias are often seen in the fingernails. Figure 458 shows the thin paper-like atrophic fingernails described as "spoon nails" or koilonychia. They are often seen in syphilis and also in chronic hypochromic anemia, in lichen planus, rheumatic fever and in acanthosis nigricans. Ridges and furrows in the nails, either longitudinal or transverse, are often seen in constitutional diseases and in infectious diseases (Fig. 459).

"Splinter hemorrhages," small linear extravasations of blood under the fingernails, are almost pathognomonic of sub-acute infectious endocarditis. They may be present before petechiae are discovered on the skin and mucous membranes. Splinter hemorrhages are also seen in the migratory stage of trichinosis. It is stated that these splinter hemorrhages are seen beneath the fingernails and toenails of 50 to 70 per cent of patients with active trichinosis.

Developmental anomalies of the fingers and hands are occasionally encountered. Figure 460 shows a congenital absence of the hand with four rudimentary fingers attached to the arm. The x-ray picture showed no carpal or metacarpal bones. Supernumerary fingers or thumbs are not rare (Fig. 461). Fusion of two or more fingers is sometimes observed, as in Figure 462.

WRISTS

The wrists are often involved in chronic arthritis, producing swelling, tenderness and limitation of movement. Ganglia are large, relatively painless swellings over the backs of the wrists, cystic tumors which grow from the tendon sheaths and are filled with clear fluid. A somewhat similar appearance may be produced by a tuberculous tenosynovitis (Fig. 463).

The wrists and forearms may be the seat of rheumatic nodules in rheumatic fever (Fig. 464). These small, subcutaneous nodules vary in size from a small shot to a pea and may also occur on the fingers, hands, elbows and knees. They are not tender and usually appear

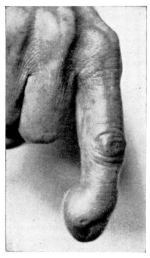

FIG. 456. Osteoma of index finger.

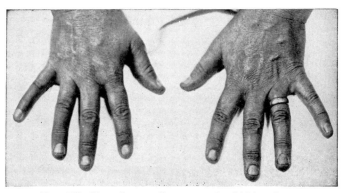

FIG. 457. Short fingernails as a result of biting them.

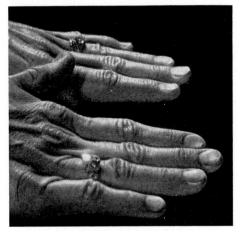

FIG. 458. Spoon nails.

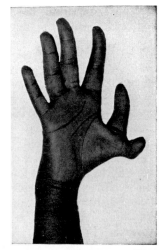

FIG. 461. Supernumerary fingers.

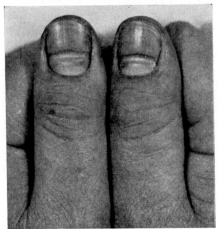

FIG. 459. Furrows in fingernails after typhoid fever.

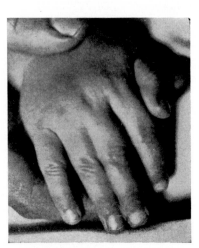

FIG. 462. Fusion of fingers.

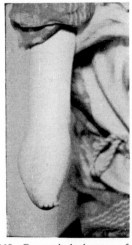

FIG. 460. Congenital absence of hand.

after the decline of the fever. On microscopical examination they often show Aschoff bodies.

Infections with pathogenic fungi may produce their characteristic lesions on the skin or in the subcutaneous tissues of the hands and arms. Figure 465 shows a hand with numerous abscesses resulting from a sporotrichosis infection.

ARMS

The size, color and temperature of the arm should be carefully noted. Figure 438 shows a marked edema of one arm in a patient with chronic nephritis and cardiac failure. A similar picture

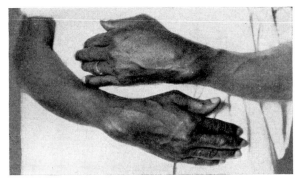

FIG. 463. Tuberculous tenosynovitis.

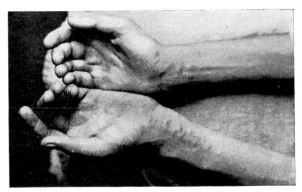

FIG. 464. Rheumatic nodules on wrists.

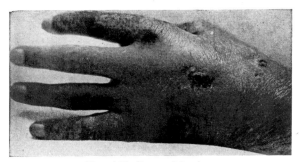

FIG. 465. Sporotrichosis.

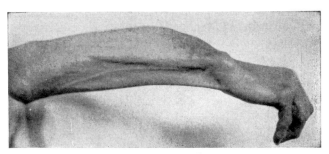

FIG. 466. Paget's disease.

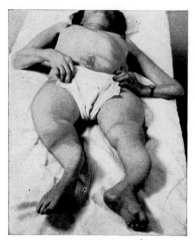

FIG. 467. Osteogenesis imperfecta.

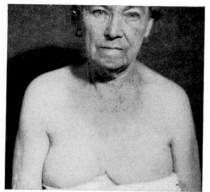

·FIG. 469. Subdeltoid bursitis. Atrophy of left shoulder.

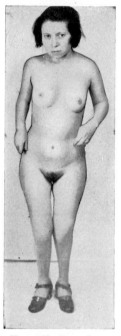

FIG. 468. Dwarfism.

who was the victim of osteogenesis imperfecta. She was accompanied by a child, aged eight, who was also suffering from the same disease. The marked deformities of the arms and legs are obvious. The bones in this disease are abnormally brittle and fragile. This patient had suffered more than 200 fractures, fractured ribs resulting in one occasion from an attack of coughing. The blue sclerae seen in this disease have been previously mentioned on page 68.

The arms may be abnormally short (Fig. 468). Such a condition is the result of a growth abnormality, and in this patient was associated with dwarfism.

The elbows may be the seat of arthritis. The skin over the elbows is a point of predilection for certain cutaneous diseases, notably psoriasis and diabetic xanthomata (Fig. 59).

THE SHOULDERS

The shoulders may be involved in chronic arthritis. Usually there is little swelling visible, but, commonly, there is atrophy of the muscles of the shoulder girdle from disuse. A similar disuse atrophy is often seen in subdeltoid bursitis (Fig. 469). In this the patient is unable to abduct the arm without causing pain. This failure to use the arm in normal movements leads to atrophy of the deltoid muscle.

Tumors of the head of the humerus, usually sarcomata or osteomata, cause marked enlargement of the shoulder.

(Fig. 439) was due to a mediastinal tumor which caused marked venous congestion of the right arm. Infections of the arm produce a similar picture.

Certain diseases associated with disturbances of bone growth often cause striking deformities both of the arms and legs. Figure 466 shows the arm of a patient suffering from osteitis deformans (Paget's disease of the bone). The patient shown in Figure 467 is a woman

LEGS

The importance of the movements of the legs in locomotion has already been discussed under gait (p. 35).

Size. The size of the legs is profoundly influenced by the state of the patient's nutrition. Obese persons usually have large legs, while emaciated people have thin legs. Fat men often, however, have most of their excess fat on the abdomen, with the result that their legs are relatively small and thin.

Enlargement of the legs along with enlargement of the arms due to a pathological deposit of fat is seen in pituitary dysfunction with involvement of the anterior lobe (Fig. 470).

Edema is one of the commonest causes of enlargement of the legs. A characteristic feature of edema of the legs is that the legs *pit on pressure* (Fig. 471). Bilateral edema of the legs is most commonly due to cardiac failure, chronic nephritis and to pressure on the abdominal veins by ascites, an enlarged organ or an intra-abdominal mass. It is often seen in diabetes mellitus, especially in severe diabetics who have just begun insulin therapy.

Unilateral edema of the leg is seen

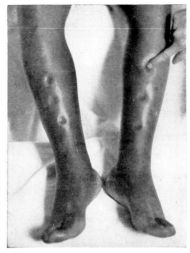

FIG. 471. Edema of legs in cirrhosis of liver.

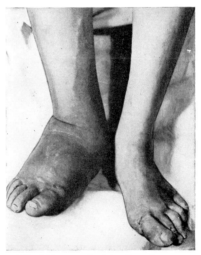

FIG. 472. Edema of right leg from venous thrombosis.

in thrombosis of the femoral vein in typhoid fever and puerperal infection— the *phlegmasia alba dolens,* the painful white swelling of the obstetricians. Figures 472 and 473 show the markedly swollen and edematous leg of a patient suffering from thrombosis of the femoral vein caused by an infection of the leg.

Edema of the legs may result from pressure of enlarged inguinal glands upon the femoral veins. Metastasis from carcinoma of the prostate may produce such enlargement.

A marked unilateral swelling of one leg is seen in a rather rare familial dis-

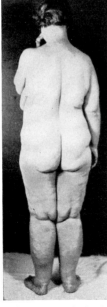

FIG. 470. Hypopituitarism.

ease known as *Milroy's disease* (Fig. 474). This disease, also known as chronic hereditary edema, may last from early childhood to advanced old age and often involves both legs. The edema varies little and is followed by hyperplasia of the skin and subcutaneous tissues.

An aneurysm of the popliteal artery shows a pulsation in the popliteal space and often enlarged veins over the posterior aspect of the leg, the result of an active collateral circulation about the knee (Fig. 475).

The classical example of *elephantiasis* is that seen in the tropics due to infection with the *Wuchereria bancrofti,* which produces blocking of the lymph channels. A similar condition, due to obstruction of the lymph vessels, is seen from time to time in this country (Fig. 476). The enormous size of the legs is responsible for the name "elephantiasis." The slow, lumbering gait of these patients resembles also the gait of an elephant. This enlargement is due largely to a hyperplasia of the skin and subcutaneous tissues.

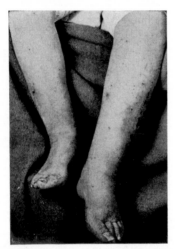

FIG. 473. Edema of left leg from venous thrombosis.

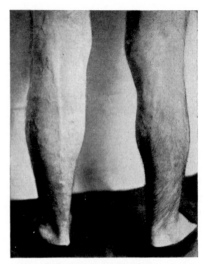

FIG. 475. Aneurysm of left popliteal artery.

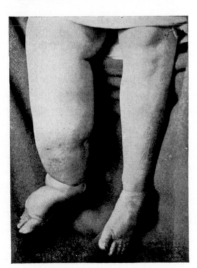

FIG. 474. Milroy's disease.

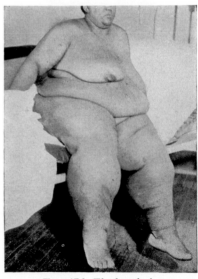

FIG. 476. Elephantiasis.

Position. The position in which the leg is held is influenced by changes in the hip joint. In anterior dislocations of the hip the foot is turned outward, in posterior dislocations inward. In inflammations of the hip joint, commonly tuberculous, the thigh is held flexed against the body with outward rotation of the leg (Fig. 477).

Shape. The shape of the legs is profoundly altered by certain bone diseases, particularly rickets, osteomalacia, osteitis deformans and osteogenesis imperfecta.

Rickets, which produces a softening of the bones, commonly causes *genu varum* (bowlegs) and *genu valgum* (knock knees) (Fig. 478). It may also produce a bowing of the leg forward, the so-called *saber shin.*

Osteitis deformans usually produces genu varum (Fig. 479) and the saber shin as well (Fig. 480).

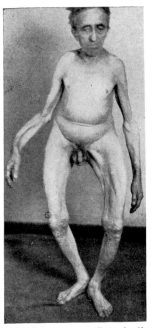

FIG. 479. Genu varum, Paget's disease.

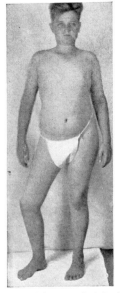

FIG. 477. Disease of right hip.

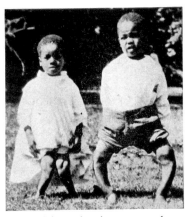

FIG. 478. Rickets showing genu valgum and genu varum.

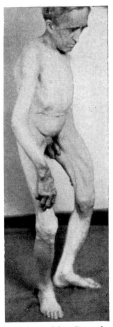

FIG. 480. Saber shin, Paget's disease.

Genu varum (Fig. 479) is also associated with achondroplasia, and genu valgum is a common complication of a birth injury (Fig. 481).

Syphilitic periostitis, or gummata of the shins, may produce local areas of swelling and tenderness. Figure 482 shows a patient with gummata on both shins.

Fractures of the leg which have badly set often cause a marked deformity of the leg (Fig. 483).

Appearance of the Skin. The skin of the leg usually reflects the condition beneath or any general skin condition.

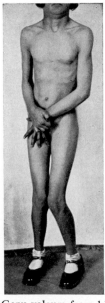

FIG. 481. Genu valgum from birth injury.

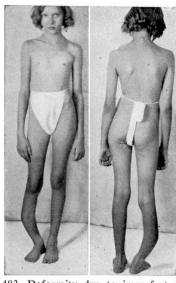

FIG. 483. Deformity due to imperfect union of fractured tibia.

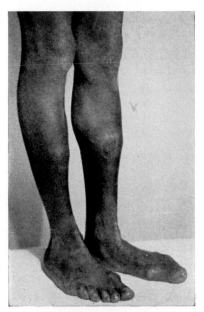

FIG. 482. Gummata of the legs.

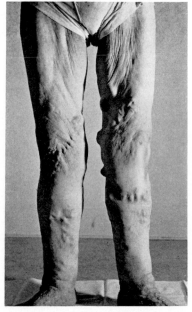

FIG. 484. Varicose veins.

Purpura haemorrhagica is common over the legs, and petechiae are often seen (Fig. 485). Figure 486 shows numerous petechiae in a patient suffering from lymphatic leukemia.

Embolism of the popliteal artery commonly produces a large, irregular circumscribed area, reddish-blue in color (Fig. 487). Varicose veins are a common cause of large purplish areas of discoloration about the ankles, because of the sluggish venous circulation which later produces varicose ulcers (Figs. 484, 488, 489, 490).

Erythema nodosum causes small subcutaneous nodules with reddening of the skin over them. These small nodules are usually tender, bilateral and rarely larger than 2 inches in diameter. The patients have some fever and malaise before the appearance of the nodules, which come out in crops. The etiology of the condition is uncertain, some

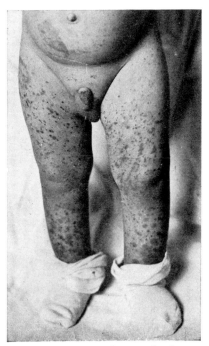

FIG. 485. Purpura haemorrhagica.

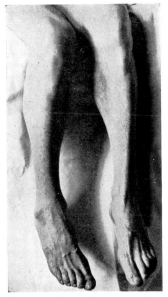

FIG. 486. Petechiae in lymphatic leukemia.

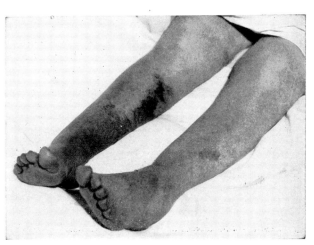

FIG. 487. Embolism of right popliteal artery.

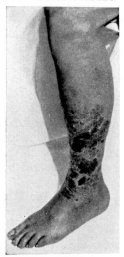

FIG. 488. Discoloration due to varicose veins.

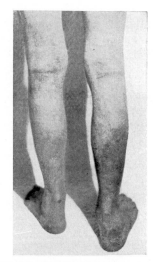

FIG. 489. Discoloration due to varicose veins.

workers regarding it as a rheumatic infection, others considering it tuberculous in origin (Fig. 491). It is also seen in coccidioidal granuloma. Closely allied to it is erythema multiforme (Fig. 492).

Cutis marmorata is a curious marble-like mottling of the skin which some persons show upon exposure to cold. The patient shown in Figure 493 had this condition when her legs hung down for a time. It indicates vasomotor instability. The patient shown in Figure 494 suffered from glomerular nephritis.

Buerger's disease, (Fig. 495) or thrombo-angiitis obliterans, is now recognized with increasing frequency. In this disease, which predominates in males of middle age, there is an inflammatory lesion of the arteries and veins with thrombus formation. The legs are

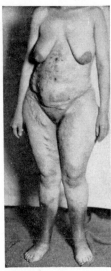

FIG. 490. Varicose veins of thigh and abdomen.

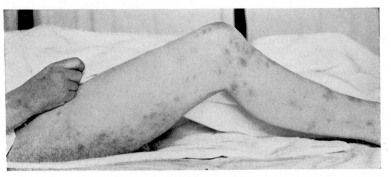

FIG. 491. Erythema nodosum.

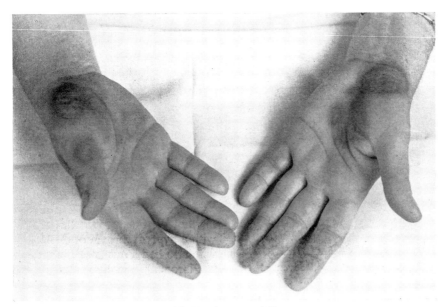

FIG. 492. Erythema multiforme.

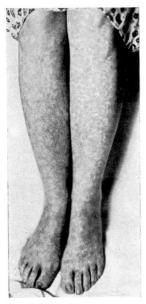

FIG. 493. Cutis marmorata.

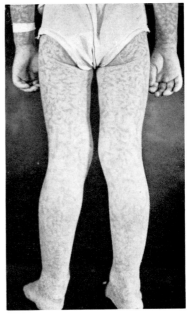

FIG. 494. Cutis marmorata in a child of five years suffering from acute glomerulo-nephritis.

most commonly involved, although the arms may be affected. When it is present in the lower extremities, the legs are deep red when hanging down, but blanch as soon as they are elevated. The leg feels cold, pulsation in the arteries is feeble or absent, and there is intermittent claudication on walking; the patient walks a short distance and then is com-pelled by the severe pains in the calves to stop. Excruciating pain in the extremities, often at night, is a common and striking symptom. Many patients note the pain first in the feet and think it is due to "fallen arches."

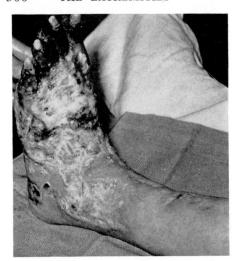

FIG. 495. Buerger's disease, advanced case showing gangrene of the foot.

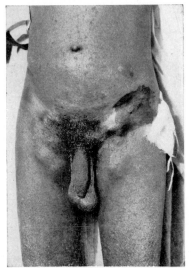

FIG. 496. Tuberculosis of inguinal lymph nodes.

Buerger's disease is sometimes confused with Raynaud's disease. In Buerger's disease, however, the findings are constant; in Raynaud's disease, paroxysmal. Buerger's disease appears predominantly in males, Raynaud's disease almost exclusively in females.

The inguinal region should be examined with special care. An aneurysm of the femoral artery is readily visible as an expansile, pulsating mass. Enlarge-

ment of the inguinal lymph glands may be seen or felt in tuberculosis (Fig. 496), syphilis, leukemia, Hodgkin's disease and lymphogranuloma inguinale. Enlargement of the femoral glands often indicates an infection of the leg or foot on the same side as an enlargement.

Tumors. Tumors of the leg may arise from the bones or from the skin and subcutaneous tissues. The most common primary bone tumors are sarcomata (Fig. 497), osteomata and osteosarcomata. Tumors of the thyroid gland, breast and kidneys often show metastases in the legs. Figure 498 shows a patient with a hypernephroma of the left kidney who also had a metastasis in the left leg.

Fibromata and lipomata are seen in the leg. Figure 499 shows a large tumor of the left thigh which proved to be a lipoma. The patient shown in Figure 500 had a ganglion arising from the tendon of the gastrocnemius muscle.

Leg ulcers are often seen in patients with varicose veins, syphilis, hemolytic icterus (Fig. 501) and sickle cell anemia (Fig. 502).

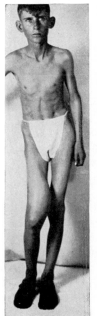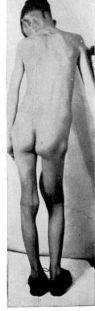

FIG. 497. Osteogenic sarcoma of femur.

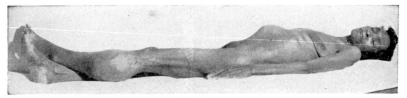

FIG. 498. Hypernephroma of left kidney with metastasis to left leg.

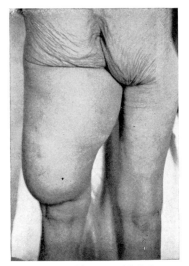

FIG. 499. Lipoma of left leg.

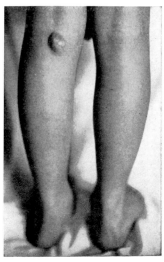

FIG. 500. Ganglion of left leg.

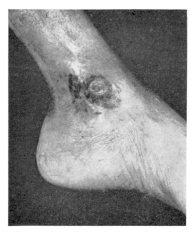

FIG. 501. Ulcer in leg in hemolytic icterus.

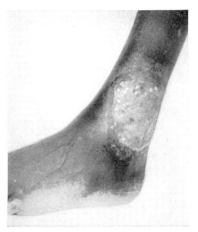

FIG. 502. Ulcer in leg in sickle cell anemia.

THE FEET

Diminution or absence of the vibration sense over the tibia is a common finding in pernicious anemia. When a tuning fork is struck and its handle placed against the bone, the patient is unaware of the vibrations.

The shape and size of the feet attract our attention first. The clubfoot, talipes, is a well-known acquired or congenital deformity which requires surgical intervention. Four types are recognized. In talipes equinus the patient walks on his toes; in talipes calcaneus he walks on his heels; in talipes varus he walks on the outside of his foot; and in talipes valgus he walks on the inside of his foot.

The most common variety is *talipes varus* (Fig. 503), which is usually congenital and bilateral.

Hallux valgus (Fig. 504) is a common foot deformity in which the great toes turn outward and often the other toes override each other. This condition is commonly due to faulty footwear, but may also be present in arthritis and in myositis ossificans.

In congenital heart disease and in chronic pulmonary infections with bron-

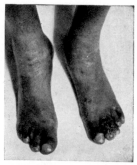

FIG. 505. Drumstick toes in congenital heart disease.

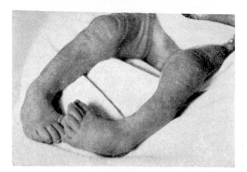

FIG. 503. Congenital clubfoot.

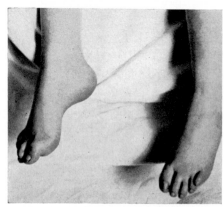

FIG. 506. Feet in Friedreich's disease.

chiectasis we may have *clubbed toes* (Fig. 505) as well as clubbed fingers.

In hereditary spinal ataxia (Friedreich's disease) the shape of the foot is characteristic. The dorsum is high, the arch deeply hollowed, and the great toe flexed at the phalangeal joint (Fig. 506). This deformity is bilateral. Flatfoot, or *pes planus* (Fig. 507), is a com-

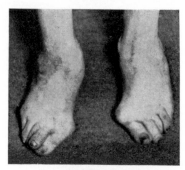

FIG. 504. Hallux valgus.

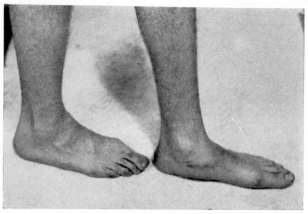

FIG. 507. Pes planus or flatfoot.

mon deformity often causing pain on walking.

Gangrene of the toes is seen in arteriosclerosis and in diabetes mellitus. In some cases only one toe is involved; in others two or more toes are involved (Figs. 508, 509). In such patients palpation of the foot commonly shows absence of pulsation in the dorsalis pedis or plantar arteries and occasionally in both.

Osteomyelitis causes sinuses from which fluid oozes, and at times spicules of bone are discharged (Fig. 510).

In *tabes dorsalis,* deep indolent painless ulcers sometimes form on the soles of the feet, usually beneath the great toe

—the so-called *mal perforant* (Fig. 511). Ulcers of the plantar surface of the feet are occasionally seen in diabetes (Fig. 512) although gangrene of the toes is a far commoner lesion.

In severe circulatory disease, excessive numbness, coldness, pain of the feet, and in gangrene of the toes, it is important to know the condition of the arterial circulation of the foot. Palpation of the dorsalis pedis artery (Fig. 513) and of the posterior tibial artery

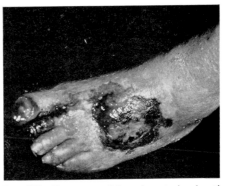

Fig. 509. Gangrene of foot in arteriosclerotic obliterating endarteritis.

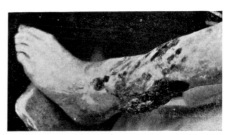

Fig. 510. Osteomyelitis of leg.

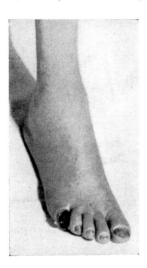

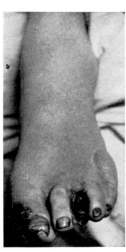

Fig. 508. Gangrene of toes in diabetes.

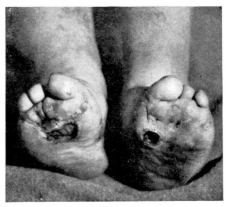

Fig. 511. *Mal perforant* in tabes.

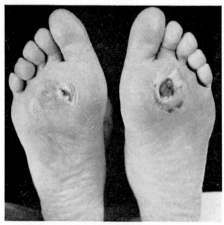

FIG. 512. Ulcers of the plantar surface of the feet in diabetes mellitus.

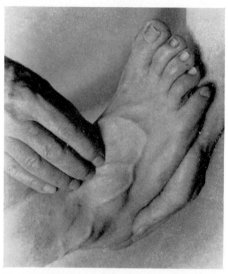

FIG. 513. Palpation of dorsalis pedis artery.

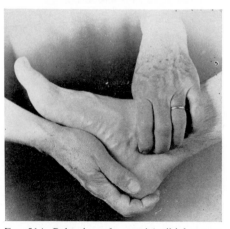

FIG. 514. Palpation of posterior tibial artery.

(Fig. 514) shows good pulsation when the circulation is adequate.

ARTHRITIS

The following types of arthritis are most commonly seen in the practice of medicine.

1. **Rheumatic Fever.** In rheumatic fever the joints most commonly involved are the wrists, elbows, knees and ankles. This type of arthritis has two characteristics that are pathognomonic. First, the arthritis is migratory, involving one joint and causing marked pain, redness, swelling and local heat, then suddenly leaving this joint and appearing in another joint and then in another. The second characteristic is that, after the arthritis leaves one joint and passes on to another joint, the first joint is perfectly normal in every respect. After the arthritis has subsided, the joints are normal.

The pain in this type of arthritis is severe. Even the accidental jarring of the bed of a patient by a passerby produces intense pain in the affected joints.

2. **Atrophic Arthritis.** This type of arthritis is called atrophic because it produces atrophy of the ends of the bone that form the joint, and not because the joint when inspected appears atrophic. On the contrary, the joint is usually swollen, hot and tender. This swelling is due to the markedly thickened periarticular tissues, often associated with an effusion into the joint. As the process advances, the articular cartilages are destroyed and a true ankylosis or fusion of the ends of the bones occurs.

Atrophic arthritis is believed to be infectious in origin. It is often seen in youthful persons and commonly causes atrophy of the muscles about the joints. "Haygarth's nodosities" may be seen in the later stages of this type of arthritis. Atrophic arthritis is also called rheumatoid arthritis.

3. **Hypertrophic Arthritis.** Hypertrophic arthritis is so termed because hypertrophy of the bone, in the form of bony spurs or outgrowths, is present.

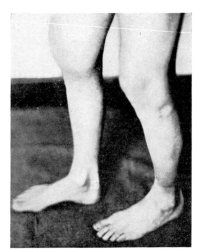

FIG. 515. Chronic arthritis of knees.

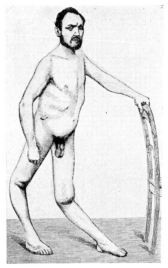

FIG. 516. Charcot's knee. (Westphal.)

The classical "Heberden's nodes" represent a mild form of this type. Because of the early bone involvement, this type of arthritis is often called osteo-arthritis.

Hypertrophic arthritis is thought by many observers to be metabolic in origin. It is commoner in persons of middle age or in advanced age than in youthful persons. It does not form a true ankylosis as does atrophic arthritis, but the bony outgrowths may interfere with the movements of a joint and lock it as effectually as if a true fusion of the bones had occurred.

This type of arthritis often involves the knee, where it may cause some thickening and hypertrophy of the villous processes of the synovial membrane (Fig. 515). This causes a grating sensation when the palm of the examiner's hand is held over the knee and the leg is alternately flexed and extended. Small cartilaginous tumors sometimes form in these villi and, if they become free in the joint cavity, are called "joint mice."

4. **Gonorrheal Arthritis.** The clinical picture of a gonorrheal arthritis is much like that of an atrophic arthritis. Some observers stress its tendency to involve the knees. The diagnosis is usually established by the recent history of a gonorrheal urethritis or the presence of this disease at the time the arthritis develops.

5. **Charcot's Joint.** This is a disease of the joint occurring as a complication usually but not exclusively of tabes dorsalis. The joints most commonly involved are the knee joint and the foot. The arthritis is painless, develops slowly and produces a marked destruction of

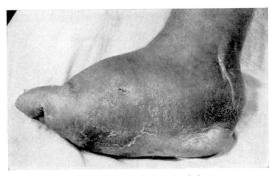

FIG. 517. Charcot's joint of foot.

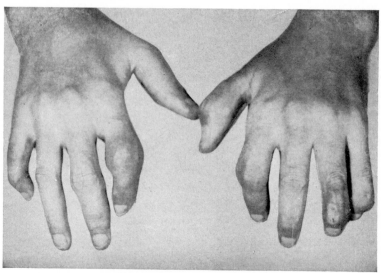

FIG. 518. Gouty arthritis of the hands.

bone. When it involves the knee, the knee is swollen and shows such a marked mobility that the patient often can neither stand nor walk. The knee can be flexed or hyperextended with equal ease (Fig. 516).

In the foot this condition produces a marked swelling of the ankle and foot which become converted into a rather shapeless mass unable to carry out the normal functions (Fig. 517).

6. **Gout.** An attack of gout most commonly involves the first joint of the great toe, then the ankles, knees and joints of the hands and wrist. Thomas Sydenham, a famous sufferer from this disease, wrote a classic account of an attack of acute gout, which every medical student should read. "The victim goes to bed and sleeps in good health. About two o'clock in the morning, he is awakened by a severe pain in the great toe; more rarely in the heel, ankle or instep. The pain is like that of a dislocation, and yet the parts feel as if cold water were poured over them." Sydenham describes how the patient awakens later and finds the toe swollen.

The presence of tophi deposits of sodium monourate in the joints of the feet or elsewhere, as in the cartilages of the ear, is diagnostic. Sydenham's statement that "more wise men than fools

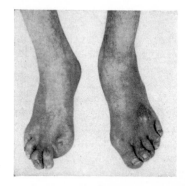

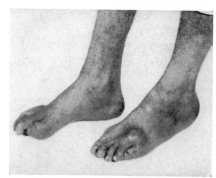

FIG. 519. Gouty arthritis of foot.

are victims," as Osler remarks, does not hold good today.

Hemarthrosis, an effusion of blood into a joint cavity, is rarely seen. It may follow trauma and is at times present in blood diseases showing disturbances in coagulation time.

Intermittent hydrarthrosis is a disease characterized by recurring effusions into the affected joints: It usually involves one or both knees, but other joints may be involved. Its cause is unknown, but its similarity to angioneurotic edema suggests that it is an allergic disease.

BIBLIOGRAPHY

Babcock, W. Wayne: A Textbook of Surgery. 2d ed. Philadelphia, W. B. Saunders Co., 1935.

Brown, George E.: Thrombo-angiitis Obliterans. Philadelphia, W. B. Saunders Co., 1928.

Buerger, Leo: The Circulatory Disturbances of the Extremities. Philadelphia, W. B. Saunders Co., 1924.

Castex, Mariono, and Mazzei, Egidio: L'hippocratisme digital unilatéral. Presse méd. 48:931, 1940.

Duke, W. W.: Palm color test. Arch. Int. Med. 42:533, 1928.

Heberden, William: Commentaries on the History and Cure of Diseases. Boston, Wells & Lilly, 1818, p. 119.

Hurwitz, S. H.: Osteitis deformans, Paget's disease. Bull. Johns Hopkins Hosp. 24:263, 1913.

Jaffe, Henry L.: Paget's disease of bone. Arch. Path. 15:83, 1933.

Kramer, David W.: Manual of Peripheral Vascular Disorders. Philadelphia, The Blakiston Co., 1940.

McNaught, James B.: The diagnosis of trichinosis. Am. J. Trop. Med. 19:181, 1939.

Major, Ralph H.: Charcot's foot. J.A.M.A. 90:846, 1928.

Nichols, B. H., and Raines, J. R.: Paget's disease of bone. Cleveland Clin. Quart. 8:139, 1941.

Pullen, Roscoe L.: Medical Diagnosis, Applied Physical Diagnosis. 2nd ed., Philadelphia, W. B. Saunders Co., 1950.

Sutton, R. L., and Sutton, R. L., Jr.: Diseases of the Skin. St. Louis, C. V. Mosby Co., 1939, p. 482.

Witherspoon, J. Thornwell: Congenital and familial clubbing of the fingers and toes. Arch. Int. Med. 57:18, 1936.

CHAPTER 16

EXAMINATION OF THE NERVOUS SYSTEM

THE EXAMINATION OF the nervous system of patients proceeds along somewhat different lines from those we have thus far considered. In this examination we depend largely upon inspection, aided by palpation, and not at all upon percussion and auscultation. In examining the nervous system the patient's cooperation is very important; indeed, many neurologic examinations cannot be carried out without it. This chapter should be considered merely an outline for a neurologic examination and not an exhaustive consideration. No type of examination requires more attention to a variety of small details, more careful examination or more searching analysis of findings obtained.

PSYCHE

Consciousness. The examiner notes whether the patient is conscious, unconscious, semiconscious, delirious or stuporous. The patient may be suffering from a delirium due to certain fevers, or to intoxication from alcohol or drugs. Stupor may be the result of mental disease, of an injury, of narcotic drugs or of alcohol. Coma, or complete loss of consciousness, is seen in diabetes, in cerebral hemorrhage, in nephritis, after an overdose of drugs, after too much alcohol or after an injury to the head.

Comprehension. We note early whether the patient has a full realization of his surroundings, recognizes his friends, comprehends words that are spoken to him, and is able to understand the meaning of written words. Failure of a patient to comprehend his surroundings or recognize his friends and companions may be due to lesions of the frontal lobe and of the corpus callosum. Similar disturbances are seen in patients suffering from certain psychoses without demonstrable anatomic lesions, and in patients suffering from alcoholic or drug intoxication. A lack of comprehension of spoken words occurs in "word deafness," in lesions of the first and second temporal convolutions. Patients with word deafness have perfectly normal hearing, but the words are as strange as if spoken in a foreign language with which the patient is not familiar. A lack of comprehension of written words occurs in "word blindness," or visual aphasia, a condition usually due to a lesion of the left angular gyrus. The patient can see words,

308

letters and signs, but cannot interpret them. He is much like the person who looks at a page printed in a language which he does not understand.

FACIES

We should always study the facies of nervous patients. Many of the points to be noted have been discussed in Chapter 4. We note whether a patient appears intelligent or stupid, emotional or phlegmatic, apprehensive or sanguine, timid or bragging, lethargic or restless. These differences in facial expression are often pathognomonic in the diagnosis of nervous and constitutional diseases. The masklike, immobile face of the patient with paralysis agitans is highly characteristic. In acute mania the expression is one of agitation, and the psychoneurotic patient often is emotional. In depressive psychoses the patient frequently is apprehensive.

The mental state of a patient can often be determined by a brief but well-directed conversation. It is important to investigate the mood of the patient. Euphoria is a feeling of unusual well-being which the patient seems desirous of communicating to his friends. Euphoria is common in general paresis, in multiple sclerosis and often in the manic stage of manic depressive insanity. The "flight of ideas" is very marked in maniacal patients, who never reach the end of their thought processes because they are constantly diverted by other stimuli. Some patients have delusions, illusions and hallucinations. Delusions are false beliefs which cannot be corrected by argument, persuasion or experience. Illusions are sensations which are falsely interpreted. There is an actual stimulus producing an illusion, but the interpretation of this stimulus is incorrect. Hallucinations are sensations or perceptions which have no external stimulus. Thus the voices that are heard, and the visions that are seen, by the patient suffering from hallucinations are purely imaginary and are not produced by any external stimulus.

EXAMINATION OF THE CRANIAL NERVES

After we have formed some ideas of the psychic state of the patient, we should next proceed with an examination of the cranial nerves.

First Nerve. The olfactory nerve is entirely sensory, so that lesions of it are detected by examining the sense of smell in each nostril. Such an examination should be preceded by a careful inspection of the nostril to exclude the presence of local disease or polyps. The sense of smell is tested by closing one nostril and allowing the patient to smell the test substance through the other. The test substances usually used are vanilla, peppermint and cloves. Disturbances in the sense of smell may be due to lesions anywhere between the nasal mucous membrane and the uncinate and hippocampal gyri in the brain. The common causes of such lesions are syphilis, brain tumor, cerebral hemorrhage and fracture of the skull. In lesions of the uncinate gyrus, hallucinations of smell are commonly encountered. Such hallucinations are also seen in mental diseases and in psychoneurotics.

Second Nerve. The examination of the optic nerve is one of the most important features of the neurological examination. The eye should first be studied with an ophthalmoscope, and the state of the media, optic disk, retina and the retinal blood vessels carefully noted (Fig. 520). *Choked disk,* or optic papillitis, is present in conditions causing increased intracranial pressure, particularly in brain tumors, as well as frequently in hypertensive cardiovascular disease. In the early stage of an optic papillitis the optic disk is congested and reddened, the margins becoming blurred and indistinct (Fig. 521). Later it is swollen, hemorrhages may appear, the cupping disappears and the disk appears to protrude. In glaucoma the optic cupping, instead of being almost obliterated as in papillitis, is accentuated.

In primary *optic atrophy* the disk is white, grayish or bluish-white, the edges

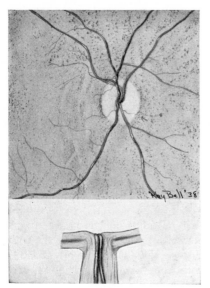

FIG. 520. Normal fundus of the eye.

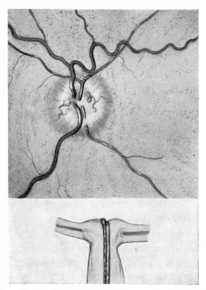

FIG. 521. Moderately advanced choked disk.

are sharply defined, and it is somewhat diminished in size. In secondary atrophy the disk is dense white or grayish, its margins irregular and hazy, and it may be covered with connective tissue from the organization of a previous exudate. Primary optic atrophy is most frequently seen in tabes dorsalis and paresis, and also in multiple sclerosis in which the temporal half of the disk shows pallor as compared with the rest of the disk. It

may also be due to acromegaly, or intoxication with poisons, especially wood alcohol. It occurs in Leber's disease or hereditary optic neuritis. Secondary optic atrophy follows choked disk, brain tumors, pigmentary degenerations of the retina, embolisms and thrombosis of the central artery, choroiditis and glaucoma. It may result from injury of the optic nerve due to fracture of the orbital canal.

Hemorrhages in the retina are seen in chronic nephritis, arterial hypertension, leukemia, pernicious anemia, diabetes and subacute infectious endocarditis.

The condition of the blood vessels should be carefully noted, since marked arteriosclerosis of the retinal arteries may be accompanied by generalized cerebral arteriosclerosis. Usually choroiditis is readily recognized by the patches of black pigment in the retina, and is commonly the result of syphilitic infection, although it may be produced by other causes.

The *fields of vision* should be carefully studied (Fig. 522). This may be

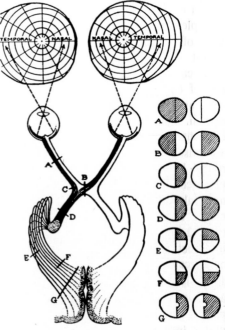

FIG. 522. Optic pathway showing how lesions at various points appear on the field of vision. (Homans.)

done roughly with the finger, but accurately only with a perimeter. The confrontation test is a simple eye-to-eye test for defects in the visual field. The examiner faces the patient, whose right eye is closed. The examiner then closes his left eye, and his finger is moved in the periphery of the fields in order to detect visual loss. The same procedure is then carried out with the patient's left eye and the examiner's right eye closed. This simple maneuver is readily carried out and is of great value. A more accurate outline of the visual fields can be made, of course, with the perimeter. Hemianopsia, or blindness in one half of the field of vision in one or in both eyes, is usually readily made out. Two types are recognized: homonymous hemianopsia (D), or blindness of the corresponding halves of the visual field, and heteronymous hemianopsia (B), or blindness of the opposite halves. Heteronymous hemianopsia is more commonly referred to as binasal or bitemporal hemianopsia. Hemianopsia may be restricted to one eye (C) or may affect both eyes (B and D). If the blindness is unilateral and complete in one eye, the lesion is in the optic nerve of the affected eye (A). In homonymous hemianopsia (D) the lesion is above the optic chiasm, while in bitemporal hemianopsia (B) the lesion is in the central part of the optic chiasm. Tumors of the pituitary gland produce bitemporal hemianopsia (B). Brain tumors and cerebral hemorrhage cause homonymous hemianopsia (D and G). A lesion of the optic radiation in the occipital lobe near the cortex produces homonymous hemianopsia with, however, intact central vision (G).

Perimetric examination may also demonstrate a contraction in the field of vision, which may be due to optic neuritis, optic atrophy, hysteria, retinitis, choroiditis and multiple sclerosis. Other less frequent causes are acromegaly, paresis, embolism of the central artery of the retina, syringomyelia and cerebellar ataxia.

Inversion of the fields of color is often seen in hysteria.

Amaurosis, or *blindness,* may be transient or permanent. Permanent blindness may follow optic atrophy, wood alcohol poisoning, sympathetic ophthalmitis, retinitis pigmentosa or any purulent inflammation of the eyeball. A transitory amaurosis is seen in hysteria, uremia, diabetes mellitus, malaria, quinine poisoning and after the excessive use of tobacco and alcohol.

Night blindness, or *nyctalopia,* is a condition in which objects are clearly seen by daylight or by a strong artificial light, but are invisible at twilight. William Heberden, who described and named this disease, relates of a patient, "on board of a ship in the river, he observed at sunsetting, that all objects began to look blue, which blueness gradually thickened into a cloud; and not long after he became so blind, as hardly to perceive the light of a candle. The next morning about sunrising his sight was restored as perfectly as ever. When the next night came on, he lost his sight again in the same manner." Nyctalopia is observed in vitamin A deficiency, in retinitis pigmentosa, occasionally in jaundice, and in hereditary axial neuritis (Leber's disease).

A *scotoma,* or blind spot, may be observed by the patient as a black spot in his field of vision, or may be present as a blind spot of which the patient is aware only upon examination. A scotoma of which the patient is aware is called a positive scotoma; that of which he is unaware is spoken of as a negative scotoma. Scotoma is seen in migraine, cataract, choroiditis, neuritis, retinitis, optic neuritis, optic atrophy, detached retina, and tumors of the pituitary gland. One of the most common varieties of scotoma is the *muscae volitantes,* which appear as small grayish dots which move with each change in position of the eye. They have no particular significance, and most normal persons see them at some time. They may be more numerous and particularly obvious during a febrile attack or in diseases of the liver.

The patient should also be tested for his visual acuity and for the presence or absence of color blindness.

Third Nerve. The third nerve supplies the levator palpebrae and the muscles of the eyeball with the exception of the external rectus, the superior oblique and the dilator of the pupil (Fig. 523). Branches of the oculomotor nerve pass to the ciliary muscle and to the constrictor of the iris. It is convenient to group the different findings produced by lesions of the oculomotor nerve.

1. *Abnormalities of the eyelids. Ptosis,* or drooping of the upper eyelid, due to paralysis of the levator palpebrae, produces a striking appearance. It is seen in tabes dorsalis, in diphtheria and in aneurysms of the basilar arteries.

2. *Abnormalities of the Pupils.* In lesions of the oculomotor nerve the pupil is usually dilated because of paralysis of the constrictor of the iris. There is also *cycloplegia,* or paralysis of the ciliary muscle, which produces a loss of the power of accommodation, because there is inability to alter the surface of the lens. Distant vision may be clear, but near vision is indistinct.

3. *Abnormalities of the Extrinsic Movements of the Eyes.* A lesion of the oculomotor nerve causes a divergent strabismus due to paralysis of the internal rectus muscle, deviation of the eyeball upward and outward due to paralysis of the inferior rectus muscle, and deviation of the eyeball downward and inward due to paralysis of the superior rectus muscle.

In summary, paralysis of the third nerve causes ptosis, deviation of the eyeball outward and downward, mydriasis, and complete loss of pupillary action both during accommodation and to light.

Lesions of the nuclei of the oculomotor nerve occur in encephalitis, anterior poliomyelitis, amyotrophic lateral sclerosis, multiple sclerosis, syringomyelia, tabes dorsalis, botulism, cerebral syphilis, brain tumors and in cerebral hemorrhage or thrombosis. Occasionally, lesions occur in exophthalmic goiter, myasthenia gravis and in migraine. The nerve itself may be affected in meningitis, diphtheria, pneumonia, diabetes and in poisoning with alcohol, lead or nicotine. Fractures of the skull and cerebral neoplasms may produce paralysis of the nerve by pressure.

Argyll Robertson Pupil. This characteristic sign of cerebrospinal syphilis has been described elsewhere. It is a pupil which reacts during accommodation and convergence, but sluggishly or not at all to light. It is nearly always bilateral, and miosis, or contraction of the pupil, is often present. Anisokoria and irregularities in the outlines of the pupils are frequently present.

In carrying out this test it should be remembered that in the aged, and in alcoholics, response of the pupils to light is feeble, and also that morphine

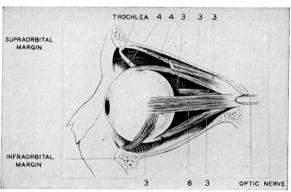

FIG. 523. The nerve supply to the muscles of the eyeball. Numbers refer to the cranial nerves. (Corning.)

and some of its derivatives produce miosis with fixed pupils.

Hippus, or rhythmic contractions of the pupil, is seen in epilepsy, hysteria and meningitis.

A *paradoxical pupil,* in which the pupil dilates instead of contracting on exposure to light, is not infrequently seen in tabes dorsalis.

Blepharospasm is a spasmodic contraction of the orbicularis palpebrarum. This is most commonly due to errors of refraction or to chronic conjunctivitis. It may also be seen in hysteria. Blepharospasm may lead later to the development of a definite tic.

Fourth Nerve. Isolated paralysis of the trochlear nerve is rare. It is occasionally found in meningitis. Usually, when the trochlear nerve is involved, the oculomotor is involved as well. In paralysis of the trochlear nerve the affected eye is turned upward and inward, a defect which is noted particularly by the patient when descending stairs. Vertical homonymous diplopia (double vision) may be present, the image of the affected eye being lower than that of the normal eye.

Sixth Nerve. The abducens nerve, although not following strictly in numerical order, is usually considered after the trochlear, since both nerves are concerned with the extrinsic movements of the eyes. The abducens nerve supplies only the external rectus muscle of the eye. A lesion of this nerve produces internal strabismus with diplopia, or double vision.

Lesions of the abducens nerve are encountered most often in brain tumors, meningitis, tabes dorsalis and multiple sclerosis.

Fifth Nerve. The trigeminal nerve is a mixed nerve containing both motor and sensory fibers, although the sensory fibers predominate. The trigeminal nerve is divided into three branches (Fig. 524).

1. *The Ophthalmic Nerve* (*Ramus Ophthalmicus*). This branch is entirely sensory and carries sensation from the eyeball, from the conjunctiva (with the

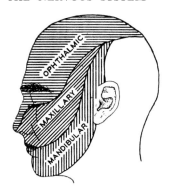

Fig. 524. The branches of the trigeminal nerve.

exception of the lower lid) and from the forehead, scalp, cornea and nose. It also carries secretory fibers to the lacrimal gland. The corneal reflex (p. 69) is an important test for lesions of the fifth nerve.

2. *The Maxillary Nerve* (*Ramus Maxillaris*). This nerve carries sensation from the upper lid, the sides of the nose, cheeks, lower eyelid and lower part of the temple, as well as from the upper teeth, mucous membrane of the lower lid, upper jaw, hard palate, uvula, tonsil, nasal pharynx, lower ear and lower part of the nasal cavity.

3. *The Mandibular Branch* (*Ramus Mandibularis*). This carries the sensory fibers from the jaw, external ear, lower part of the temple, mucous membrane of the cheek, tongue and lower lip, and from the lower teeth.

The motor branch of the mandibular branch supplies the muscles of mastication—the temporal, masseter and pterygoid muscles. When this nerve is paralyzed, there is inability to use the muscles of mastication on the affected side. It can be recognized by placing the fingers on the temple and masseter muscles and asking the patient to close his jaws. Feebleness of the contraction on the affected side is readily perceived. If the lesion is bilateral, chewing is impossible.

The lesion of the trigeminal nerve most commonly seen is trifacial neuralgia. This disease is associated with intense pain, the distribution of pain depending upon whether the first, second, third, or all three of these branches are involved. It commonly involves the maxillary and mandibular branches of the trigeminal nerve and, because of the location, is falsely diagnosed as dental disease. In herpes labialis the fibers of the maxillary or mandibular branches are involved. The ophthalmic division, however, also may be involved, producing severe pain and often scarring of the cornea.

Seventh Nerve. The facial nerve is largely motor and supplies the frontal muscle, the orbicularis oculi, orbicularis oris and most of the other muscles of the face (Fig. 525). Paralysis of the frontal muscle produces inability to frown; paralysis of the orbicularis oculi, inability to close the eyelids; paralysis of the orbicularis oris, inability to smile or show the teeth on the affected side. The condition known clinically as *Bell's palsy,* which has been described elsewhere (pp. 63 and 71), is due to a lesion of the facial nerve. In Bell's palsy the affected side is flaccid and expressionless, the nasolabial furrow is obliterated, the corner of the mouth droops, the eye can only be partly closed, the lower lid is lax, and tears flow over the cheek. An attempt to close the eyelids causes rotation of the eyeball upward and outward. Because of the paralysis of the muscles about the mouth saliva often trickles out and food lodges between the teeth and cheek. The patient is unable to whistle or blow.

Supranuclear paralysis due to lesions of the cortex or of the facial fibers is associated with hemiplegia. In nuclear lesions there is generally bilateral paralysis of the face, and when the lesion is basal, the sixth and eighth cranial nerves are often involved and cross paralysis with hemiplegia of the opposite side of the body appears. When the nerve is affected in the fallopian aqueduct, hearing is usually disturbed and there may be loss of taste in the anterior two-thirds of the paralyzed half of the tongue.

The irritability of the seventh nerve is greatly increased in tetany. This can be demonstrated by tapping the cheek just in front of the ear. This procedure stimulates the facial nerve, producing contraction of the muscles on this side of the face (*Chvostek's sign*).

The chorda tympani, a branch of the facial nerve, also carries taste fibers coming from the anterior two-thirds of

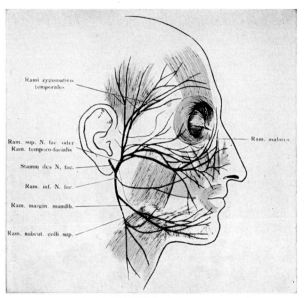

Fig. 525. Distribution of facial nerve. (Corning.)

the tongue. A lesion of its fibers produces insensibility of taste, which is readily tested by applying acid, salt or sugar to the anterior two-thirds of the tongue on the suspected side. The tongue should be protruded in carrying out these tests.

Eighth Nerve. The auditory nerve consists of two branches which differ in their peripheral endings and in their functions: the cochlear nerve and the vestibular nerve.

Disease of the cochlear nerve causes disturbance of hearing, usually *deafness* or *tinnitus*. Deafness or impairment of hearing can readily be tested by holding a watch at stated distances from each ear. This distance at which the ticking can be heard depends upon the watch, but ordinarily it can be heard from 30 to 40 inches from the ear. By this simple method differences in acuity of hearing in the two ears may be tested. It is important to close one ear with the finger while testing the other ear.

When there is deafness, it is important to find out whether the deafness is due to a lesion of the cochlear nerve itself or to disease of the middle ear. This is determined by the following tests.

Weber's Test. When a vibrating tuning fork is held against the forehead, the sound is best heard in the normal ear if the disease is due to a lesion of the auditory nerve, but better by the affected ear if there is an obstruction in the ear passages.

Rinne's Test. A tuning fork is first held in front of the ear and then placed on the mastoid process. If the sounds are not heard when the tuning fork is held near the ear, but are heard when it is placed over the mastoid process, the lesion is probably in the middle ear and not in the nerve itself.

The vestibular nerve plays an important role in controlling the balance of the body and in appreciation of our position in space. Disease of the vestibular branch of the auditory nerve often causes nystagmus, horizontal, vertical or rotary. Vertigo or dizzy attacks are commonly the result of disturbances in the vestibular apparatus. Sea sickness is a classic example. Another well-known example of this is Menière's disease, a disease accompanied by tinnitus and recurring attacks of intense vertigo, often ending in vomiting and sometimes in loss of consciousness. Nystagmus may or may not be present in this affection.

Bárány Test. Disease of the vestibular apparatus is tested by means of the Bárány tests, the simplest of which consists in irrigating the ear first with warm water and then with cold water. When the normal ear is irrigated with warm water (110° to 120° F.), a rotary nystagmus develops with the quick movement away from the irrigated ear. With cold water (68° F.) the quick movement is toward the irrigated ear. In disease of the labyrinth, no nystagmus appears. The details of carrying out the other tests are somewhat complicated and are described in detail in treatises on nervous diseases.

Pointing Test. Another test for vestibular disease is the pointing test. In carrying out this test the patient, with his eyes closed, sits opposite the examiner, extends his forearm and touches his forefinger to the examiner's finger. He is then requested to raise his arm vertically, then bring it down and again touch the examiner's finger with his forefinger. A normal person does this readily, but a patient with vestibular disorder is unable to do so and misses the examiner's finger often as much as several centimeters.

Ninth Nerve. The glossopharyngeal nerve contains both motor and sensory fibers, the motor branches supplying the stylopharyngeus muscle and sending fibers through the pharyngeal plexus to the constrictors of the pharynx, while the sensory fibers supply the upper part of the pharynx and the posterior third of the tongue. Isolated lesions of the glossopharyngeal nerve rarely occur. A lesion of this nerve produces difficulty in swallowing, anesthesia of the upper part of the pharynx, soft palate, absence of the pharyngeal reflexes and loss of the sensation of taste over the posterior third of the tongue.

The ninth nerve is liable to neuralgia, producing a syndrome comparable in every way to trigeminal neuralgia, the "trigger point" being in the tonsillar region and the pain radiating into the ear.

Tenth Nerve. The vagus nerve has a wide distribution, supplying the pharynx, larynx, lungs, heart, esophagus and stomach. Lesions of this nerve may be produced by pathological change in the nucleus, an example of which is seen in bulbar paralysis. It may be compressed by tumors, by aneurysms, and by exudates as in meningitis, and may be affected by an inflammatory process. In examining for lesions of the vagus nerve, it is desirable to consider each division separately.

Pharyngeal Branch. In unilateral lesions of this branch the soft palate does not move on the affected side and the arch is lower on this side. The uvula, which normally hangs in the midline, is deviated toward the normal side. Bilateral lesions of the pharyngeal branch produce difficulty in swallowing with regurgitation of foods and liquids through the nostrils. In bulbar palsy the paralysis is bilateral; in diphtheria, unilateral or bilateral.

Laryngeal Branch. The superior laryngeal nerve supplies the mucous membrane of the larynx above the cord and the cricothyroid muscle. The inferior, or recurrent, laryngeal nerve supplies all the muscles of the larynx except the cricothyroid. The recurrent laryngeal nerve curves around the arch of the aorta on the left side and around the subclavian artery on the right side, before ascending upward to innervate the larynx. The long course of these nerves renders them particularly liable to injury, and they are frequently involved in aneurysm of the aorta or of the right subclavian artery. Paralysis of the laryngeal and pharyngeal branches causes a marked nasal quality of the voice and difficulty in swallowing.

Examination of the larynx with a laryngoscope may show in disease of the laryngeal nerves bilateral paralysis of the abductors, unilateral abductor or adductor paralysis. In abductor paralysis the vocal cords are brought close together in the position of phonation. This condition may be produced by pressure on the vagus or upon both recurrent laryngeal nerves and is also seen occasionally in tabes, bulbar paralysis and more rarely in hysteria. Patients with abductor paralysis usually show an inpiratory stridor. Unilateral abductor paralysis is seen most frequently in aneurysms of the aorta, which press upon the left recurrent laryngeal nerve, and also in mitral stenosis, in which the hypertrophied left auricle presses upon the left recurrent laryngeal nerve. The voices of such patients are hoarse and rough, and a brassy cough may also be present. In adductor paralysis the laryngoscopic examination shows that the cords are far apart, and the patient is unable to closely approximate them in attempting to speak. This condition is often seen in hysteria, and may occur in acute laryngitis and after excessive use of the voice.

Cardiac Branch. The demonstration by the Weber brothers in 1845 that the vagus nerve contains fibers which slow the rate of the heart remains one of the striking scientific facts in physiology and in clinical medicine. Pressure or irritation of the vagus nerve slows the action of the heart. The slow pulse seen in increased intracranial pressure due to meningitis, brain tumors or cerebral hemorrhage is probably due to stimulation of the vagus nerve. With complete paralysis of the vagus, however, its inhibitory action is abolished and the pulse rate becomes rapid. This is sometimes seen in diphtheria.

The action of the pulmonary branch of the vagus is still poorly understood.

The muscular movements of the stomach and esophagus are largely regulated by the vagus. The most striking example of disturbances due to the gastric branch of the vagus are the gastric crises seen in tabes dorsalis.

Vagotonia. This condition, according to the conception of Eppinger and Hess, comprises a group of symptoms which occur in various diseases and produce certain modifications of the clinical pictures. Vagotonia, according to these authors, is the result of an excessive sensitiveness of the autonomic nervous system, particularly of the vagus. The symptoms comprise miosis, hot flushes, abundant perspiration, bluish hands, dermatographia, slow pulse, low blood pressure, eosinophilia, and tendency to spasm of the gastrointestinal tract.

Eleventh Nerve. The spinal accessory nerve innervates the sternocleidomastoid muscle and part of the trapezius muscle. Lesions of the spinal accessory nerve produce torticollis, or wryneck, although lesions of the nerve are not the sole cause of this condition. Two varieties of torticollis are recognized, the fixed and the spasmodic. In the fixed variety the spasm is constant and due to persistent contraction of the cervical muscles, particularly the sternocleidomastoid and the trapezius, the head being drawn to one side and turned so that the occiput points to the shoulder. In spasmodic torticollis there are intermittent spasmodic contractions or twitchings of the neck involving particularly the sternocleidomastoid muscle. This condition may appear suddenly, and is prone to be obstinate and of long duration.

The spinal accessory nerve may be damaged by injuries involving the neck, by diseases of the upper cervical vertebrae, tumor, enlargement of the cervical glands or abscesses in the neck.

Twelfth Nerve. The hypoglossal is a motor nerve supplying the muscles of the tongue, and diseases of the twelfth nerve are tested by asking the patient to protrude his tongue. When there is paralysis of the hypoglossal nerve, the tongue on protrusion deviates toward the paralyzed side because of the unopposed action of the geniohyoglossus muscle. Such deviation of the tongue on protrusion is a common finding in cerebral hemorrhage.

THE MOTOR SYSTEM

From the large pyramidal cells of the motor cortex axons descend by way of the pyramidal tract to terminate in contact with the anterior horn cells of the spinal cord. These are known as *upper motor neurons.* The pyramidal tract decussates at the lower end of the brain stem, so that motor impulses originating in the precentral convolution of the left cerebral hemisphere control the movements of the right side of the body, while those originating in the right hemisphere control the movements of the left side. This fact, well known to Hippocrates, is one of the oldest of medical observations. From the anterior horn cells, fibers pass to the muscles, forming the *lower motor neuron.* The distinction between upper and lower motor neurons is fundamental, for injuries to the upper motor neuron produce a spastic paralysis, with increased reflexes, a Babinski reflex, and the paralyzed muscles do not atrophy. Exactly the opposite picture results from injury to the lower motor neuron, namely, a flaccid paralysis, diminished or lost reflexes, with flabbiness and wasting of the paralyzed muscles.

Involvement of the motor system produces distressing complications to patients. This may entail either loss or impairment of motion. This loss or impairment of motion may be produced by paralysis, altered tonus, tremors or inability to carry out the finer movements. Continued disturbance in the motor functions of the nerve when the lower motor neuron is involved may lead to atrophy and contracture of the muscles.

Tonus. The tonus of a muscle after paralysis depends upon the location of the lesion. When the lower motor neuron is involved, the paralysis is flaccid and the tonus of the muscle is diminished. When the upper neuron is involved, the tonus is greatly increased and a clonus

may be present. The best-known examples are the patellar clonus and the
ankle clonus. In patients with a lesion
of the upper motor neuron, a pull downward on the patella causes rhythmic
contractions of the patella—the *patellar
clonus,* while marked dorsal flexion of
the foot produces a series of rhythmic
contractions of the tendon of Achilles—
the *ankle clonus.* The patellar clonus
and the ankle clonus are both conclusive
evidence of a disturbance of the upper
motor neuron (Fig. 533).

Another evidence of increased muscular tonus is seen in exaggerated knee
kicks and Achilles reflex. The patellar
clonus is accompanied by an exaggerated knee kick, and the ankle clonus
by an exaggerated Achilles reflex.

Disturbances in the finer movements
of the hand show evidence of alteration
of muscular tonus.

Power. The most obvious evidence
of loss of power is seen in paralysis of
an extremity. Paralysis of one extremity
is spoken of as monoplegia. Paralysis of
both the arm and the leg on the same
side is called "hemiplegia." Paraplegia
is paralysis of the lower extremities. In
lesions of the cerebral cortex, it should
be remembered that movements rather
than muscles are paralyzed.

A patient may show definite diminution in motor functions without presenting an outspoken paralysis. The
motor functions of various muscles are
readily tested. Usually we test groups
of muscles, asking the patient to resist
the movement we are making. We flex

and extend the following extremities—
ankles, knees, thighs, wrists, elbows and
shoulders. A comparison of the patient's
resistance on the two sides to these
movements of the examiner will show
a marked difference when weakness is
present on one side. A patient should
be asked to grasp as firmly as possible
with his hands both the examiner's
hands. This procedure gives one a good
idea of the strength of the muscles of
the hands as well as of the comparative
strength of the two hands.

Fibrillary Twitchings. Fibrillary
twitchings are disturbances of motor
function seen particularly in progressive
muscular atrophy. In this condition,
small bundles of muscles twitch from
time to time without the volition of the
patient and, indeed, usually without his
knowledge.

Choreiform movements are sudden,
spasmodic, purposeless movements, obviously due to motor stimulation and
probably of cortical origin. They are
seen particularly in Sydenham's chorea
and in Huntington's chorea; they usually
disappear in both diseases during sleep.

Athetosis, or twitching and bending
movements of the fingers, is also involuntary, and follows motor irritation,
usually the result of lesions in the cerebrum. It is seen in lesions involving the
basal ganglia of the brain—tumors,
hemorrhage, softening, and in lenticular
degeneration (Wilson's disease).

Tremor. The term "tremor" is usually employed to mean an involuntary
rhythmic contraction of a group of mus-

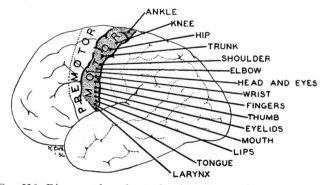

Fig. 526. Diagram of cerebrum showing motor and premotor areas.

cles. Tremors may involve only one group of muscles or may involve several sets of muscle groups. *Tremors are usually absent during sleep.*

Tremors are seen in exophthalmic goiter, Parkinson's syndrome, multiple sclerosis, alcoholism, hysteria, neurasthenia, cerebellar lesions, paresis and in certain emotional states.

It is important to note the location of the tremors. The most common locations are in the head and in the hands. We should note also the rate. In exophthalmic goiter the rate is rapid, while in paralysis agitans it is much slower. The amplitude of the tremor should also be considered as well as its relation to voluntary movements. In paralysis agitans the tremor is present during repose, becomes less marked when the patient makes a voluntary effort, and disappears during sleep. In multiple sclerosis the tremor appears only when the patient makes a voluntary movement; for this reason it is called an intention tremor.

Gait. An examination of the gait of the patient is one of the most obvious ways to determine disturbance in the motor system, although it should be emphasized that not all disturbances in the gait are due to motor system lesions. Walking, like all muscular movements, is a complicated phenomenon in which four sets of muscles, the agonists or prime movers, antagonists, synergists, and fixation muscles are concerned. Sensory stimuli which inform the person of the position and location of his legs are often as important as the motor stimuli. Gait, therefore, is a test for motor power, for sensory integrity and for coordination.

In spastic paraplegia the lower extremities are moved stiffly and the patient takes short steps.

In peripheral neuritis the gait is spoken of as the *steppage gait*. In this condition the toes cannot be raised; therefore the whole leg must be lifted in order that the feet clear the floor.

When there are bilateral cerebral lesions, an adductor spasm results and produces a so-called *scissor gait* in which the feet are placed alternately in front of each other.

In a *spastic gait*, which is due to a lesion of the upper neuron, a patient walks stiffly and the toes of the shoes are worn long before the rest of the sole.

In the *hemiplegic gait* the leg on the affected side is swung around from the hip, and the internal part of the shoe commonly drags on the floor. The arm on the affected side is usually held stiffly in flexion.

The *ataxic gait,* which is sometimes loosely called the *tabetic gait,* is seen in tabes dorsalis, occasionally in multiple neuritis, in diabetic neuritis—the so-called "tabes diabetica"—and in any disease involving the posterior columns, such as pernicious anemia. The patient walks with his feet widely apart, lifts his feet quickly, throws them too high, and then slaps them down on the ground. Motor power is here little affected, sensation and coordination markedly so.

Obviously, disturbances in gait are frequently associated with disturbance in equilibrium. Patients with Menière's disease are often unable to walk, or stagger and sway in attempting to walk. A patient with cerebellar tumor, combined system disease of the cord, multiple sclerosis or tabes dorsalis may show marked ataxia. The ataxia of tabes dorsalis is well demonstrated by asking the patient to close his eyes and bring his feet together. Usually he sways markedly—*Romberg's sign.* When a tabetic patient is lying down, ataxia can usually be demonstrated by asking him to flex his leg, place the heel of this leg on the knee of the other and run his heel down the shin of the leg which is flat. This movement is carried out with ease by the normal person, but is very difficult for the tabetic patient. In addition, the patient with tabes dorsalis commonly gives a history of difficulty in walking in the dark.

The finger and nose test will demonstrate ataxia in the upper extremities. A patient with tabetic involvement of the cervical cord will be unable to place his finger on the tip of his nose with his eyes closed.

Adiadokokinesia is inability to carry out rapidly in alternation diametrically opposite muscular actions. It is tested usually by asking the patient to sit down, place his hands on his knees with the palms down, and then rapidly pronate and supinate them. Adiadokokinesia is seen in cerebellar disease.

Patients with Sydenham's or Huntington's *chorea* have a peculiarly irregular and bizarre gait, which causes them to swing from side to side. Frequently the patient, after taking a series of normal steps, suddenly takes a very long step with one leg and a catch step with the other, pauses a moment, and then proceeds to walk normally.

A *staggering* or *drunken gait* is suggestive of cerebellar disease. If the cerebellar lesion is unilateral, the patient has a tendency to pitch toward the diseased side.

The *gait of Parkinson's disease,* described as a man running after his center of gravity, has been discussed previously (p. 36). The gait of such a patient becomes faster and faster until often he has to lay hold of something in order to stop. In spite of this striking picture, the patient with paralysis agitans rarely falls.

In the hysterical condition described as *astasia abasia,* the patient can move the lower extremities perfectly, but is unable to stand or walk.

REFLEXES

Examination of the reflexes is one of the simplest and, at the same time, one of the most important of all neurologic examinations. Information regarding the reflexes is easy to elicit and of great importance in diagnosis.

Pupillary Reflexes. *Direct Light Reflex.* Normally the eye contracts when light is shown on the eye. The extent of the contraction depends upon the amount of light which enters the eyeball. The *consensual light reflex* is the reaction of the right pupil to stimulation of the left retina by a ray of light,

and vice versa. A pupil which has lost the light reflex, but retained the reflex of accommodation and convergence, is known as the *Argyll Robertson pupil* (see page 312). An Argyll Robertson pupil is almost pathognomonic of syphilis of the central nervous system. The *ciliospinal reflex* is the term applied to the dilation of the pupil when the skin of the neck is scratched or pinched on the same side. Disturbance of this reflex is often one of the earliest signs of tabes.

The *corneal reflex* is carried out by touching the cornea gently with a wisp of cotton or some object that will not damage it. This slight pressure produces a sudden closure of the eye. The corneal reflex is familiar to the anesthetist, who considers its absence a proof of complete anesthesia. In carrying out this reflex, if there is a lesion of the trigeminal nerve, neither eye closes; if the lesion is in the facial nerve, the eye on the opposite side will close.

The **biceps reflex** is elicited by tapping the biceps tendon, thus producing flexion of the forearm.

The **triceps reflex** is produced by striking the triceps tendon, producing extension of the forearm.

The **abdominal reflex** is obtained by stroking the skin of the upper part of the abdomen parallel to the costal border and the lower part parallel to Poupart's ligament. Normally this procedure produces contractions of the recti muscles of the abdomen. Absence of abdominal reflexes is found in diseases of the anterior horn of the cord, such as poliomyelitis, involvement of the pyramidal tract, such as hemiplegia, and in multiple sclerosis.

The **cremasteric reflex** is elicited by stroking the upper and inner aspect of the thigh from above downward, causing an elevation of the testicle on the same side. It is quite active in young children, but in old people may be sluggish or absent. Unilateral absence of the cremasteric reflex may occur in organic hemiplegia.

Knee Kick. In most normal persons, when the patellar tendon is struck a sharp quick blow, the leg flies forward (Fig. 527). This reflex is usually known as the knee kick or knee jerk, and should be tested in every patient. It may be absent in conditions of great fatigue, in severe infectious diseases, during anesthesia, after epileptic convulsions, in amyotonia congenita and, for a variable time, after cerebral vascular lesions. It is usually absent in tabes dorsalis, anterior poliomyelitis, peripheral neuritis, Friedreich's ataxia, and often in diabetes mellitus. It is increased in general paresis, in lesions of the upper neuron, such as compression of the cord by tumors or bone disease above the level of the third lumbar vertebra, in multiple sclerosis, in amyotrophic lateral sclerosis and often in hemiplegia a short time after cerebral vascular lesions.

In myasthenia gravis the muscles tire easily with use and their fatigability increases until a virtual paralysis ensues. The tendon reflexes also tire; repeated tapping on the patellar tendon produces continued weakening of the knee kick and finally its complete disappearance.

The knee kick can often be more readily obtained by asking the patient to clasp his hands and pull strongly when the patellar tendon is struck. This procedure was first described by Ernst Jendrássik and is known as Jendrássik's maneuver. "I set the patient, who shows no knee kick by the ordinary method, on the edge of a table with his legs as relaxed as possible, and while I strike on his patellar tendon, I ask him to clasp together the flexed fingers of the right and left hand and with outstretched arms, to pull apart as firmly as possible." In some persons, particularly when lying down, a blow upon the patellar tendon produces a contraction of the quadriceps femoris muscle, but no knee kick. Such a contraction should be regarded as the equivalent of a knee kick.

Patellar Clonus. A patellar clonus is elicited by suddenly pulling the patella down and holding it down. This produces a series of rhythmic clonic contractions of the quadriceps muscle. It has the same significance as an exaggerated knee kick and is due to a lesion of the upper motor neuron.

Achilles Reflex. Tapping over the tendon of Achilles normally produces a flexion of the foot. It is carried out most satisfactorily when the patient kneels on a chair and extends his feet and ankles over the edge (Fig. 528).

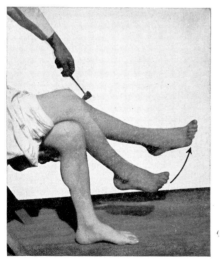

FIG. 527. Knee kick.

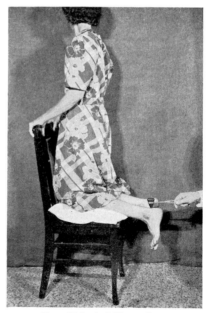

FIG. 528. Achilles reflex.

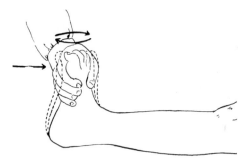

FIG. 529. Ankle clonus.

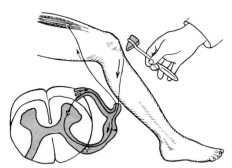

FIG. 530. Diagram of the nervous mechanism involved in a normal knee kick.

Ankle Clonus. The ankle clonus is elicited by pressing the foot sharply against the leg and holding it firmly in this position (Fig. 529). When clonus is present, the foot shows a series of rapid, rhythmical clonic movements.

An ankle clonus, like the patellar clonus, indicates a lesion of the upper neuron. It is often present in tuberculous disease of the spine, in tumors of the spinal cord and after cerebral hemorrhage.

A pseudo-ankle clonus which is seen especially in neurasthenia may cause confusion. However, a pseudoclonus consists in irregular, uneven movements which soon disappear, while a true clonus consists in rhythmic regular contractions which can usually be produced at will.

Babinski Reflex. This is an extremely important sign and, with certain unimportant exceptions, *always* indicates an organic lesion of the pyramidal tract. It is elicited by stroking firmly but not roughly the *outer part* of the sole of the foot with a moderately sharp instrument. This procedure produces plantar flexion of the smaller toes, but dorsal flexion of the great toe (Figs. 531 and 532). In normal persons plantar flexion of the great toe occurs. This sign may be present in babies at birth, but is never observed in normal children after the second year. It is sometimes present for a short time after an epileptic seizure. It has also been observed during insulin reactions and in hyperinsulinism. In severe exhaustion a temporary Babinski phenomenon may be seen.

Another reflex which is important as indicating lesions in the pyramidal tract is the **Trömner or Hoffmann reflex.** In eliciting this reflex, the examiner, with one hand, supports the forearm of the

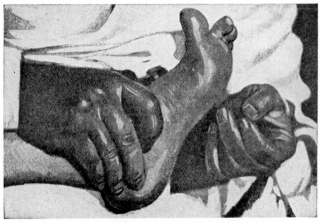

FIG. 531. Babinski reflex. (Babinski's original illustration.)

patient, and with the other strokes the nail of the middle finger gently outward or flicks its tip toward the ball of the finger. In lesions of the pyramidal tract the thumb of this hand is flexed and adducted; in normal persons no movement occurs. This reflex was first described by Trömner, who noted: "If one holds the hand comfortably and strikes gently on the slightly flexed finger of the patient with his own fingers; then follows flexion not only of the finger but also of the thumb."

Oppenheim's sign consists in a similar hyperextension of the great toe induced by drawing the back of the fingernail forcibly along the skin of the shin from the knee to the internal malleolus. **Gordon's sign** is again similar hyperextension of the great toe produced by kneading the muscles of the calf with the fingers while the patient is lying

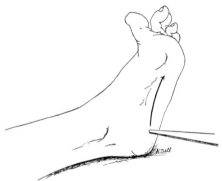

FIG. 532. Diagram of method of producing Babinski reflex.

down and relaxed. Oppenheim's sign and Gordon's sign have the same significance as a Babinski reflex.

Kernig's sign is the inability to extend the leg of a patient who is lying on his back with the thigh flexed (Fig. 534). It is usually present in cerebrospinal meningitis.

Brudzinski's Sign. Brudzinski's sign is often present in meningitis and is of considerable value. In reality there are two Brudzinski signs. The first is elicited by making passive flexion of one leg, which produces a similar flexion of the leg which is not touched. The other sign is elicited by raising the patient up by his neck when there is a flexion of the legs, the knees and the hips, and at times of all four extremities. The first of these signs is often referred to as contralateral reflex, while the second is referred to as Brudzinski's neck phenomenon. The second sign is more commonly present than the first.

SENSORY FUNCTIONS

In testing for sensation, numerous bits of complicated apparatus have been devised from time to time. A satisfactory examination can, however, usually be carried out with a pin, a wisp of cotton and two test tubes, one containing hot and the other containing cold water. Testing a patient for sensation is a tedious and painstaking process which requires much patience on the part of

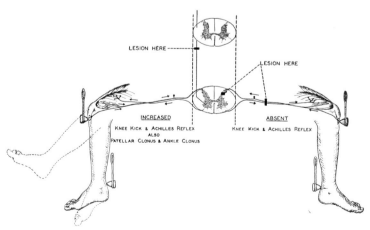

FIG. 533. Diagram illustrating lesions affecting reflexes.

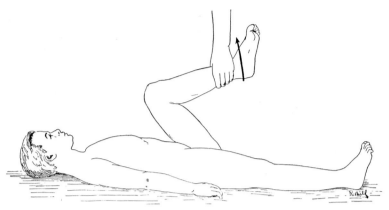

FIG. 534. Kernig's sign.

the examiner and of the patient. It is also important that both the patient and the examiner be as little fatigued as possible. For this reason a sensory examination is usually best carried out during the early morning hours. It is also imperative that the patient either be blindfolded or close his eyes tightly while the tests are being carried out.

Touch can be tested by stroking with a wisp of cotton, a camel-hair brush or a feather. This procedure will reveal anesthesia, or impaired sensation; hyperesthesia, or increased sensitiveness of the skin; and paresthesia, or a perverted sensation. Deep pressure pain is produced by pressure on an area until the patient complains of discomfort. Sensitiveness to heat and cold is usually tested by using test tubes filled with hot or cold water. This test may also be carried out by blowing on the area, blowing closely to produce a hot sensation, and blowing from a distance to produce a cold one.

Stereognosis is the ability of a person to recognize an object by touch, and is tested by placing a certain object in the patient's hand and asking him to identify it. Vibratory sense is tested with a tuning fork.

It would lead us too far to attempt to discuss all the types of disturbance in sensation which may be encountered.

Areas of anesthesia can be made out in tabes dorsalis, multiple neuritis, transverse myelitis, trauma of the nerve,

tumor of the spinal cord, and multiple sclerosis, herpes zoster, leprosy and hysteria. In herpes zoster the anesthesia follows the attack of zoster. In hysteria the anesthesia is commonly a hemianesthesia, but is usually characteristic because the area of anesthesia does not follow the distribution of any peripheral nerve.

In *syringomyelia* the sense of touch may be retained, while anesthesia to pain and temperature is present. In Brown-Séquard's syndrome, a unilateral lesion of the cord, there is a spastic paralysis on the side of, and below the lesion, while on the opposite side there is loss of sensation for pain, heat and cold and often for touch and pressure. This syndrome may be caused by a stab or bullet wound producing hemisection of the spinal cord, or by syphilis or tumors.

Hyperesthesia is seen in trigeminal neuralgia, in the early stages of multiple neuritis, herpes zoster, over the affected areas, in the arms or over the chest in coronary insufficiency, over the right iliac region in appendicitis, over the legs after "lightning pains" and sometimes in psychoneuroses.

Paresthesia in the form of burning, itching, formication and numbness is seen in myelitis, tabes dorsalis, cerebral thrombosis, arteriosclerosis, pernicious anemia, Raynaud's disease and endarteritis obliterans, multiple sclerosis and in psychoneuroses. The feeling of constriction, the "girdle sensation" of tabes dorsalis, is a classic example of paresthesia.

With advanced or complete destruction of a nerve, there is a loss of all sensation. In syringomyelia there is complete loss of sensation to heat, cold and pain with retention of sensitiveness to light touch.

SPEECH

The speech centers, according to the older authorities, are located in the cortex in the left side of the brain in a right-handed person, in the right side of the brain in a left-handed person. The most important areas concerned with speech are the posterior part of the inferior frontal gyrus, Broca's area, the posterior part of the first and second temporal convolutions, Wernicke's area and the angular gyrus (Fig. 535). This older anatomical conception has been attacked by Marie and by Head. Marie denied that Broca's area has anything to do with speech and believes that aphasia is produced only by lesions of Wernicke's zone, while Head does not believe there are any centers for use of language. For a fuller discussion of this problem the student is referred to textbooks on neurology.

Aphasia. Aphasia (a = without + φάσις, phasia = speech) is one of the most obvious speech defects. It is an impairment or loss of speech caused by loss of memory for vocal, written, manual and other signs or symbols by which we communicate with other men. Speech requires both a motor and a sensory apparatus, which are under the control of higher centers dominating intellectual processes. These centers are concerned in the mechanism of speech. According to the classic conception, there is an auditory speech center, a visual speech center and a motor speech center. Accordingly, there may be an auditory aphasia, a visual aphasia and a motor aphasia, corresponding to lesions of these speech centers. Though there is much doubt as to the accuracy of this anatomical localization, clinically these three types of aphasia can usually be differentiated.

In *auditory aphasia* a patient is unable to comprehend spoken words, although the sound of them is perfectly heard. He cannot read aloud or write, but can speak. He is unable to understand his own speech, and he is likely to misplace words and talk a jargon.

In *visual aphasia* the patient is unable to read printed or written characters, is unable to write and cannot copy, but his understanding of spoken words is good and his speech is almost normal. Visual aphasia is also called word blindness or *alexia*.

In *motor aphasia* the patient may understand what is said to him, but be entirely dumb and read aloud poorly. The patient cannot speak spontaneously or repeat words, read aloud or to himself, or write spontaneously or from

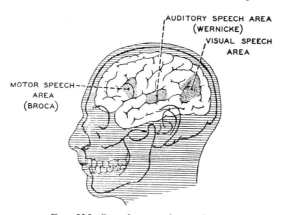

FIG. 535. Speech areas in cerebrum.

dictation. He understands spoken words and can write from copy.

In testing for aphasia we use the following tests:

1. Ability to recognize the nature and the use of objects
2. Ability to recall names of familiar objects
3. Ability to understand spoken words
4. Ability to understand printed or written words
5. Ability to speak
6. Ability to read aloud and understand words
7. Ability to write and to read aloud what has been written
8. Ability to copy
9. Ability to write what is dictated
10. Ability to repeat spoken words.

Closely related to aphasia is *apraxia* (*a* = neg. + πράσσειν, prassein = to do), which is the inability to perform coordinated movements with the extremities, although these extremities show no motor or sensory disturbances. For instance, the patient with apraxia, if given a cigarette and a match, may put the match in his mouth and attempt to strike the cigarette. Lesions of the corpus callosum and of the frontal lobes are prone to produce apraxia.

Other disturbances in speech which are important in diagnosis should be mentioned.

Scanning speech is often seen in multiple sclerosis. Here the enunciation is slow, and the patient hesitates at the beginning of words and then rushes on with his sentences.

Slurring speech is seen in paresis, in which the patient speaks in a slovenly fashion and seems to stick, as it were, at certain consonants.

Echolalia (ἠχώ = echo + λαλιά, lalia = babble) is an interesting condition in which the patient involuntarily repeats over and over words or phrases that he has heard.

Another striking speech defect is *palilalia* (πάλιν, palin = backward + λαλεῖν, lalein = to babble), in which a patient repeats a great many times a word, phrase or sentence which he has just spoken. In one instance, described by MacDonald Critchley, a patient, accompanied by his wife to a moving picture theatre, was noted to be reading the caption over and over. His wife, becoming annoyed, poked him in the ribs and said, "For God's sake, Bob, shut up." The patient replied, "I can't shut up. I can't shut up. I can't shut up," and continued to repeat this phrase until his speech became inaudible. This patient proved to be suffering from the results of an attack of epidemic encephalitis, which developed later into a typical parkinsonian syndrome. Palilalia has been frequently described as a sequel of epidemic encephalitis.

Disturbances of Articulation. Articulation is not a function of the cortex. In disturbances of articulation a patient is unable to speak clearly, but has no lesion of the speech centers. Such disturbances are seen especially in bulbar palsy and in pseudobulbar palsy. The most advanced disturbance of articulation is *anarthria,* a condition in which a patient is unable to say a word or make a sound. *Dysarthria* is a disturbance in speech, usually due to involuntary tremors or to muscular movements affecting the mechanism of articulation. Anarthria and dysarthria may be due to a lesion of the internal capsule, corpus striatum bulb, or cerebellum or may be due to disease of the affected muscles.

Stuttering and Stammering. Stuttering and stammering are two of the commonest speech defects and are frequently confused. In stuttering there are spasmodic contractions of some of the speech muscles interfering with articulation; in stammering such contractions are absent. In stuttering the difficulty often disappears when the words are sung.

AUTONOMIC FUNCTIONS

The autonomic system shows certain changes in the course of various diseases. There are, however, certain diseases which apparently are themselves due to disturbances of the autonomic nervous system. In examination of the autonomic nervous system we should be alert for the following changes.

1. **Vasomotor.** The most obvious changes of vasomotor origin are those in the color of the skin—the change from pallor to flushing. Fainting and dizziness on change of position are evidences of a lack of vasomotor control. Some patients on rising from a stooping position become dizzy, owing to poor vasomotor control. *Urticaria,* or hives, is a well-known vasomotor disturbance. *Dermatographia* is proof of vasomotor instability. Classic examples of vasomotor disease with serious consequences are *Raynaud's disease, erythromelalgia* and *angioneurotic edema. Raynaud's disease,* which has been described previously, is produced by the constriction of blood vessels of the hands or feet, leading to a persistent ischemia of the fingers or toes. *Erythromelalgia,* first described by Weir Mitchell, was referred to by him as "a chronic disease in which a part or parts—usually one or more extremity —suffered with pain, flushing, and local fever, made far worse if the parts hang down." *Angioneurotic edema* is an edema which appears suddenly, is usually circumscribed, and involves most commonly the face, eyelids, hands, legs or throat. It is usually transient and of little moment, although a sudden edema of the larynx may prove fatal.

2. **Secretory Disturbance.** Disturbance in the secretory functions of the vasomotor system is shown most commonly in the tendency to profuse sweating, often seen in nervous persons during examination.

Paralysis of the sympathetic nerves on one side of the face or trunk may be followed by unilateral sweating, the affected side remaining dry, while the opposite is drenched with perspiration (Fig. 536). In Horner's syndrome there is often a disturbance of the secretion of sweat, the area on the side of the lesion showing no perspiration.

3. **Trophic.** The genesis of trophic disturbances is not well understood, but they are probably due to alterations in

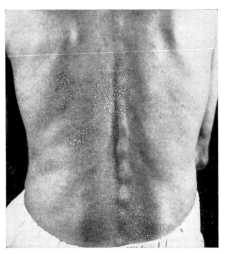

FIG. 536. Unilateral sweating over left side of back, crossing to right side at the level of the fifth lumbar vertebra.

the vasomotor system which affect the vascular supply of the organ or extremity in question. The late changes of scleroderma are probably of this origin. Other examples of trophic changes are seen in mutilation and the gangrene of the extremities encountered in leprosy and in the "mal perforant" of tabes dorsalis.

SEXUAL FUNCTIONS

The sexual functions are closely related to the nervous system, and many diseases, particularly functional nervous diseases, lead to a disturbance of the sexual function. The best-known example of disturbance in the sexual function of the male is *impotence,* which is the inability to perform the act of coitus because of the absence of erection at the proper moment. Impotence is most commonly of psychic origin, but is frequently present in diabetes mellitus, chronic pulmonary tuberculosis, multiple sclerosis, chronic prostatitis, tabes dorsalis, paresis, and in pernicious anemia with cord changes.

BIBLIOGRAPHY

Bedell, Arthur J.: The ophthalmoscopic signs of constitutional disease. J.A.M.A. *112:* 1052, 1939.
Bing, Robert: Compendium of Regional Diagnosis in Affections of the Brain and

Spinal Cord. 3rd ed. St. Louis, C. V. Mosby Co., 1929.

Brain, W. Russell: Diseases of the Nervous System. London, Oxford, 1933.

Corning, H. K.: Lehrbuch der topographischen Anatomie. 5th ed. Wiesbaden, J. F. Bergmann, 1914.

Critchley, MacDonald: Palilalia. J. Neurol. & Psychopath. *8:*23, 1927.

Dana, Charles L.: Text-book of Nervous Diseases. 4th ed. New York, Wm. Wood & Co., 1900.

Grinker, Roy R.: Neurology. Springfield, Ill., Charles C Thomas, 1934.

Head, Henry: Studies in Neurology. London, Oxford University Press, 1920.

Jelliffe, Smith E., and White, William A.: Diseases of the Nervous System. Philadelphia, Lea & Febiger, 1929.

Jendrássik, Ernst: Zur Untersuchungsmethode des Kniephänomens. Neurol. Zentralbl. *4:*412, 1885.

Kraepelin, Emil: Einführung in die Psychiatrische Klinik. Leipzig, Johann Ambrosius Barth, 1921.

Kuntz, Albert: The Autonomic Nervous System. Philadelphia, Lea & Febiger, 1929.

Lewandowsky, M.: Handbuch der Neurologie. Berlin, Julius Springer, 1911–14.

Pullen, Roscoe L.: Medical Diagnosis, Applied Physical Diagnosis. 2nd ed. Philadelphia, W. B. Saunders Co., 1950.

Spurling, R. Glen: Practical Neurological Diagnosis. Springfield, Ill., Charles C Thomas, 1935.

Stewart, Sir James Purves: The Diagnosis of Nervous Diseases. 6th ed. London, Edward Arnold & Co., 1924.

Tilney, Frederick, and Riley, Henry A.: The Form and Functions of the Nervous System. New York, Paul B. Hoeber, Inc., 1923.

Trömner, E.: Einige neue Reflextatsachen. Deutsche med. Wchnschr. *1:*1020, 1912.

Wilson, S. A. Kinnier: Modern Problems in Neurology. New York, Wm. Wood & Co., 1929.

Yakovlev, Paul I.: Plantar reflex as a criterion of endurance. J. Lab. & Clin. M. *28:*606, 1943.

INDEX